Patient Care Skills

Sixth Edition

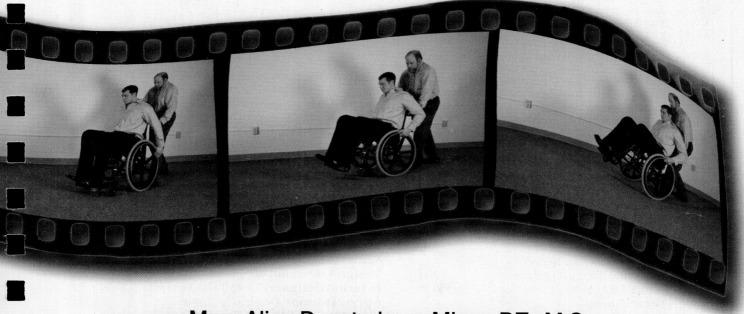

Mary Alice Duesterhaus Minor, P.T., M.S.
Clinical Assistant Professor of Physical Therapy
Clarkson University, Potsdam, New York

Scott Duesterhaus Minor, P.T., Ph.D.
Associate Dean for Health Science
Associate Professor and Chair
Department of Physical Therapy
Clarkson University, Potsdam, New York

Photography

Sarah Ruth Minor
Minor Manor Enterprises, Incorporated, Potsdam, New York

Pearson

Boston   Columbus   Indianapolis   New York   San Francisco   Upper Saddle River
Amsterdam   Cape Town   Dubai   London   Madrid   Milan   Munich   Paris   Montreal   Toronto
Delhi   Mexico City   Sao Paulo   Sydney   Hong Kong   Seoul   Singapore   Taipei   Tokyo

Library of Congress Cataloging-in-Publication Data

Minor, Mary Alice D.
  Patient care skills / Mary Alice Duesterhaus Minor, Scott Duesterhaus
Minor.—6th ed.
    p. ; cm.
  Includes bibliographical references and index.
  ISBN-13: 978-0-13-208234-1 (alk. paper)
  ISBN-10: 0-13-208234-9 (alk. paper)
 1. Transport of sick and wounded.   2. Patients—Positioning.   3. Physical therapy assistants.   I. Minor, Scott Duesterhaus.   II. Title.
  [DNLM: 1. Physical Therapy Modalities.   2. Asepsis—methods.   3. Nursing Care—methods.   4. Orthopedic Equipment.
5. Transportation of Patients—methods. WB 460 M666p 2010]
  RT87.T72M56 2010
  610.73—dc22

                                                                                                2009017898

Notice: The authors and the publisher of this volume have taken care that the information and technical recommendations contained herein are based on research and expert consultation, and are accurate and compatible with the standards generally accepted at the time of publication. Nevertheless, as new information becomes available, changes in clinical and technical practices become necessary. The reader is advised to carefully consult manufacturers' instructions and information material for all supplies and equipment before use, and to consult with a healthcare professional as necessary. This advice is especially important when using new supplies or equipment for clinical purposes. The authors and publisher disclaim all responsibility for any liability, loss, injury, or damage incurred as a consequence, directly or indirectly, of the use and application of any of the contents of this volume.

Publisher: Julie Levin Alexander
Publisher's Assistant: Regina Bruno
Editor-in-Chief: Mark Cohen
Associate Editor: Melissa Kerian
Assistant Editor: Nicole Ragonese
Development Editor: Stephanie Kelly, Triple SSS Press
  Media Development
Director of Marketing: Karen Allman
Executive Marketing Manager: Katrin Beacom
Marketing Specialist: Michael Sirinides
Marketing Assistant: Judy Noh
Managing Production Editor: Patrick Walsh
Production Liaison: Yagnesh Jani
Production Editor: Kate Boilard, Laserwords Maine
Senior Media Editor: Amy Peltier

Media Project Manager: Lorena Cerisano
Manufacturing Manager: Ilene Sanford
Manufacturing Buyer: Pat Brown
Senior Art Director: Maria Guglielmo
Design Coordinator: Chris Weigand
Interior Designer: Nesbitt Graphics Inc.
Cover/Interior Design: Jill Little
Manager, Rights and Permissions: Zina Arabia
Manager, Visual Research: Beth Brenzel
**Manager, Cover Visual Research
  and Permissions:** Karen Sanatar
Image Permission Coordinator: Debbie Latronica
Composition: Laserwords India
Printing and Binding: Q.G. Taunton
Cover Printer: Lehigh Phoenix

10 9 8 7 6 5

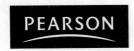

www.pearsonhighered.com

ISBN-13: 978-0-13-208234-1
ISBN-10:   0-13-208234-9

This book is dedicated
to better care
for all patients

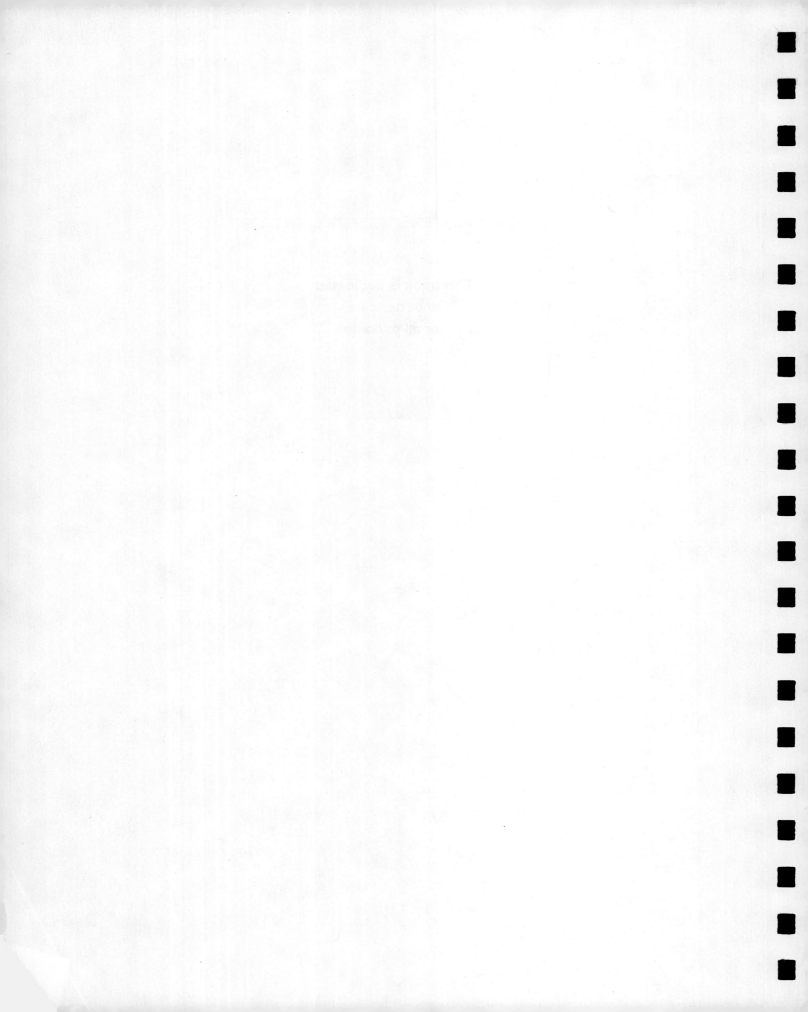

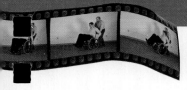

Contents

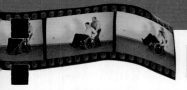

Preface

As the authors of the first text in physical therapy on these topics, first published in 1982, it is exciting to see a sixth edition come to fruition 27 years later. This effort continues to be truly a family project. Our daughter, Sarah, born during the first year of publication, has been a photographic subject in earlier editions and has become the photographer for this sixth edition as well as for the fifth edition.

We feel extremely fortunate for the continued acceptance of this text. We have worked diligently to meet the responsibility of the faith our colleagues have given us by the addition of new elements in this sixth edition that build on the strengths of the previous five editions and by updating information. We appreciate the faith our colleagues have demonstrated by allowing us to assist them in teaching new generations of physical therapists and physical therapist assistants over the past three decades. We have been fortunate to have received, and we continue to seek, critical commentary and counsel from students and colleagues who have used previous editions of this text. The video presentation of selected procedures from the text has been acclaimed and supported by numerous readers and continues in this edition. We extend our appreciation and thanks to those who have provided information and critical commentary that assisted us as we have moved forward through six editions.

As in previous editions, a large number of procedures and variations are included in this text, although it is not all inclusive. There are numerous choices to make in all patient interventions. When choosing among alternative methods or procedures, the most important consideration is to use the safest and most beneficial method for patients and physical therapists/assistants. In some cases, this will require modification of previously learned procedures. In all cases, practice will develop safe and efficient performance.

We find that when teaching these procedures, instructors can help students learn both the specifics of the procedures as well as general rules of good body mechanics, patient handling, and safety for patients and physical therapists/assistants. Students may require assistance in problem solving when applying procedures in a variety of patient-care situations. To assist student learning and problem solving, *Suggested Activities* and *Case Studies* continue to be included in the text.

For this sixth edition we have reordered some chapters. The material related to the Americans with Disabilities Act (previously Chapter 10) has been moved to Chapter 1. The purpose of this change was to promote consideration of the environment in which our patients/clients must function, which influences our choices when selecting procedures to be taught. Chapters 7–10 in this edition were reordered to follow a sequence of transferring (Chapter 7) patients/clients so they may be in the proper environment for appropriate positioning and turning (Chapter 8), which then may lead to range of motion exercises (Chapter 9), and then to ambulation with assistive devices (Chapter 10). We hope the new order of chapters provides a sequence of thinking that will be of use to students beyond the details of included procedures.

Each chapter and major section is introduced by a general explanation of the basis for performing the procedures to be described and by a presentation of general rules or guidelines that are generic to a series of procedures. Wording of instructions in the text are repeated in similar format to enhance generic application when appropriate. For each procedure presented, step-by-step illustrations are accompanied by brief written explanations. Following the sequence of illustrations for a specific procedure decreases the need for extensive text explanations and provides students with a visual reference to determine if the sequence of steps they are performing matches the sequence of steps presented. We recognize that there may be a need to adapt procedures to meet the abilities and needs of patients and physical therapists/assistants. Each chapter concludes with Review Questions that provide students an opportunity to test newly acquired knowledge. Review Questions can also be used as a study guide by reviewing the questions *before* beginning study of a chapter's content.

Finally, we wish to comment on the terms "patient" and "physical therapist/assistant." We have used the term "patient" throughout the text to designate the individual receiving care. This term has been used for its general sense of meaning for consistency throughout the text. We have used the term "physical therapist/assistant" throughout the text to designate the potential individuals providing care. In cases where decision making is to be performed (from our perspective) by a physical therapist before delegating care to a physical therapist assistant, we have used only the term physical therapist.

We expect that in addition to physical therapists and physical therapist assistants, many health-care providers, including home health aides, medical assistants, nurses, nurses' aides, nursing home attendants, occupational therapists, occupational therapy assistants, and orderlies will perform these procedures. Therefore, we hope this text will be useful to the practitioners providing, and the many individuals receiving care.

Mary Alice Duesterhaus Minor
Scott Duesterhaus Minor
Potsdam, NY

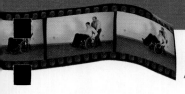

Acknowledgments

No authors can create a text and then perform by themselves all the additional tasks required to transform the text into a book and place it before the public. Having created five previous editions, we are very aware that this is not possible.

The five previous editions acknowledge significant numbers of people who contributed to each of those editions, and the numbers increase as we acknowledge those who have contributed significantly to this sixth edition.

First, we thank our daughter, Sarah Minor, photographer, for the photographic illustrations on which this book depends. We are grateful to Sarah for her critical eye, suggestions, attention to detail, and diligent work in creating the photographic illustrations. We are also grateful to Sarah for willingly putting her education and training as a professional photographer at our disposal.

For the sixth edition we thank, and acknowledge our appreciation to, Anne Gilbert, Kelly McGuire, and Michael Richards as new participants in photography sessions.

We must acknowledge our appreciation to the Pearson Education personnel who have provided patience, support, and assistance as we have prepared this sixth edition. We are grateful to Mark Cohen, Editor-in-Chief, and Melissa Kerian, Associate Editor, for guiding this project from inception to completion and for their perseverance in continuing the existence of this text. We are most grateful to Stephanie Kelly, Development Editor, Triple SSS Press Media Development, Inc., for her support and assistance while providing the prodding any author will agree is necessary for a successful text. We are fortunate that her prodding has been low key and friendly. Her work has been indispensible to this sixth edition.

Finally, to acknowledge that this is the sixth edition of a successful text, we wish to remember those who contributed to the first five editions. This list is long, as we are fortunate to have created so many editions. For their participation and contributions to the first two editions, we thank Jim York, photographer, Gary Bergner, Freda Bowden, Mary Edna Harrell, Marvin Levand, Julie Leidecker, and Jennifer McFarland. We thank Cheryl L. Mehalik, Editor, and Sondra Greenfield, Production Editor, for their contributions to the third edition. For their participation and contributions to the fourth edition, we thank Lin Marshall, Editor, Robert Morrison, photographer, Arnie Berger, Deborah Bosse, Jeffrey Bosse, Bettina Brown, Suzanne Cornbleet, Kathleen Dixon, Mustafa Koluman, Janice Loudon, and Sarah Minor. For their participation and contributions to the fifth edition we thank Ruth Ann Bosse, Christin Cavoretto, Michelle Deslauriers, Jason Garner, Pradip Grosh, Chuck Gulas, Buddy Heimburger, Nick Heimburger, Kristen Hobgood, Bonnie Hogenkamp, MaryClare Krusing, Chrysta Lloyd, Lewis Mueller, Patty Navarro, Jason Rubel, Abby Schilly, Debbie Schilly, Kathryn Schopmeyer, Joe Shapiro, Tina Shapiro, Sarah Stawizynski, and Michelle Unterberg for their participation in photography sessions, and to Gerald Bunker, Heather Caswell, George Fulk, Natalie Gilbert, Justin Hetu, Ellie O'Neill, and King Wilcox for their participation in videography sessions for the companion website that accompanies the sixth edition. We thank Kate Boilard of Laserwords Maine for her work as Production Editor and Yagnesh Jani, John Jordan, Anne Lukens, Hector Grillone, and Karen Holmes of Pearson Education for their advice, technical savvy, and support for the videographic aspect.

For arranging the loan and use of patient care equipment we thank Joe Neels of Provider Plus Inc. (St. Louis, MO) and Philip Lyons of Orthotic Mobility Systems, Inc. (Kensington, MD).

For their contributions of facilities and equipment for our work for all editions we acknowledge and express our appreciation to Wichita State University, Maryville University–St. Louis, Washington University–St. Louis, and Clarkson University.

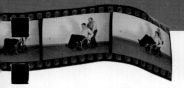

Reviewers

Barbara J. Behrens, PTA, MS
Coordinator, Physical Therapist Assistant
  Program
Mercer County Community College
Trenton, New Jersey

Farica Bialstock, PT MS
Professor, Allied Health Sciences
Nassau Community College
Garden City, New York

Tracey L. Collins PT, PhD, MBA, GCS
Assistant Professor, Physical Therapy
University of Scranton
Scranton, Pennsylvania

Susan Cotterman, PT
Director, Physical Therapist Assistant Program
Marion Technical College
Marion, Ohio

Susan Denham, OTR/L, CHT
Associate Professor, Occupational Therapy
Alabama State University
Montgomery, Alabama

Charles G. Fitzgerald, PTA
Academic Coordinator of Clinical Education,
  Physical Therapist Assistant Program
El Paso Community College
El Paso, Texas

Melissa Gill, MPT
Instructor, Physical Therapy
Anoka Ramsey Community College
Coon Rapids, Minnesota

Lois Harrison, PT, DPT, MS
Director of Clinical Education
Assistant Professor, Physical Therapy
Concordia University Wisconsin
Mequon, Wisconsin

Maria Holodak, PTA, MEd
Assistant Professor, Physical Therapist Assistant
  Program
Broward Community College
Coconut Creek, Florida

Jeffrey Krug, PT
Instructor, Physical Therapy
University of Missouri
Columbia, Missouri

Andrew Priest, EDD, PT
Chair, Physical Therapy
Clarke College
Dubuque, Iowa

Jeffrey Rothman, PT, EdD
Professor and Chair, Physical Therapy
College of Staten Island
Graduate Center City University of New York
Staten Island, New York

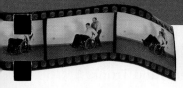

Procedures

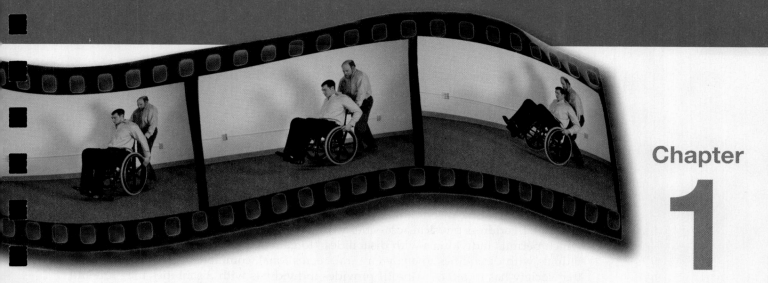

Americans with Disabilities Act

Learning Objectives

Upon completion of this chapter, you will be able to:

1. State the purpose of the Americans with Disabilities Act (ADA).
2. List the government agencies responsible for developing rules and regulations and enforcing the ADA law.
3. List sources of updated information on ADA.
4. Locate specific requirements for an accessible environment: accessible routes, alarms, assembly and auditorium areas, business and mercantile areas, clear space areas, control mechanisms, curb ramps, doors and doorways, drinking fountains, elevators, grab bars, ground and floor surfaces, handrails, hotels, libraries, parking spaces, platform lifts, ramps, reach heights, restaurant and food service areas, restrooms and bathrooms, signage, stairs, telephones, and transportation facilities.
5. Discuss how requirements of the ADA affect the education and training of clients or support staff who will use wheelchairs and assistive devices.
6. Integrate requirements of the ADA in teaching patients and support staff about the use of wheelchairs and assistive devices.

Key Terms

Accessible route	Grab bars
Americans with	Guidelines
Disabilities Act	Nosing
(1990) (ADA)	Platform lifts
Architectural Barriers	Ramp
Act (1968) (ABA)	Reach ranges
Clear-space areas	Regulations
Control mechanisms	Riser
Curb cut	Rules
Department of Justice	Transitions
(DOJ)	Tread
Equal Employment	United States Access
Opportunity	Board (USAB)
Commission (EEOC)	

Introduction

The goal of physical therapy is to provide a patient/client with the highest level of function possible. In many cases function is limited by the physical environment and not just patient/client impairments. This aspect of function is amplified in the International Classification of Function (ICF),[1] which is discussed in Chapter 2.

Laws have been passed, and regulations issued, to reduce such barriers, providing potential for higher levels of function. In this chapter, we present selected basic components of the physical environment that may impede patient/client function, as well as the regulations that require accommodation.

In 1990, Congress passed the **Americans with Disabilities Act (ADA)** (public Law 101–336). The law contains five titles:

Title I—Employment
Title II—Public Services and Transportation
Title III—Public Accommodations
Title IV—Telecommunications
Title V—Other Provisions

The purpose of the ADA is to provide "a clear and comprehensive national mandate for the elimination of discrimination against individuals with disabilities."[1] First, Title II and Title III address physical accessibility. Title II provides for accessible transportation, which permits individuals with disabilities "to gain employment,"[1] and "allows individuals with disabilities to enjoy cultural, recreational, commercial and other benefits that society has to offer."[1] Title III provides individuals with disabilities the "full and equal enjoyment of the goods, services, facilities, privileges, advantages, or accommodations of any place of public accommodation."[1]

Second is the use of wheelchairs for physical accessibility. The ADA provides standardized space requirements for accessibility in hallways, in front of elevator doors, and in elevators. These standards provide for the ability to pass other wheelchairs in hallways and for patients using wheelchairs to maneuver around, in, and out of elevators. Activities of such a nature mandate that the patient care skills of educating and training patients and staff on how to use wheelchairs must include specific maneuvering techniques and not just the abilities required for patient transfers into and out of wheelchairs.

It is true that many buildings and other structures still retain areas that are not compliant with the ADA. Public buildings undergoing significant renovation and new public structures must comply with ADA standards. Construction of ramps and interior facilities for private residences also are guided by the Uniform Guidelines. Therefore it is important that practitioners know the Uniform Guidelines, assist in employing Uniform Guidelines whenever necessary, and provide patient care skills aligned with ambulatory devices that match the environment in which patients/clients will function. It is for this purpose that at least basic knowledge of ADA standards must be considered by students and practitioners as they learn and as they teach clients.

The ADA was passed on July 2, 1990. Phased implementation of Titles II and III has been completed, and the ADA is now fully implemented. Initial development of guidelines for accessibility was distributed among several public and professional organizations, such as United States Access Board, Building Officials and Code Administrators International, Inc. (BOCA), Council of American Building Officials (CABO), and American National Standards Institute (ANSI). These organizations provided expertise as the requirements known as the Uniform Federal Accessibility Standards (UFAS) and the Americans with Disabilities Accessibility Guidelines (ADAG) were developed.

In July 2004, the **United States Access Board** (USAB) issued updated accessibility guidelines for new or renovated facilities. During this review, USAB combined requirements of the ADA and of the **Architectural Barriers Act** (ABA) of 1968. Combining the requirements of the ADA and the ABA represents an effort to ensure consistency of accessibility guidelines for a wide range of facilities in the private and public sectors. The USAB guidelines now appear as *The New ADA–ABA Accessibility Guidelines.*

The language of the law cannot possibly or appropriately contain provisions for every potential situation intended to be covered by the law. Therefore, **rules, regulations**, and **guidelines** for implementation of laws are issued following passage of a new law. In the case of the ADA, the government agencies primarily responsible for developing rules and regulations and enforcing the law are the **Equal Employment Opportunity Commission (EEOC)** and the **Department of Justice (DOJ)**. More specific interpretation of the law and its rules, regulations, and guidelines occurs as the result of administrative rulings and legal opinions in response to complaints and lawsuits filed by those who believe they have been subjected to discrimination as defined by the ADA. Definitive interpretations of specific requirements of the ADA become known as the result of such administrative rulings or legal opinions.

Resources

USAB material, including *A Guide to the New ADA–ABA Accessibility Guidelines* and the full text and diagrams of the *Guidelines,* are available from the USAB. The text and diagrams can be downloaded directly from the Internet:

United States Access Board

1331 F Street, N.W., Suite 1000

Washington, DC 20004–1111

(800) 872–2253 (voice)

(800) 993–2822 (TTY)

www.access-board.gov

In addition to access to the USAB, several private reporting services provide monthly updates regarding changes and recent legal opinions. The listing of one such service follows. This is a proprietary service with which the authors are most familiar. The listing of this service does not imply an endorsement of this service by the authors. The cost of a service such as this is higher than the cost for government or quasi-government publications. The benefits of such services are more timely and in-depth research and information.

Thompson Publishing Group, Inc.

Americans with Disabilities Act—ADA Compliance Guide

805 15th Street N.W., 3rd floor

Washington, D.C. 20005

(800) 677–3789

www.thompson.com

General Considerations for Accessibility

Requirements for accessibility must take into account a variety of disabilities resulting from a range of impairments. For example, requirements for ground- and floor-surface guidelines must take into account their effect on patients in wheelchairs and those who are visually impaired. Curb cuts may be advantageous for people in wheelchairs but may present a hazard to patients who are visually impaired. Accessibility designs must accommodate a broad spectrum of disabilities, rather than identifying each barrier to accessibility with a single impairment.

Specific Requirements

Within each area of public accommodation, such as an office or a restroom, there are specific components that must be examined and criteria that must be met for each component. For example, when a public accommodation encompasses a collection of areas, such as both an office and a restroom, then the criteria for doorways must be applied to both areas, but the criteria for toilets need only be applied to the restroom. In the case of door widths, the clear open width of a door must be no less than 32 inches. This requirement is true of all doors, whether they are for an entry into an office or restroom.

Listed on the following pages are the requirements for the many specific areas of accessibility that may be encountered in public accommodations. Each area is listed as a heading. Specific components and criteria for a given area are listed under the area heading. The list of area headings is alphabetical. Under each area heading, specific components, and criteria for each component, also are listed alphabetically.

In the following list, reference may be made to areas previously listed or to areas that follow later in the list. These are areas that appear in a number of environments and have common criteria, regardless of the area in which they are required. This method reduces redundancy but is limited to avoid the need for constant cross-reference searching. While certain components or criteria are applied in a variety of circumstances, there are some components or criteria that are not applied very often. For this reason, and because of space considerations, the following list does not include every individual requirement for accessibility.

The following guidelines are taken from the USAB *Guide*.[2] For a list of every requirement, and additional details concerning each requirement, referencing the USAB *Guide* is strongly recommended.

Accessible Route

A minimum of one **accessible route** within the path from public access via public transportation, accessible parking spaces, and public streets must be available. Such a route also must be available to connect additional accessible buildings at the same site. Stairs, steps, ramps, or escalators are separate considerations from an accessible route and have their own specific requirements.

■ **Take Note**

Guidelines to provide when home access ramps are required.

An accessible route may not have a grade (slope) greater than 1:20 (5 percent) in the direction of travel. Its cross slope shall not be greater than 1:48.

The vertical distance from floor to ceiling may be not less than 80 inches. When vertical clearance along an accessible route is less than 80 inches, a warning barrier must be provided. The required floor dimensions of an accessible route are presented in ■ **Figure 1–1**.

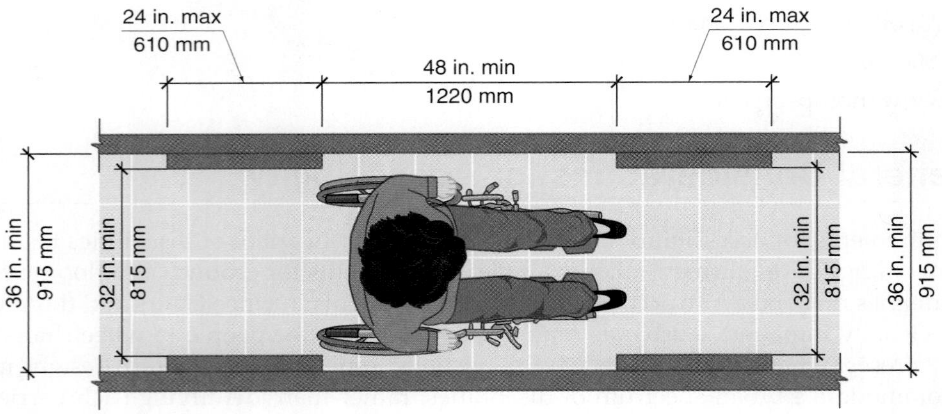

■ **Figure 1–1** Clear width of an accessible route.

In all cases, protrusions along an accessible route may not reduce the minimum required clear width as previously presented. Because of the potential for injury, even protrusions that do not limit clear width to less than 36 inches may not be greater than 4 inches in the horizontal dimension and are limited to specific areas in the vertical dimensions.

When 180-degree turns are encountered on an accessible route, guidelines for clear areas must be followed. These dimensions are presented in ■ **Figure 1–2**.

Assembly and Auditorium Areas for Wheelchair Seating

Clear areas that provide seating for patrons using wheelchairs are presented in the following two figures. ■ **Figure 1–3** presents the width of seating areas.

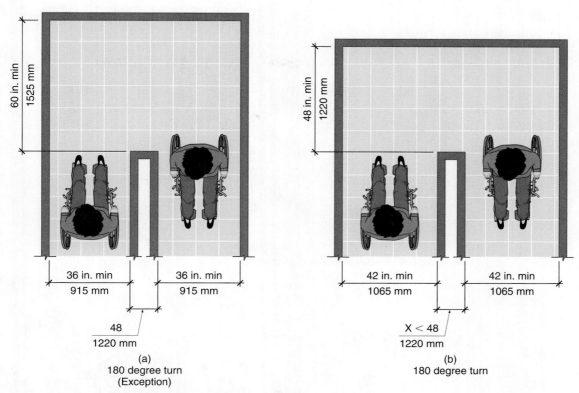

60 in. min
1525 mm

48 in. min
1220 mm

36 in. min
915 mm

36 in. min
915 mm

42 in. min
1065 mm

42 in. min
1065 mm

48
1220 mm

X < 48
1220 mm

(a)
180 degree turn
(Exception)

(b)
180 degree turn

■ **Figure 1–2**   Clear width for turning 180 degrees on an accessible route.

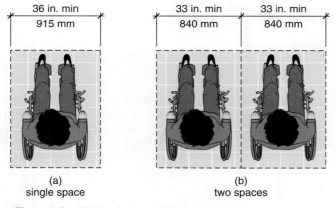

36 in. min
915 mm

33 in. min
840 mm

33 in. min
840 mm

(a)
single space

(b)
two spaces

■ **Figure 1–3**   Width of wheelchair spaces.

■ **Figure 1–4** presents the depth of seating areas, which is dependent upon the direction of wheelchair access to the seating area.

Wheelchair seating locations must be configured in conjunction with assistive listening systems, must be on (but not overlap with) an accessible route with access to accessible emergency exits, and must have access to accessible restrooms. In assembly areas with capacity greater than 300 people, accessible wheelchair areas must be located in more than one location.

Appropriate lines of sight must be provided for patrons using wheelchairs. In areas where patrons are expected to remain seated, elevations must provide lines of sight either over the heads of patrons (■ **Figure 1–5**) or via alternate spacing to provide lines of sight over the shoulders but between the heads of patrons in the row immediately in front.

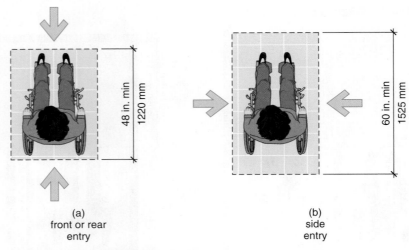

(a)
front or rear
entry

(b)
side
entry

■ **Figure 1–4**   Depth of wheelchair spaces.

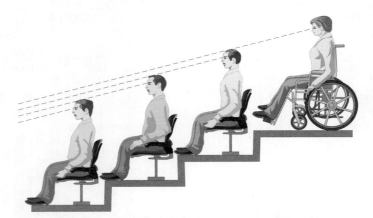

■ **Figure 1–5**   Sight-line elevation over the heads of seated patrons.

In areas where patrons are expected to rise from their seats, elevations must provide lines of sight either over the heads or via alternate spacing to provide lines of sight over the shoulders but between the heads of patrons (■ Figure 1–6), in the row immediately in front when patrons are standing.

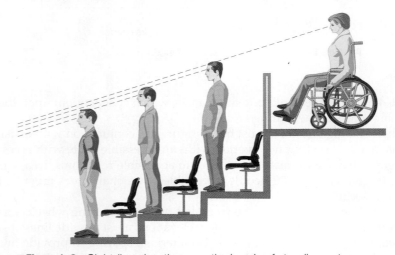

■ **Figure 1–6**   Sight-line elevation over the heads of standing patrons.

Check-Out Counters

Check-out counters must be situated on accessible routes within the business or commercial facility. Security barriers used to prevent shopping carts from being removed from stores may not prevent access for users of wheelchairs. Vertical dimensions of check-out counter surfaces and protective edges are presented in ▪ Figure 1–7.

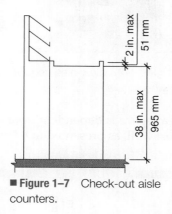

▪ **Figure 1–7** Check-out aisle counters.

Clear-Space Areas

Clear-space areas include the floor dimensions of an accessible route and clearances for use of certain facilities, such as toilet stalls and drinking fountains. For accessible routes, the minimum width for passing is 60 inches. If the width of an accessible route is less than 60 inches, then a passing area must be provided. A passing area shall be not less than 60 inches by 60 inches and must be provided not less than every 200 feet along the accessible route.

Landings on an accessible route also must have a clear area of not less than 60 inches by 60 inches. Such landings provide a clear space for turning and other maneuvers. Dimensions for a T-shaped turning space are presented in ▪ Figure 1–8.

▪ **Take Note**
Clear spaces ensure ease of mobility.

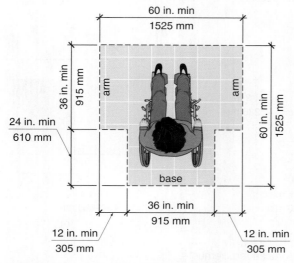

▪ **Figure 1–8** T-shaped turning spaces.

Clear-space areas for positioning of wheelchairs must be not less than 30 inches by 48 inches, as presented in ▪ Figure 1–9.

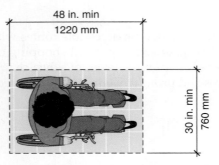

■ **Figure 1–9**   Clear-area requirements for wheelchairs.

The orientation of such clear space is dependent upon position of wheelchair placement with respect to the closest wall, as presented in ■ **Figure 1–10**.

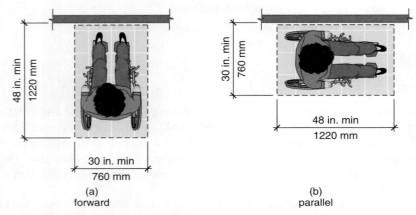

■ **Figure 1–10**   Orientation of clear area for wheelchairs.

Toe clearances shall be between 17 and 25 inches deep under an element and a minimum width of 30 inches, as presented in ■ **Figure 1–11**.

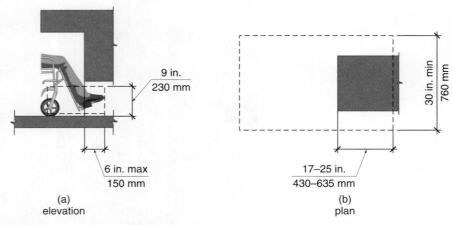

■ **Figure 1–11**   Toe clearance requirements.

Knee clearance height (vertical dimension) generally is not less than 27 inches from the floor (■ Figure 1–12). Knee clearance depths must be not less than 11 inches in the horizontal dimension at a point 9 inches above the floor and not less than 8 inches in the horizontal dimension at a point 27 inches above the floor. This takes into account angulation of wheelchair leg rests, which extend farther from a wheelchair as they extend toward the floor. Maximum knee clearance in the horizontal dimension must be no greater than 25 inches under any element at a point 9 inches above the floor.

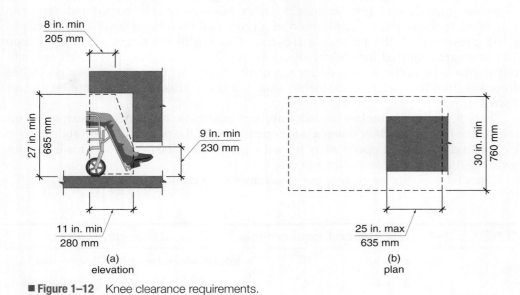

■ **Figure 1–12**   Knee clearance requirements.

Control Mechanisms

Control mechanisms must be easy to grasp with one hand and must not require tight grasping, tight pinching, or twisting of a wrist to operate.

Curb Cuts

Curb cuts may not have a grade greater than 1:12 (8.3 percent) for new construction, with a vertical rise of not greater than 30 inches. For existing sites, a grade may not be greater than 1:10 (10 percent), with a vertical rise of not greater than 6 inches if space does not permit construction of a grade of 1:12 or less, or not greater than 1:8 (12.5 percent) for existing sites, with a vertical rise of not greater than 3 inches if space does not permit construction of a grade of 1:12 or less. In all cases, the width of the curb cut, exclusive of the flared sides, must be not less than 36 inches, the same width as an accessible route.

Doors and Doorways

Access to all facilities requires that entrances be accessible. Revolving doors and turnstiles shall not be part of an accessible route and may not be the only method of entrance. Gates must meet requirements when on an accessible route. For double-leaf doorways, at least one leaf must meet the requirements, and this leaf must be the active leaf.

Handles must be easy to grasp; must not require tight grasping, tight pinching, or twisting of wrist to operate; and must be mounted not higher than 48 inches above the floor. When automatic door mechanisms are used for opening, the time to open must not be greater than 3 seconds, and the force to stop movement must not be greater than

■ **Take Note**

Information for families for moving within a house.

15 pounds. When automatic door mechanisms are used for closing, the time to close must not be less than 3 seconds for closing from 70 degrees open to a point where the leading edge of the door is 3 inches from the latch.

Fire-door opening forces must be the minimum required by the local administrative entity (i.e., Fire Department, Department of Public Safety, etc.) and not greater than 5 pounds of force for interior hinged doors, sliding doors, or folding doors. Latches or other hardware do not come under these force requirements.

The depth of an opening in which a door is placed should not be greater than 24 inches. If the depth is greater than 24 inches, this area must be considered part of an accessible route, requiring application of all minimal width and depth requirements.

As presented in the following figures, clear width openings of not less than 32 inches are required for almost all doorways. No projections into the clear opening width may occur within 34 inches of the floor or ground. Between 34 inches from the floor to a height of 80 inches from the floor, projections may not be greater than 4 inches.

There are a large number of doorway configurations. In all cases, clear space for maneuvering a wheelchair when a door opens toward the person and the ability to get close to a door when it opens away from the person must be provided. This is true for swinging doors, gates, and sliding doors.

■ Table 1–1 presents the clear-space requirements for manual swinging doors.

TABLE 1–1 Clear-Space Requirements for Manual Swinging Doors

Type of Use		Minimum Maneuvering Clearance	
Approach Direction	Door or Gate Side	Perpendicular to Doorway	Parallel to Doorway (beyond latch side unless noted)
From front	Pull	60 inches (1525 mm)	18 inches (455 mm)
From front	Push	48 inches (1220 mm)	0 inches (0 mm)[1]
From hinge side	Pull	60 inches (1525 mm)	36 inches (915 mm)
From hinge side	Push	54 inches (1370 mm)	42 inches (1065 mm)
From hinge side	Push	42 inches (1065 mm)[2]	22 inches (560 mm)[3]
From latch side	Pull	48 inches (1220 mm)[4]	24 inches (610 mm)
From latch side	Push	42 inches (1065 mm)[4]	24 inches (610 mm)

1. Add 12 inches (305 mm) if closer and latch are provided.

2. Add 6 inches (150 mm) if closer and latch are provided.

3. Beyond hinge side.

4. Add 6 inches (150 mm) if closer is provided.

■ Figure 1–13 presents eleven clear-area configurations for maneuvering at swinging doors.

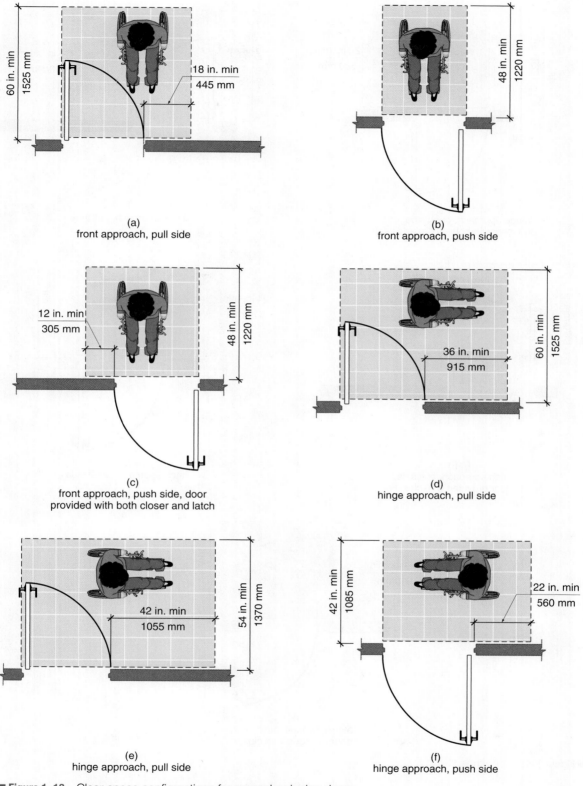

(a)
front approach, pull side

(b)
front approach, push side

(c)
front approach, push side, door
provided with both closer and latch

(d)
hinge approach, pull side

(e)
hinge approach, pull side

(f)
hinge approach, push side

■ Figure 1–13   Clear-space configurations for manual swinging doors.

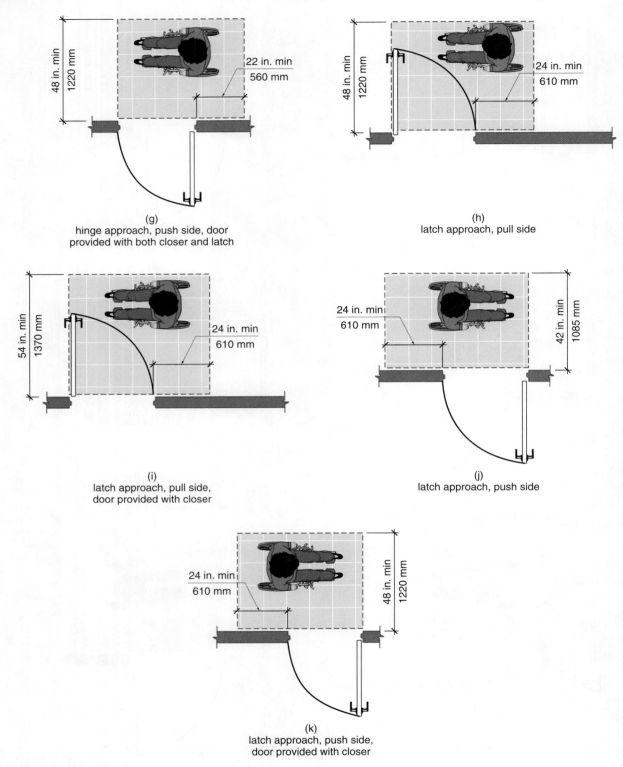

(g)
hinge approach, push side, door
provided with both closer and latch

(h)
latch approach, pull side

(i)
latch approach, pull side,
door provided with closer

(j)
latch approach, push side

(k)
latch approach, push side,
door provided with closer

■ **Figure 1–13** (continued)

■ Table 1–2 presents the clear-space requirements for sliding and folding doors.

■ Figure 1–14 presents four clear-area configurations for maneuvering at sliding and folding doors. ■ Figure 1–15 presents three clear-area configurations for maneuvering at recessed doors.

When swinging doors are in series, specific dimensions, as presented in ■ Figure 1–16, are required. These dimensions permit the opening of doors in series while maintaining clear space for maneuvering without hindrance from opening/closing doors.

TABLE 1–2 Clear-Space Requirements for Sliding and Folding Doors

	Minimum Maneuvering Clearance	
Approach Direction	**Perpendicular to Doorway**	**Parallel to Doorway (beyond stop/latch side unless noted)**
From front	48 inches (1220 mm)	0 inches (0 mm)
From side[1]	42 inches (1065 mm)	0 inches (0 mm)
From pocket/hinge side	42 inches (1065 mm)	22 inches (560 mm)[2]
From stop/latch side	42 inches (1065 mm)	24 inches (610 mm)

1. Doorway with no door only.

2. Beyond pocket/hinge side.

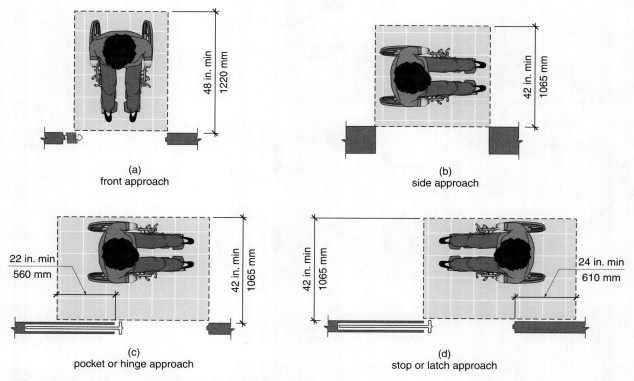

(a)
front approach

(b)
side approach

(c)
pocket or hinge approach

(d)
stop or latch approach

■ Figure 1–14   Clear-space configurations for sliding and folding doors.

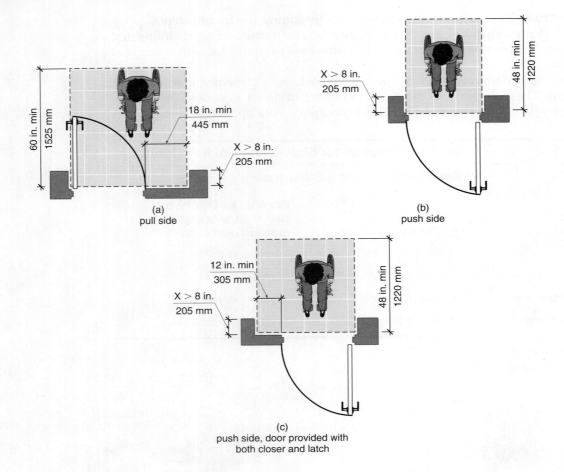

■ **Figure 1–15** Clear-space configurations for recessed doors.

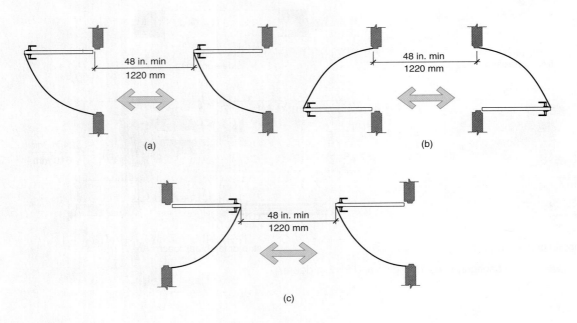

■ **Figure 1–16** Clear-space configurations for doors in series.

Drinking Fountains

Spout outlet height for drinking fountains must not be greater than 36 inches, with not less than 27 inches vertical clear space beneath the unit (■ Figure 1–17). Spout location should be not less than 15 inches from the fountain's vertical support and not greater than 5 inches from the front edge of the fountain unit. Water ejection must be at least 4 inches high. Toe and knee clearances must conform to dimensions provided previously in *Clear-Space Areas*. Controls must be mounted on the front of the unit, or on the side of the unit near the front, and must conform to the requirements previously presented for *Control Mechanisms*.

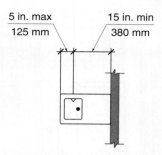

■ **Figure 1–17** Positioning requirements for drinking fountains.

Elevators

To be considered accessible, an elevator must be on an accessible route. Unless freight elevators are used for the general public as combination passenger and freight elevators, freight elevators may not be used to meet the requirement of an accessible elevator. All elevators considered accessible must be automatic-control elevators.

Elevator car controls must be placed in readily accessible locations and within the reach dimensions presented later in this chapter under *Reach Ranges*. For elevator cars with the door opening in the center of the front wall, controls must be on a front wall. For cars with the door opening set to one side of the front wall, controls must be located on the front wall or on the side wall nearest the door.

Elevator dimensions are presented in ■ Table 1–3, with five possible configurations presented in ■ Figures 1–18.

The center point of hall elevator call buttons must be 42 inches above the floor and must not be recessed. Projections greater than 4 inches in the horizontal dimension mounted below hall elevator call buttons must be avoided. The up button must be on top. All buttons must have both raised and Braille signage.

Hall elevator signals must contain visual and audible signal at each hoistway, centered not less than 72 inches above the floor level. An audible signal must sound once for up and twice for down or must have verbal annunciators capable of saying "up" or "down." Signals within the elevator also must be audible, either tone or annunciator, indicating the passage of each floor.

TABLE 1–3 Elevator Car Dimensions

	Minimum Dimensions			
Door Location	Door Clear Width	Inside Car, Side to Side	Inside Car, Back Wall to Front Return	Inside Car, Back Wall to Inside Face of Door
Centered	42 inches (1065 mm)	80 inches (2030 mm)	51 inches (1295 mm)	54 inches (1370 mm)
Side (off-centered)	36 inches (915 mm)[1]	68 inches (1725 mm)	51 inches (1295 mm)	54 inches (1370 mm)
Any	36 inches (915 mm)[1]	54 inches (1370 mm)	80 inches (2030 mm)	80 inches (2030 mm)
Any	36 inches (1525 mm)[1]	60 inches (1525 mm)[2]	60 inches (1525 mm)[2]	60 inches (1525 mm)[2]

1. A tolerance of minus 5/8 inch (16 mm) is permitted, which provides a door clear width of only 35 3/8 inches.

2. Other elevator car configurations that provide a turning *space* complying with guidelines with the elevator door closed are permitted.

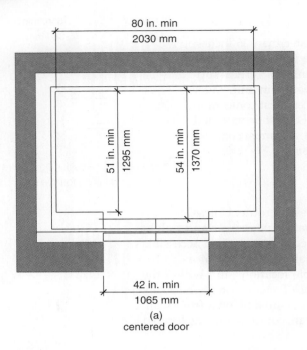

80 in. min
2030 mm

51 in. min
1295 mm

54 in. min
1370 mm

42 in. min
1065 mm

(a)
centered door

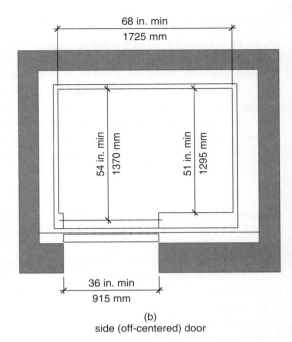

68 in. min
1725 mm

54 in. min
1370 mm

51 in. min
1295 mm

36 in. min
915 mm

(b)
side (off-centered) door

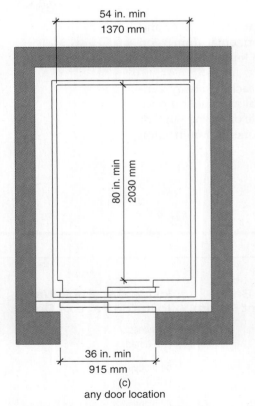

54 in. min
1370 mm

80 in. min
2030 mm

36 in. min
915 mm

(c)
any door location

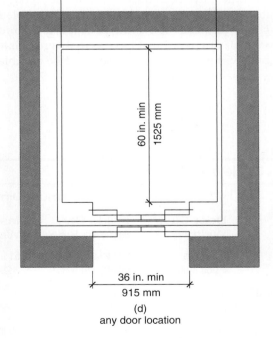

60 in. min
1525 mm

60 in. min
1525 mm

36 in. min
915 mm

(d)
any door location

■ **Figure 1–18** Elevator car configurations.

Grab Bars

Circular **grab bars** must have a diameter not less than 1.25 inches and not more than 2 inches. Noncircular grab bar dimensions, both cross section and perimeter, are presented in ■ **Figure 1–19**. The horizontal distance between grab bars and wall, or vertical distance between grab bars and vertical projections below grab bars, must be 1.5 inches. The vertical distance between grab bars and horizontal projections above grab bars must be not less than 12 inches.

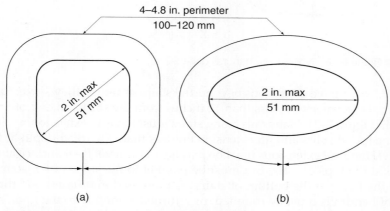

■ **Figure 1–19**   Noncircular grab bar dimensions.

Ground and Floor Surfaces

Ground and floor surfaces must be stable, firm, and slip resistant. Carpet must be securely attached, with exposed edges fastened to the floor, and have trim along the full length of exposed edges. Pile thickness must not be greater than .5 inch.

Grating spaces must be no greater than .5 inch in any dimension. If elongated openings are used, the long dimension of the opening must be oriented perpendicular to the dominant direction of travel.

Transitions between connected surfaces up to .25 inch may be left untreated. Transitions between .25 inch and .5 inch must have a beveled edge with a slope no greater than 1:2 (50 percent). Ramp guidelines, presented later in the chapter, must be used to accommodate transitions greater than .5 inch.

■ Take Note
Information for safe movement within a building.

Handrails

Circular handrails must have a diameter not less than 1.25 inches and not more than 2 inches. Noncircular handrail dimensions, both cross section and perimeter, are presented in ■ **Figure 1–20**. The horizontal distance between handrails and wall and vertical distance between handrails and horizontal projections below handrails must be 1.5 inches. The top gripping surface of handrails must not be less than 34 inches or greater than 38 inches in the vertical dimension from the floor or stair tread.

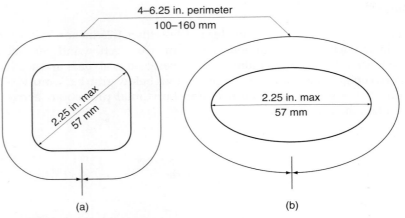

■ **Figure 1–20**   Noncircular handrail dimensions.

Handrails must have extensions beyond the stairs or ramps they serve. Ramps must have handrail extensions not less than 12 inches from the start and end of the ramp, as presented in Figure 1–21. Handrails along stairs must have an extension not less than 12 inches at the top of stairs and an extension not less than one tread depth at the bottom of the stairs. Handrail extensions must be parallel to the level floor surface at the ends of ramps and at the tops of stairs but must be parallel to the slope of the stair flight (not parallel to the floor) at the bottom of stairs, as presented in ■ Figures 1–21 through 1–23. The ends of handrails must be rounded, or returned smoothly to the floor, a wall, or a post. All handrails must be secured and must not rotate within fittings.

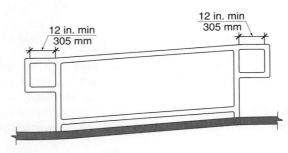

■ **Figure 1–21**   Handrail extensions for ramps.

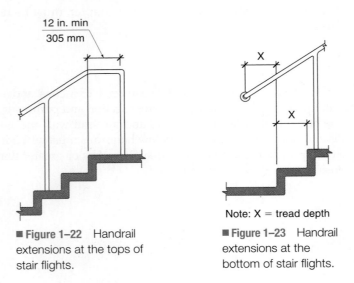

■ **Figure 1–22**   Handrail extensions at the tops of stair flights.

■ **Figure 1–23**   Handrail extensions at the bottom of stair flights.

Hotels (Transient Lodging)

Hotel accommodations must meet general accessibility guidelines for public areas. Complete specifications for each component area are available in the *USAB Guide.* Accessible areas must include the guest room and bathroom, public restrooms, dining and meeting facilities, entrances, hallways and accessible routes, and elevators. Units made available to guests requiring accommodation must be dispersed among the entire range of units available to the general public in terms of facilities and size, cost, and number of beds provided.

A unique guideline for guest rooms is that there must be not less than 36 inches clear space on each side of a bed. In rooms with two beds, a common clear space between them may be shared, maintaining the 36-inch clear space on the unshared side of each bed.

Medical Facilities

In general, each specific area of a medical facility must comply with the appropriate requirements for the designated type of area. There are some specific differences, however. The bathroom in each patient room must comply with the requirements for an accessible toilet and sink. Clear-space areas must not be less than 36 inches along each side of a bed, with an accessible path to each side of the bed that allows for a parallel approach to the bed and includes a maneuvering area (preferably between the two beds in a double room) of not less than 60 inches in width.

Parking Spaces

Accessible parking spaces must be designated to be on the shortest possible path from the parking area to an accessible entrance via an accessible route. Access to parking spaces should not be behind other parked cars. Such spaces must be designated with a posted sign not less than 60 inches high, measured from the ground to the bottom of the sign. A sign or symbol painted on the ground alone is not acceptable.

Car parking spaces must not be less than 96 inches wide, and van parking spaces must not be less than 132 inches wide. Access aisles between vehicles must not be less than 60 inches wide. An exception is that a van parking space may be only 96 inches wide if the access aisle is not less than 96 inches wide. Access aisles must run the full length of the marked parking space and be not less than 240 inches long. Vertical clearance for vehicle access routes to accessible spaces, and the vertical clearance for such parking spaces, must be not less than 98 inches. Vertical clearance for vehicle access routes to passenger loading zones must be not less than 114 inches. Accessible curb ramps that are not obstructed by a parking space also must be available when necessary.

■ **Take Note**
Information for getting from vehicle to destination.

Platform Lifts

Platform lifts are used for building entrances, in building interiors, and with transportation vehicles. Clear-space areas for approaches and landings adjacent to platform lifts must meet the requirements previously presented in *Clear-Space Areas.* Controls must be placed within the dimensions presented later in this chapter in *Reach Ranges.* The minimum dimensions and configuration of platform lifts are presented in ■ **Figure 1–24.**

■ **Take Note**
Information for families creating access to a house.

Ramps

Any portion of an accessible route with a grade greater than 1:20 (5 percent) must be considered a **ramp.** Any transition between two connected surfaces greater than .5 inch must be considered a ramp. Ramps must use the least slope possible, must not exceed

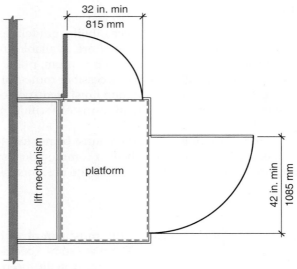

■ **Figure 1–24** Dimensions and configuration of platform lifts.

the guidelines previously presented for curb cuts, must have a cross slope no greater than 1:50 (2 percent), and must not exceed a rise of 30 inches in any single run. Ramp width must not be less than 36 inches.

Landings must be provided at the top and bottom of each run. They must be not less than 60 inches in length and at least as wide as the ramp. If a change in ramp direction or doorway occurs at a landing, the landing must meet the required landing clear space of 60 inches by 60 inches.

Handrails are required for a rise of 6 inches or more or for a horizontal run of 72 inches or more. They must be provided along both sides of the ramp and must meet the general requirements listed previously under *Handrails.*

Reach Ranges

■ **Take Note**

Information for remodeling bathrooms.

Reach ranges, within which control mechanisms must be placed, are dependent upon the direction of reach, forward or side, and whether a reach is obstructed or unobstructed. Specific requirements for each type of reach are presented in ■ **Figures 1–25** through **1–28.**

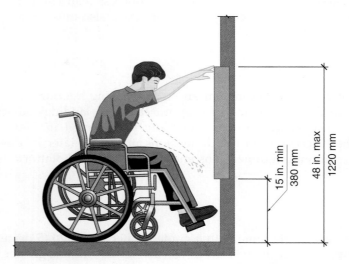

■ **Figure 1–25** Reach range—unobstructed forward reach.

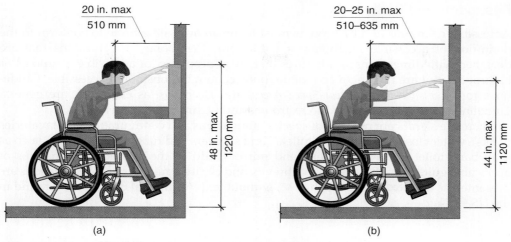

■ **Figure 1–26**   Reach range—obstructed high forward reach.

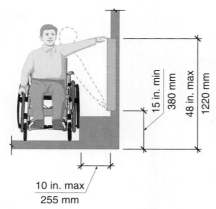

■ **Figure 1–27**   Reach range—
unobstructed side reach.

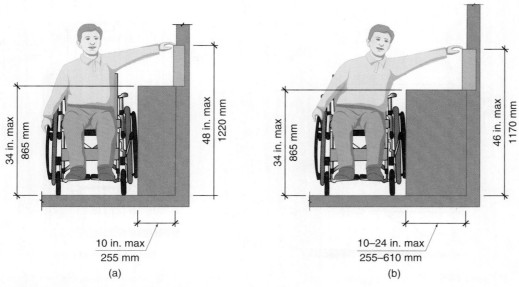

■ **Figure 1–28**   Reach range—obstructed high side reach.

Restrooms and Bathrooms

Accessible restrooms and bathrooms must be on an accessible route to conform to the definition of accessible restrooms or bathrooms. Restrooms or bathrooms that are designed with dimensions and fixtures that are appropriate for accessible restrooms or bathrooms, but are not on an accessible route, cannot be considered accessible. Guidelines for *Accessible Route, Clear-Space Areas,* and *Doorways,* as examples, are general guidelines that must be applied to restrooms and bathrooms in general.

There is a significant number of specific dimensions and configurations for lavatories (sinks), water closets and urinals (toilets), and showers and tubs. Other fixtures, such as grab bars, toilet paper dispensers, and mirrors, add to the myriad combinations of applicable guidelines. For the sake of brevity and clarity, a number of configurations are presented as ■ **Figures 1–29** through **1–46,** without text. Additional detail can be found in the *USAB Guide.*

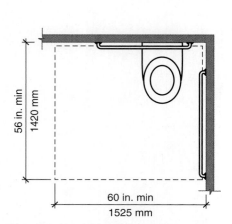

■ **Figure 1–29** Clearance for water closets.

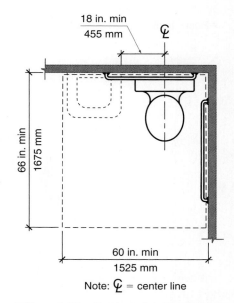

Note: ℄ = center line

■ **Figure 1–30** Overlap of water closet clearance in residential bathrooms.

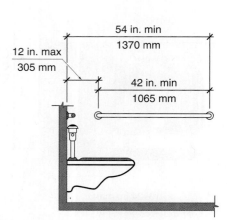

■ **Figure 1–31** Sidewall placement of grab bars in water closets.

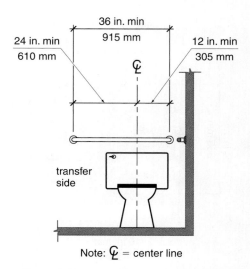

Note: ℄ = center line

■ **Figure 1–32** Rear wall placement of grab bars in water closets.

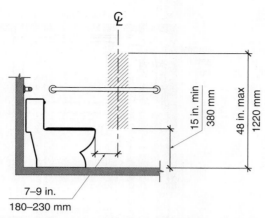

■ **Figure 1–33** Placement of toilet paper dispenser in water closets.

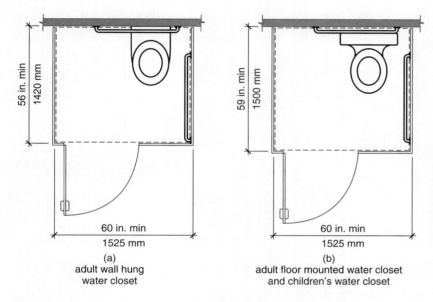

(a)
adult wall hung
water closet

(b)
adult floor mounted water closet
and children's water closet

■ **Figure 1–34** Dimensions of wheelchair-accessible water closets.

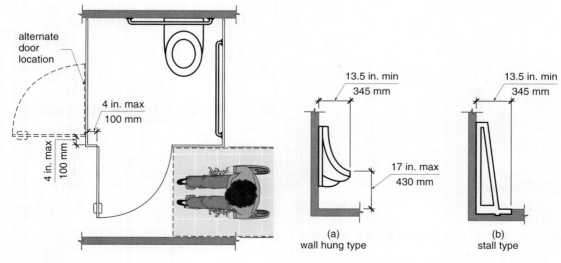

(a)
wall hung type

(b)
stall type

■ **Figure 1–35** Door dimensions of wheelchair-accessible water closets.

■ **Figure 1–36** Placement dimensions for urinals.

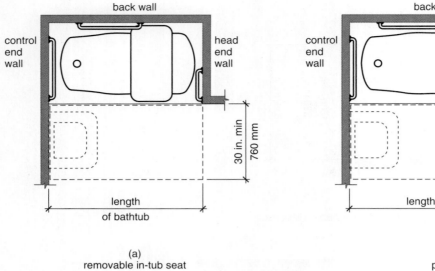

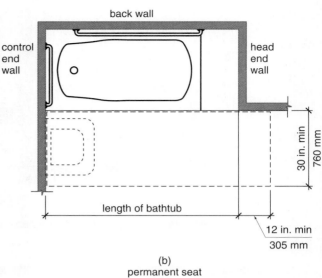

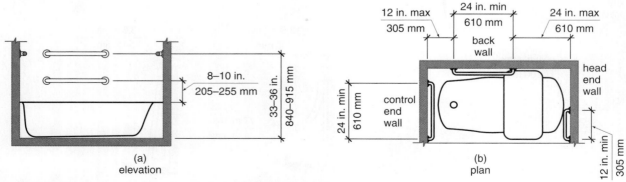

(a)
removable in-tub seat

(b)
permanent seat

■ **Figure 1–37** Clearance dimensions for bathtubs.

(a)
elevation

(b)
plan

■ **Figure 1–38** Placement of grab bars for bathtubs with permanent seats.

(a)
elevation

(b)
plan

■ **Figure 1–39** Placement of grab bars for bathtubs with removable seats.

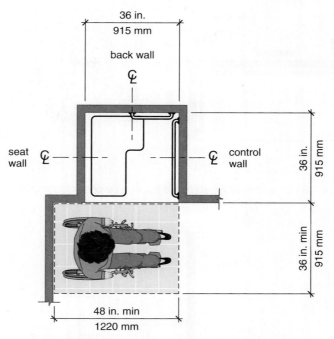

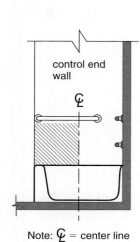

Note: C_L = center line

■ **Figure 1–40** Placement of water controls in bathtubs.

Note: inside finished dimensions measured at the center points of opposing sides

C_L = center line

■ **Figure 1–41** Dimensions for transfer-type shower compartments.

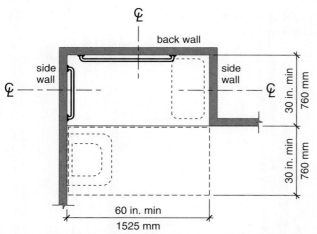

Note: inside finished dimensions measured at the center points of opposing sides

C_L = center line

■ **Figure 1–42** Dimensions for standard roll-in-type shower compartments.

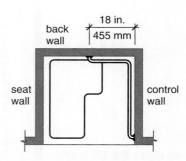

■ **Figure 1–43** Placement of grab bars in transfer-type shower compartments.

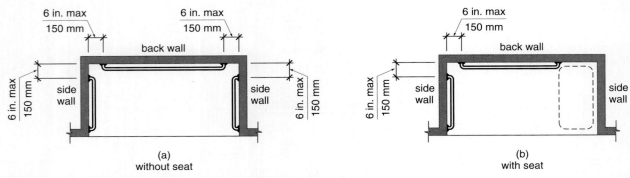

■ **Figure 1–44**   Placement of grab bars for standard roll-in-type shower compartments.

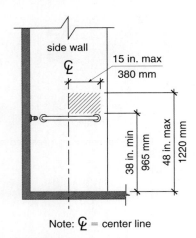

Note: ℄ = center line

■ **Figure 1–45**   Placement of water controls for transfer-type shower compartments.

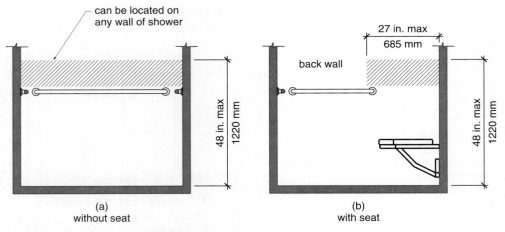

■ **Figure 1–46**   Placement of water controls for roll-in-type shower compartments.

Stairs

Riser (the vertical dimension that separates one stair tread from the next stair tread) height must be not less than 4 inches or greater than 7 inches. Angulation of risers (lowest point to highest point for each stair) must not exceed 30 degrees. Open risers, a lack of the vertical board at the back of each stair, are not permitted. Tread (horizontal dimension) must be not less than 11 inches. Tread nosing, the front edge of a tread, must not project greater than 1.5 inches, with a radius of curvature for the nosing of not greater than .5 inch. For any given set of stairs, dimensions and configuration must be consistent for all stairs. Outdoor stairs and paths must be designed to avoid accumulation of moisture. Handrails must be provided along both sides of the stairway, except in assembly areas, and must conform to the guidelines presented previously under *Handrails*.

Transportation Facilities

Many areas and components within municipal and intercity transportation facilities appear elsewhere on this list, such as *Accessible Routes, Reach Ranges,* and *Restrooms,* and must meet all individually listed criteria.

Clear-space areas must be on an accessible route. For entry onto buses, a clear-space area of not less than 96 inches in length parallel to the path of bus travel is required. The width of such a clear-space area must be not less than 60 inches in width from the curb, although this may be limited by site constraints.

Fare gates must be on an accessible route, and automatic fare gates may not prohibit accessible entry to a transit system. At least one accessible fare gate must be available. Accessible fare gates must be not less than 32 inches in width at fare collection. Controls for such fare gates must conform to *Reach Range* requirements presented earlier.

To the greatest extent possible, accessible routes should follow paths comparable to paths used by the general public, with distances along the accessible route minimized to the greatest extent possible. Platform edges must be protected by screens or guard rails. When not protected by screens or guard rails, detectable warnings must be in place. Shelters must be on an accessible route, with clear-space areas of not less than 30 inches by 48 inches available entirely within the shelter.

■ Take Note
Information for safe stairs and families creating access to, and within, a house.

Chapter Review

Review Questions

1. What is the purpose of the Americans with Disabilities Act (ADA)?

2. What are the years in which the ADA, the ABA, and the most recent USAB guidelines were issued?

3. List general considerations and specific requirements of the ADA.

4. How does the ADA improve accessibility of facilities for people with physical impairments?

Suggested Activities

1. Access the USAB website and find the *New ADA–ABA Accessibility Guidelines*.

2. Examine specific areas for accessibility at your campus. Suggested areas are classrooms, restrooms, the library, building entryways, the cafeteria, dormitory rooms, and access to floors other than the ground floor.

3. Examine assigned areas playing the role of physical therapist or patient. Suggested modes of ambulation when role-playing as patient include using crutches, a wheelchair, or a walker.

4. Spend at least 2 hours in a public area while using an assistive device for ambulation. Consistently and appropriately role-play the need for the assistive device. Observe and write a report about the public reaction to your presence, your own reaction to using assistive devices in a public place, and any architectural barriers encountered.

Case Study

You have been tasked with providing the characteristics of an entrance ramp into a building. The rise from grade level (the ground) to entry level is 22 inches. The clear space for the ramp is 15 feet along the front of the building and 8 feet between the front of the building and the sidewalk.

1. Is this enough clear space to build a ramp that meets ADA requirements?
2. How would the ramp be configured with respect to
   a. Length
   b. Landings if necessary
   c. Width
   d. Handrails?

References

1. United States Congress (101st), Americans with Disabilities Act (PL 101–336), 1990.
2. United States Access Board, A Guide to the New ADA-ABA Accessibility Guidelines. www.access-board.gov; July 23, 2004.

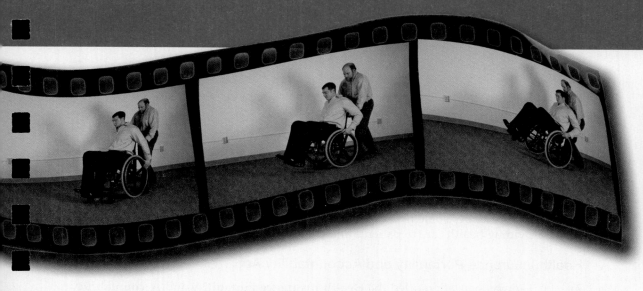

Patient/Client Management Process

Learning Objectives

Upon completion of this chapter, you will be able to:

1. Describe the Health Insurance Portability and Accountability Act (HIPAA) with respect to protection of patient confidentiality.

2. Describe the nineteen Health Insurance Portability and Accountability Act (HIPAA) identifiers in medical records.

3. Describe why these patient identifiers are protected by HIPAA.

4. Describe the Nagi and International Classification of Function (ICF) models of the continuums of health to disability.

5. Describe the elements of the Patient/Client Management process presented in the *Guide to Physical Therapist Practice.*

6. Describe the purposes of an initial interview with the patient.

7. Describe the two styles of questions, and when they are used, in an interview.

8. List and provide examples of the content included in an initial patient interview.

9. List the purposes of documentation in the health-care system.

10. Describe two formats of medical records: Discipline Specific and Problem Oriented Medical Record.

11. Describe two formats of documentation within the medical record: SOAP note and Patient/Client Management.

12. Describe the sections of the SOAP note format, and provide an overview of material included in each section.

13. Describe the elements of the Patient/Client Management note format, and provide an overview of material included in each section.

Key Terms

Active pathology
Analysis (SOAP note)
Audit
Closed-ended question
Daily note
Database
Diagnosis
Disability
Discharge note
Documentation
Evaluation
Examination
Functional limitation
Health Insurance
  Portability and
  Accountability Act
  (HIPAA)
Identifiers
Impairment
Initial note
Intervention
Interview

Long-term goals (LTGs)
Narrative note
Objective (SOAP note)
Open-ended question
Outcome
Patient/client management
  note
Plan (SOAP note)
Plan of care
Preferred practice patterns
Problem list
Problem-oriented medical
  record (POMR) method
Prognosis
Progress (interim) notes
Short-term goals (STGs)
Signs
SOAP note
Source-oriented method
Subjective (SOAP note)
Symptoms
Systems review

14. State where Medicare requirements for documentation can be found.

15. Write examples of patient goals, using appropriate criteria for content and format.

16. Discuss the requirements of adequate documentation.

17. List the information provided by the medical records audit.

Introduction

This chapter describes some of the processes, responsibilities, and requirements of clinicians providing health care to patients and clients.

Health Insurance Portability and Accountability Act

In 1996, Federal legislation titled the **Health Insurance Portability and Accountability Act (HIPAA)**[1] became law. Its effective date of compliance was April, 2002. The purpose of HIPAA requirements is to protect confidentiality of patient medical information and records when stored, when discussed by health-care providers, and as they are conveyed between health-care providers or between health-care providers and insurers. The requirements of HIPAA were established to avoid confidential patient medical information being revealed and used inappropriately. An example of revealing patient medical information inappropriately can occur when health-care providers discuss patient care in public venues, such as hallways or elevators, or when medical records are left accessible to persons who do not have a right to view such information. Inappropriate use of patient medical information might be obtained by disregard of, or insensitivity to, HIPAA. HIPAA rules are mandates that health-care providers protect patient confidentiality by how they store and disseminate patient medical information in written and oral format.

Within HIPAA, eighteen specific **identifiers** (the first eighteen listed) and one general (the last listed) identifier are listed. These identifiers could allow identification of an individual and the individual's medical information and thus are to be protected to prevent inappropriate use of this information. The nineteen identifiers are

- Name/initials
- Street address, city, county, precinct, zip code, and equivalent geocodes
- All elements of dates (except year) directly related to an individual
- All ages over 89
- Telephone number
- Fax number
- E-mail address
- Social Security number
- Medical record numbers
- Health plan identification numbers
- Account numbers
- Certificate/license numbers
- Vehicle identifiers and serial numbers, including license plate numbers
- Device identifiers and serial numbers
- Web (Internet) addresses (uniform resource locators [URLs])
- Internet provider (IP) addresses
- Biometric identifiers, including finger and voice prints
- Full face photographic images and any comparable images
- Any other unique identifying number, characteristic, or code (a code is an identifier if the person holding the coded data can re-identify the individual).

HIPAA identifiers are data that might be used to identify a specific person and any health conditions that person may have. Protecting these data from intentional or unintentional dissemination avoids identifying a person and his/her medical history. While a direct connection may not be able to be made between health information and a specific person without additional effort, knowledge of any one of the nineteen identifiers can allow others to connect a person and his or her medical history.

To provide confidentiality, the nineteen identifiers must not be released without a patient's express written permission. Permission must be requested by each facility with which a patient has a relationship. Facilities also are required to provide each patient with written notification of policies and procedures relating to patient confidentiality under HIPAA regulations, and each patient must sign a statement indicating that he or she has been informed of such policies. To ensure that expectations of privacy encompassed by HIPAA regulations are met successfully, health-care professionals' conversations concerning patients must be conducted in appropriate areas to avoid being overheard by others. Discussion in certain areas such as cafeterias, elevators, and hallways, when others can overhear the conversation, is *not* appropriate.

■ **Take Note**

Permission to release or share patient medical information is required and must be in writing.

Institutions are required to inform patients/clients as to how medical information will be shared. Typically, a brochure that provides a short synopsis of the institution's confidentiality policies is given to the patient for information. A second form, which may be called a *Patient Authorization Form, Informed Consent Form,* or *Release Form,* then is provided to patients/clients for signature. The institution retains a copy of the form the patient/client has signed in the patient's/client's file as an indication that the patient/client was informed and gave his or her consent.

The brochure provided to patients includes the institution's name, effective date of the information, and an office name and telephone number for contact if there are questions or if issues arise. Subsequent portions of the informational notice include, but are not limited to, (1) the institution's statement of why it provides this information; (2) who will be following these practices; (3) how a patient's/client's medical information can be used under stated policies, including insurance companies that provide reimbursement and law enforcement agencies; (4) special circumstances that may arise; and (5) how the patient's/client's medical information can/will be shared in the event of disputes and lawsuits that may arise from the cause of an illness/injury or as a result of care by the institution. The informational brochure might be two sides of a legal-size piece of paper, while the form to be signed is usually a half page or full page. The forms for signature typically state that the patient/client has been given the information, the information is understood, and the patient/client agrees to the scenarios under which confidential medical information may be shared.

Models for Describing the Continuum of Health to Disability

Models are methods that assist thinking on a topic. A number of models exist to describe a person's state of health. Nagi[2-4] describes a model with four sequential phases: (1) active pathology, (2) impairment, (3) functional limitation, and (4) disability (see ■ **Figure 2–1**). The first phase, **active pathology**, is the interruption of normal body function at the cellular level. The second phase, **impairment**, results when the body cannot compensate or heal itself, with the result that the individual sustains loss of normal function of a system. The third phase, **functional limitation**, occurs when the loss of a system is sufficient to prevent the performance of routine tasks by an individual, such as performing activities of daily living (ADLs), independently and in a timely manner. The fourth phase, **disability**, occurs when functional limitations prevent an individual from fulfilling his/her life roles.

■ **Take Note**

An example of the Nagi model—active pathology = osteoarthritis of the hip; impairment = decreased hip extension; functional limitation = decreased distance of ambulation; disability = inability to do grocery shopping.

Pathology → *Impairment* → *Functional Limitation* → *Disability*

■ **Figure 2–1** The Nagi Model of Disability.[2-4]

In the International Classification of Function (ICF)[5] model (■ Figures 2–2 and ■ 2–3), emphasis is placed on what an individual is able to do and how the environment influences participation in life roles. The ICF model is more complex because it accommodates more variables. The shifting of emphasis from pathology and disability (NAGI model) to activities and participation (World Health Organization's ICF) is ongoing and is increasingly being incorporated as the framework for the provision of health care.

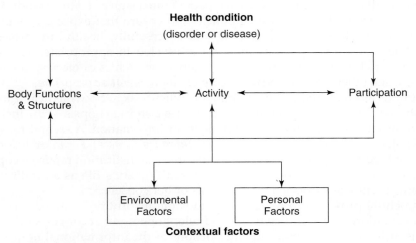

Health condition
(disorder or disease)

Body Functions & Structure ⟷ Activity ⟷ Participation

Environmental Factors   Personal Factors

Contextual factors

■ **Figure 2–2** The International Classification of Function.[5]

	Part 1: Functioning and Disability		Part 2: Contextual Factors	
Components	Body functions and structures	Activities and participation	Environmental factors	Personal factors
Domains	Body functions and structures	Life areas (tasks, actions)	External influences on functioning and disability	Internal influences on functioning and disability
Constructs	Change in body functions (physiological) Change in body structures (anatomical)	Capacity executing tasks in a standard environment Performance executing tasks in the current environment	Facilitating or hindering impact of features of the physical, social, and attitudinal world	Impact of attributes of the person
Positive aspect	Functional and structural integrity	Activities and participation	Facilitators	Not applicable
	Functioning			
Negative aspect	Impairment	Activity limitation and participation restriction	Barriers/hindrances	Not applicable
	Disability			

■ **Figure 2–3** Overview of International Classification of Function.[5]

Guide to Physical Therapist Practice

The American Physical Therapy Association developed an evolving document, the *Guide to Physical Therapist Practice (Guide)*,[6] based in part on the Nagi model. The *Guide* describes physical therapy practice and defines the physical therapy patient/client management process (see ■ Figure 2–4). *Guide* contents describe preferred practice patterns in four categories in the scope of physical therapy practice: (1) musculoskeletal, (2) neuromuscular, (3) cardiovascular/pulmonary, and (4) integumentary. In many cases we have quoted directly from, or paraphrased, the *Guide* to illustrate connections between general concepts and how physical therapists apply those concepts.

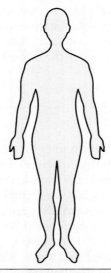

DIAGNOSIS
Both the process and the end result of evaluating examination data, which the physical therapist organizes into defined clusters, syn-dromes, or categories to help determine the prognosis (including the plan of care) and the most appropriate intervention strategies.

PROGNOSIS (Including Plan of Care)
Determination of the level of optimal improvement that may be attained through intervention and the amount of time required to reach that level. The plan of care specifies the inter- ventions to be used and their timing and frequency.

EVALUATION
A dynamic process in which the physical therapist makes clinical judgments based on data gathered during the examination. This process also may identify possible problems that require consultation with or referral to another provider.

INTERVENTION
Purposeful and skilled interaction of the physical therapist with the patient/client and, if appropriate, with other individuals involved in care of the patient/client, using various physical therapy methods and techniques to produce changes in the condition that are consistent with the diagnosis and prognosis. The physical therapist conducts a reex-amination to determine changes in patient/client status and to modify or redirect intervention. The decision to reexamine may be based on new clinical findings or on lack of patient/client progress. The process of reexamination also may identify the need for consultation with or referral to another provider.

EXAMINATION
The process of obtaining a history, performing a systems review, and selecting and administering tests and measures to gather data about the patient/client. The initial examination is a comprehensive screening and specific testing process that leads to a diagnostic classification. The examination process also may identify possible problems that require consultation with or referral to another provider.

OUTCOMES
Results of patient/client management, which include the impact of physical therapy interventions in the following domains: pathology/pathophysiology (disease, disorder, or condition); impairments, functional limitations, and disabilities; risk reduction/prevention; health, wellness, and fitness; societal resources; and patient/client satisfaction.

■ **Figure 2–4**   Elements of Patient/Client Management Leading to Optimal Outcomes. Reprinted with permission from the American Physical Therapy Association.

Preferred practice patterns describe elements of evidence-based patient management for specific diagnoses. Preferred practice patterns guide management of patients but do not prescribe specifics of patient/client management. Each health-care discipline has its own preferred practice patterns. A physical therapy preferred practice pattern is a detailed description of the elements that comprise physical therapy patient/client management of impairments, functional limitations, activity limitations, or participation restrictions. Physical therapy patient/client management must be within the scope of physical therapist

■ **Take Note**
PT patient/client management process—examination, evaluation, diagnosis, prognosis, intervention, and outcomes.

practice. Physical therapy patient/client management is individualized through implementation of six elements: (1) examination, (2) evaluation, (3) diagnosis, (4) prognosis (including plan of care), (5) intervention, and (6) outcomes. **Examination** is the process of generating a patient/client history, reviewing all physiologic systems, and applying tests and measures. Some of the tests and measures selected by a physical therapist may be performed by a physical therapist assistant under the direction and supervision of a physical therapist. **Evaluation** is the process whereby physical therapists use examination data, professional knowledge, and clinical judgment to identify impairments and functional limitations and generate diagnoses, prognoses, and a plan of care. **Diagnosis** is assignment of a label that states the categorization or classification of problems identified and is selected from the practice pattern or diagnostic category that most closely describes a patient's impairments and functional limitations as presented in the *Guide*. A physical therapist's diagnosis is related to the impairments and functional limitations. Diagnosis directs the development of prognosis, plan of care, and selection of interventions. When a physical therapist cannot place a patient in a diagnostic category, the patient's active pathology is not within the scope of physical therapy practice. In such cases, physical therapists refer patients to appropriate health-care practitioners. **Prognosis** is the determination of an optimal level of improvement and the time necessary to achieve projected outcomes. An **outcome** is the functional capacity of a patient/client. A **plan of care** is a statement that specifies outcomes, interventions to be provided to achieve the stated outcomes, and a timeline for reaching the stated outcomes. An **intervention** includes treatment, communication, education, and planning. Some aspects of treatment, communication, and education may be performed by a physical therapist assistant under the direction and supervision of a physical therapist.

Examination

Chart Review

A patient's medical information may be available in either paper or electronic form. Access to medical information in either format is subject to HIPAA requirements. Complete charts are available for inpatient care in hospitals and residential environments. Complete charts may not be available in outpatient environments, with outpatient charts containing information specific to only the outpatient clinic. Initial reviews of patient charts are performed by physical therapists prior to the first contact with patients. Subsequent review(s), prior to treatment sessions, may be performed by physical therapist assistants. Chart reviews prior to each treatment are necessary to determine any relevant changes in patient status or orders. When chart reviews are conducted by a physical therapist assistant, and changes in patient status or orders are noted, the physical therapist must be informed as soon as such changes are noted. Periodically, charts are reviewed by physical therapists to ensure appropriate clinical decision making and continuity of care.

Intake history in medical charts usually contains information about (1) general demographics, (2) current condition or chief complaint, (3) medical/surgical history, (4) general health status, (5) social history, (6) family history, (7) social health habits, (8) previous and present functional status, (9) medications, and (10) clinical tests ordered and their results. When the patient is a child, development is also reviewed. While initial information related to patient status is in the intake history, continually updated information concerning patient status, medications, and other orders will be recorded in specific sections of the chart.

Interview

Patient **interviews** (■ **Figure 2–5**) are a component of the patient/client management process. Physical therapists introduce themselves to patients by full name and profession and address patients by their full name. Only when a patient indicates that less for-

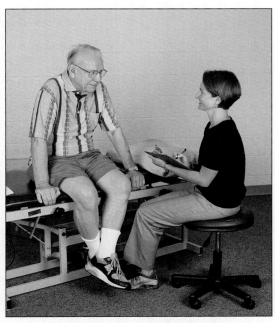

■ **Figure 2–5**   Physical therapist interviewing a patient.

mality is acceptable or desired should a patient be addressed by his/her first name. The physical therapist should request and receive permission to conduct an interview. Patient comfort, safety, and eye contact with the patient, when possible, are established. Types of data necessary for the patient/client management process that may be obtained by a chart review and patient/client interview are presented in ■ **Figure 2–6**.

A physical therapist's relationship with a patient/client usually begins with an initial interview. Experienced physical therapists initiate collection of information about patients as soon as a patient is observed. Patients begin judging therapists when they are first observed and introduced. Dress, body language, and general demeanor convey a message that may be more powerful than a therapist's words. Health-care professionals are responsible for establishing an appropriate environment and interactions with patients/clients based upon mutual trust.

Information gathered during chart reviews is discussed with patients to determine accuracy and completeness. Specifics of the chief complaint(s) are explored. A survey of all physiologic systems is completed by questioning the patient. An example of a format for recording information, reproduced from the *Guide*, is included in ■ **Figure 2–7**. Brief patient interviews should be conducted prior to each treatment to determine if the patient perceives any relevant changes in his or her status. These subsequent brief interviews should be conducted by physical therapists whenever possible but may be conducted by physical therapist assistants. As with chart reviews, when follow-up patient interviews by physical therapist assistants reveal significant changes in patient status, the physical therapist must be informed as soon as possible.

Two types of questions are used during interviews. **Open-ended questions** allow a patient to tell his or her story in his or her own words. Examples of open-ended questions are:

- "What are the problems you are having?"
- "Tell me about your injury."

Closed-ended questions are used to obtain or confirm specific information. An example of a closed-ended question is: "Have you ever had this pain before?" Closed-ended questions often are answered with a single word or a brief phrase, such as "Yes," "No," or "Yes, once or twice before."

■ **Take Note**
Confirms chart information, obtains subjective information.

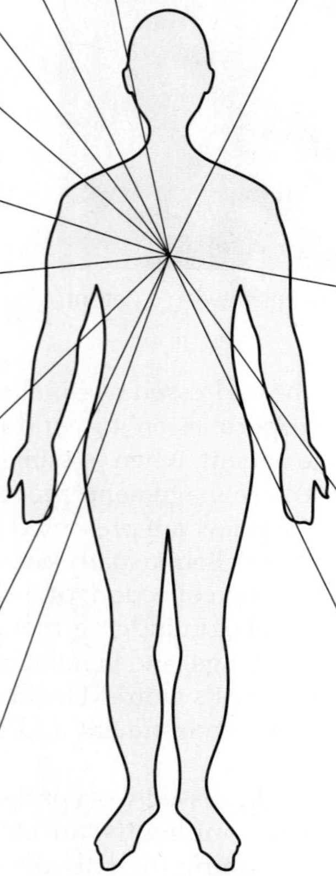

General Demographics
- Age
- Gender
- Race/ethnicity
- Primary language
- Education

Social History
- Cultural beliefs and behaviors
- Family and caregiver resources
- Social interactions, social activities, and support systems

Employment/Work (Job/School/Play)
- Current and prior work (job/school/play), community, and leisure actions, tasks, or activities

Growth and Development
- Developmental history
- Hand dominance

Living Environment
- Devices and equipment (e.g., assistive, adaptive, orthotic, protective, supportive, prosthetic)
- Living environment and community characteristics
- Projected discharge destinations

General Health Status (Self-Report, Family Report, Caregiver Report)
- General health perception
- Physical function (e.g., mobility, sleep patterns, restricted bed days)
- Psychological function (e.g., memory, reasoning ability, depression, anxiety)
- Role function (e.g., community, leisure, social, work)
- Social function (e.g., social activity, social interaction, social support)

Social/Health Habits (Past and Current)
- Behavioral health risks (e.g., smoking, drug abuse)
- Level of physical fitness

Family History
- Familial health risks

Medical/Surgical History
- Cardiovascular
- Endocrine/metabolic
- Gastrointestinal
- Genitourinary
- Gynecological
- Integumentary
- Musculoskeletal
- Neuromuscular
- Obstetrical
- Prior hospitalizations, surgeries, and preexisting medical and other health-related conditions
- Psychological
- Pulmonary

Current Condition(s)/ Chief Complaint(s)
- Concerns that led the patient/client to seek the services of a physical therapist
- Concerns or needs of patient/client who requires the services of a physical therapist
- Current therapeutic interventions
- Mechanisms of injury or disease, including date of onset and course of events
- Onset and pattern of symptoms
- Patient/client, family, significant other, and caregiver expectations and goals for the therapeutic intervention
- Patient/client, family, significant other, and caregiver perceptions of patient's/client's emotional response to the current clinical situation
- Previous occurrence of chief complaint(s)
- Prior therapeutic interventions

Functional Status and Activity Level
- Current and prior functional status in self-care and home management, including activities of daily living (ADL) and instrumental activities of daily living (IADL)
- Current and prior functional status in work (job/school/play), community, and leisure actions, tasks, or activities

Medications
- Medications for current condition
- Medications previously taken for current condition
- Medications for other conditions

Other Clinical Tests
- Laboratory and diagnostic tests
- Review of available records (e.g., medical, education, surgical)
- Review of other clinical findings (e.g., nutrition and hydration)

■ Figure 2–6 Types of Data That May Be Generated from a Patient/Client History. Reprinted with permission from the American Physical Therapy Association.

**DOCUMENTATION TEMPLATE FOR
PHYSICAL THERAPIST PATIENT/CLIENT MANAGEMENT
Inpatient Form, Page 1**

Today's Date: _____
Patient ID#: _____

Inpatient History

American Physical Therapy Association

IDENTIFICATION INFORMATION

1 Name: _____

a Last _____

b First _____ c MI _____ d Jr/Sr

2 Admission Date: [Month □□] [Day □□] [Year □□□□]

3 Date of Birth: [Month □□] [Day □□] [Year □□□□]

4 Gender: a □ Male   b □ Female

5 Dominant Hand: a □ Right   b □ Left   c □ Unknown

6 Race
a □ Asian
b □ Native Hawaiian/
   Pacific Islander
c □ Black
d □ White

7 Ethnicity
a □ Hispanic or
   Latino
b □ Not Hispanic
   or Latino

8 Language
a □ English
   understood?
b □ Interpreter
   needed?
c □ Primary
   language:
   _____

9 Education
a Highest grade completed (Circle one): 1 2 3 4 5 6 7 8 9 10 11 12
b □ Some college/technical school
c □ College graduate
d □ Graduate school/advanced degree

10 Has patient completed an advance directive? a □ Yes b □ No

11 Referred by: _____

12 Reasons for referral to physical therapy: _____
_____
_____

SOCIAL HISTORY
13 Cultural/Religious
Any customs or religious beliefs or wishes that might affect care?
_____
_____

14 Lives(d) With

	A-Admission	B-Expected at Discharge
a Alone	□	□
b Spouse only	□	□
c Spouse and other(s)	□	□
d Child (not spouse)	□	□
e Other relative(s) (not spouse or children)	□	□
f Group setting	□	□
g Personal care attendant	□	□
h Unknown	□	□
i Other_____		

15 Available Social Supports (family/friends)
0 = No   1 = Possibly yes   2 = Definitely

	Now	Willing/Able Postdischarge
a Emotional support	□	□
b Intermittent physical support with ADLs or IADLs—less than daily	□	□
c Intermittent physical support with ADLs or IADLs—daily	□	□
d Full-time physical support (as needed) with ADLs or IADLs	□	□
e All or most of necessary transportation	□	□

16 Caregiver Status Presence of family member/friend willing and able to assist patient/client?   a □ Yes   b □ No

17 EMPLOYMENT/WORK (Job/School/Play)
a □ Working full-time outside of home
b □ Working part-time outside of home
c □ Working full-time from home
d □ Working part-time from home
e □ Homemaker f □ Student g □ Retired h □ Unemployed

i Occupation: _____

LIVING ENVIRONMENT
18 Devices and Equipment (eg, cane, glasses, hearing aids, walker)
_____
_____
_____
_____
_____
_____

19 Type of Residence

	A-Admission	B-Expected at Discharge
a Private home	□	□
b Private apartment	□	□
c Rented room	□	□
d Board and care/assisted living/group home	□	□
e Homeless (with or without shelter)	□	□
f Long-term care facility (nursing home)	□	□
g Hospice	□	□
h Unknown	□	□
i Other_____		

20 Environment

	A-Admission	B-Expected at Discharge
a Stairs, no railing	□	□
b Stairs, railing	□	□
c Ramps	□	□
d Elevator	□	□
e Uneven terrain	□	□
f Other obstacles:_____		

21 Past Use of Community Services
0 = No   1 = Unknown   2 = Yes

a Day services/programs	□	f Mental health service	□
b Home health services	□	g Respiratory therapy	□
c Homemaking services	□	h Therapies—PT, OT, SLP	□
d Hospice	□	i Other (eg, volunteer)	□
e Meals on Wheels	□	_____	

22 GENERAL HEALTH STATUS
a Patient/client rates health as:

□ Excellent   □ Good   □ Fair   □ Poor

b Major life changes during past year? (1) □ Yes (2) □ No

[OVER]

■ **Figure 2–7** Documentation Template for Physical Therapist/Client Management: Inpatient Form. Reprinted with permission from the American Physical Therapy Association.

DOCUMENTATION TEMPLATE FOR PHYSICAL THERAPIST PATIENT/CLIENT MANAGEMENT
Inpatient Form, Page 2

23 SOCIAL/HEALTH HABITS (Past and Current)

a Alcohol
   (1) How many days per week does patient/client drink beer, wine, or other alcoholic beverages, on average? _____
   (2) If one beer, one glass of wine, or one cocktail equals one drink, how many drinks does patient/client have, on an average day? _____

b Smoking
   (1) Currently smokes tobacco?
      (a) ☐ Yes
         1. ☐ Cigarettes # of packs per day _____
         2. ☐ Cigars/pipes # per day _____
      (b) ☐ No
   (2) Smoked in past?   (a) ☐ Yes   Year quit: ☐☐☐☐
                          (b) ☐ No

c Exercise
   (1) Exercises beyond normal daily activities and chores?
      (a) ☐ Yes
   Describe the exercise: _____
      1. On average, how many days per week does patient/client exercise or do physical activity? _____
      2. For how many minutes, on an average day? _____
      (b) ☐ No

24 FAMILY HISTORY

Condition:	Relationship to Patient/Client:	Age of Onset (if known):
a Heart disease	_____	_____
b Hypertension	_____	_____
c Stroke	_____	_____
d Diabetes	_____	_____
e Cancer	_____	_____
f Other: _____	_____	_____
_____	_____	_____

25 PATIENT/CLIENT MEDICAL/SURGICAL HISTORY: _____
_____
_____
_____
_____
_____

26 FUNCTIONAL STATUS/ACTIVITY LEVEL (Check all that apply.)
a ☐ Difficulty with locomotion/movement:
   (1) ☐ bed mobility
   (2) ☐ transfers
   (3) ☐ gait (walking)
      (a) ☐ on level
      (b) ☐ on stairs
      (c) ☐ on ramps
      (d) ☐ on uneven terrain
b ☐ Difficulty with self-care (such as bathing, dressing, eating, toileting)
c ☐ Difficulty with home management (such as household chores, shopping, driving/transportation)
d ☐ Difficulty with community and work activities/integration
   (1) ☐ work/school
   (2) ☐ recreation or play activity

27 MEDICATIONS (list): _____
_____
_____
_____
_____
_____
_____
_____
_____
_____
_____
_____

28 OTHER CLINICAL TESTS (list):

	Month	Year	Findings
_____	☐☐	☐☐☐☐	_____
_____	☐☐	☐☐☐☐	_____
_____	☐☐	☐☐☐☐	_____
_____	☐☐	☐☐☐☐	_____

■ **Figure 2–7**   (continued)

The types of questions used provide direction for interviews, beginning with open-ended questions to elicit the most information from the patient. During an interview, physical therapists should summarize patient responses periodically. Then, using closed-ended questions, physical therapists should ask the patient if the summary is correct. If the summary is not correct, additional questions are used to clarify details. Closed-ended questions focus the discussion and are used to elicit specific information a patient may not have thought to include. Interviews are concluded by asking the patient if there is any additional information he or she believes is relevant to his or her care.

A plan and structure for interviews permits physical therapists to elicit information in a reasonable amount of time. Data collection forms, such as those reproduced from the *Guide* (Figure 2–7 and ■ Figure 2–8) for both inpatient and outpatient environments, provide structure for interviews and assist in collection of data in an organized manner. Patients in outpatient settings can complete forms that provide information about current and prior medical conditions, including family history, prior to being seen by a physical therapist. During interviews, data supplied by patients are reviewed with the patient, and additional data are elicited to complete any missing and necessary information.

Systems Review

The last part of interviews consists of a **systems review**. A review of systems is a "brief or limited examination of (1) the anatomical and physiological status of the cardiovascular/pulmonary, integumentary, musculoskeletal, and neuromuscular systems and (2) the communication ability, affect, cognition, language, and learning style of the patient."[6] Patients/clients should be questioned as to any complaints about bodily systems not identified during the interview. ■ Figure 2–9 is a form reproduced from the *Guide* that can be used for systems review.

Following chart review, collection of interview data, and systems review, a physical therapist should organize and review patient information to choose appropriate tests and measures.

Tests and Measures

Physical therapists may perform all tests and measures selected and may delegate performance of specific tests and measures to physical therapist assistants. Examples of tests and measures for each of the four patient care patterns are aerobic endurance, integumentary integrity, joint mobility and integrity, and sensory integrity. These tests and measures generate data used in evaluation. ■ Figure 2–10 is a form reproduced from the *Guide* that can be used to select tests and measures.

Evaluation

Evaluation (■ Figure 2–11) is the synthesis and analysis of data collected during chart review, interview, systems review, and application of tests and measures. From this evaluation, physical therapists make clinical judgments with regard to diagnosis, prognosis, and plan of care. Only physical therapists may perform these functions. Inability to provide a diagnosis indicates that a patient should be referred to a different practitioner. Need for such a referral may occur because (1) additional tests and measures must be performed or (2) the health care required is not within the scope of physical therapy practice. There are cases where physical therapists refer patients to another physical therapist with expertise in the necessary domain.

DOCUMENTATION TEMPLATE FOR PHYSICAL THERAPIST
PATIENT/CLIENT MANAGEMENT
Outpatient Form 1, Page 1

Today's Date: _____

Patient ID#: _____

1 Name: _____

a Last _____

b First _____ c MI ____ d Jr/Sr ____

2 Street Address: _____

City _____ State _____ Zip _____

3 Date of Birth: Month [ ][ ] Day [ ][ ] Year [ ][ ][ ][ ]

4 Gender: a ☐ Male b ☐ Female

5 Are you: a ☐ Right-handed b ☐ Left-handed

6 Type of Insurance: a ☐ Insurer _____

b ☐ Workers' Comp c ☐ Medicare d ☐ Self-pay e ☐ Other

7 Race
a ☐ Asian
b ☐ Native Hawaiian/
  Pacific Islander
c ☐ Black
d ☐ White

8 Ethnicity
a ☐ Hispanic or
  Latino
b ☐ Not Hispanic
  or Latino

9 Language
a ☐ English
  understood?
b ☐ Interpreter
  needed?
c ☐ Language you
  speak most
  often:
  _____

10 Education
a Highest grade completed (Circle one): 1 2 3 4 5 6 7 8 9 10 11 12
b ☐ Some college/technical school
c ☐ College graduate
d ☐ Graduate school/advanced degree

SOCIAL HISTORY
11 Cultural/Religious
Any customs or religious beliefs or wishes that might affect care?

_____

12 With whom do you live?
a ☐ Alone
b ☐ Spouse only
c ☐ Spouse and other(s)
d ☐ Child (not spouse)
e ☐ Other relative(s) (not spouse or children)
f ☐ Group setting
g ☐ Personal care attendant
h ☐ Other:

13 Have you completed an advance directive?
a ☐ Yes b ☐ No

14 Who referred you to the physical therapist:

_____

15 Employment/Work (Job/School/Play)

a ☐ Working full-time
  outside of home
b ☐ Working part-time
  outside of home
c ☐ Working full-time
  from home
d ☐ Working part-time
  from home
e ☐ Homemaker f ☐ Student g ☐ Retired h ☐ Unemployed

i Occupation: _____

LIVING ENVIRONMENT
16 Does your home have:
a ☐ Stairs, no railing
b ☐ Stairs, railing
c ☐ Ramps
d ☐ Elevator
e ☐ Uneven terrain
f ☐ Assistive devices (eg,
  bathroom): _____
g ☐ Any obstacles: _____

17 Do you use:
a ☐ Cane
b ☐ Walker or rollator
c ☐ Manual wheelchair
d ☐ Motorized wheelchair
e ☐ Glasses, hearing aids
f ☐ Other: _____
  _____
  _____

18 Where do you live?
a ☐ Private home
b ☐ Private apartment
c ☐ Rented room
d ☐ Board and care / assisted living / group home
e ☐ Homeless (with or without shelter)
f ☐ Long-term care facility (nursing home)
g ☐ Hospice
h ☐ Other: _____

19 GENERAL HEALTH STATUS
a Please rate your health:
  (1) ☐ Excellent (2) ☐ Good (3) ☐ Fair (4) ☐ Poor
b Have you had any major life changes during past year? (eg, new baby, job change, death of a family member) (1) ☐ Yes (2) ☐ No

20 SOCIAL/HEALTH HABITS
a Smoking
  (1) Currently smoke tobacco? (a) ☐ Yes 1. ☐ Cigarettes
      # of packs per day _____
      2. ☐ Cigars/Pipes
      # per day _____
      (b) ☐ No
  (2) Smoked in past? (a) ☐ Yes Year quit: [ ][ ][ ][ ] (b) ☐ No

b Alcohol
  (1) How many days per week do you drink beer, wine, or other alcoholic beverages, on average? _____
  (2) If one beer, one glass of wine, or one cocktail equals one drink, how many drinks do you have, on an average day? _____
c Exercise
  Do you exercise beyond normal daily activities and chores?
      (a) ☐ Yes Describe the exercise: _____
          1. On average, how many days per week
             do you exercise or do physical activity? _____
          2. For how many minutes, on an average day? _____
      (b) ☐ No

21 FAMILY HISTORY (Indicate whether mother, father, brother/sister, aunt/uncle, or grandmother/grandfather, and age of onset if known)
a Heart disease: _____
b Hypertension: _____
c Stroke: _____
d Diabetes: _____
e Cancer: _____
f Psychological: _____
g Arthritis: _____
h Osteoporosis: _____
i Other: _____

© American Physical Therapy Association 1999; revised September 2000

Outpatient History

American Physical Therapy Association

■ **Figure 2–8** Documentation Template for Physical Therapist Patient/Client Management: Outpatient Form. Reprinted with permission from the American Physical Therapy Association.

DOCUMENTATION TEMPLATE FOR PHYSICAL THERAPIST PATIENT/CLIENT MANAGEMENT
Outpatient Form, Page 2

22 MEDICAL/SURGICAL HISTORY

a Please check if you have ever had:

(1) ☐ Arthritis		(13) ☐	Multiple sclerosis
(2) ☐ Broken bones/ fractures		(14) ☐	Muscular dystrophy
		(15) ☐	Parkinson disease
(3) ☐ Osteoporosis		(16) ☐	Seizures/epilepsy
(4) ☐ Blood disorders		(17) ☐	Allergies
(5) ☐ Circulation/vascular problems		(18) ☐	Developmental or growth problems
(6) ☐ Heart problems		(19) ☐	Thyroid problems
(7) ☐ High blood pressure		(20) ☐	Cancer
		(21) ☐	Infectious disease (eg, tuberculosis, hepatitis)
(8) ☐ Lung problems			
(9) ☐ Stroke		(22) ☐	Kidney problems
(10) ☐ Diabetes/ high blood sugar		(23) ☐	Repeated infections
		(24) ☐	Ulcers/stomach problems
(11) ☐ Low blood sugar/ hypoglycemia		(25) ☐	Skin diseases
		(26) ☐	Depression
(12) ☐ Head injury		(27) ☐	Other:_____

b Within the past year, have you had any of the following symptoms? (Check all that apply.)

(1) ☐ Chest pain		(13) ☐	Difficulty sleeping
(2) ☐ Heart palpitations		(14) ☐	Loss of appetite
(3) ☐ Cough		(15) ☐	Nausea/vomiting
(4) ☐ Hoarseness		(16) ☐	Difficulty swallowing
(5) ☐ Shortness of breath		(17) ☐	Bowel problems
(6) ☐ Dizziness or blackouts		(18) ☐	Weight loss/gain
(7) ☐ Coordination problems		(19) ☐	Urinary problems
(8) ☐ Weakness in arms or legs		(20) ☐	Fever/chills/sweats
(9) ☐ Loss of balance		(21) ☐	Headaches
(10) ☐ Difficulty walking		(22) ☐	Hearing problems
(11) ☐ Joint pain or swelling		(23) ☐	Vision problems
(12) ☐ Pain at night		(24) ☐	Other:_____

c Have you ever had surgery?   (1) ☐ Yes   (2) ☐ No
If yes, please describe, and include dates:

	Month	Year
_____	☐☐	☐☐☐☐
_____	☐☐	☐☐☐☐
_____	☐☐	☐☐☐☐

For men only: d Have you been diagnosed with prostate disease?
(1) ☐ Yes (2) ☐ No

For women only:
Have you been diagnosed with:

e Pelvic inflammatory disease?
(1) ☐ Yes   (2) ☐ No

f Endometriosis?
(1) ☐ Yes   (2) ☐ No

g Trouble with your period?
(1) ☐ Yes   (2) ☐ No

h Complicated pregnancies or deliveries?
(1) ☐ Yes   (2) ☐ No

i Pregnant, or think you might be pregnant?
(1) ☐ Yes   (2) ☐ No

j Other gynecological or obstetrical difficulties?
(1) ☐ Yes   (2) ☐ No
If yes, please describe:
_____

23 CURRENT CONDITION(S)/CHIEF COMPLAINT(S)

a Describe the problem(s) for which you seek physical therapy
_____

b When did the problem(s) begin (date)?   Month ☐☐   Year ☐☐☐☐

c What happened?_____

d Have you ever had the problem(s) before?
(1) ☐ Yes
(a) What did you do for the problem(s)?_____
(b) Did the problem(s) get better?
1. ☐ Yes 2. ☐ No
(c) About how long did the problem(s) last?_____
(2) ☐ No

23 Current Condition(s)/Chief Complaint(s) (continued)

e How are you taking care of the problem(s) now?_____

f What makes the problem(s) better?_____

g What makes the problem(s) worse?_____

h What are your goals for physical therapy?_____

i Are you seeing anyone else for the problem(s)? (Check all that apply.)

(1) ☐ Acupuncturist		(10) ☐	Occupational therapist
(2) ☐ Cardiologist		(11) ☐	Orthopedist
(3) ☐ Chiropractor		(12) ☐	Osteopath
(4) ☐ Dentist		(13) ☐	Pediatrician
(5) ☐ Family practitioner		(14) ☐	Podiatrist
(6) ☐ Internist		(15) ☐	Primary care physician
(7) ☐ Massage therapist		(16) ☐	Rheumatologist
(8) ☐ Neurologist			Other:_____
(9) ☐ Obstetrician/gynecologist			

24 FUNCTIONAL STATUS/ACTIVITY LEVEL (Check all that apply.)

a ☐ Difficulty with locomotion/movement:
(1) ☐ bed mobility
(2) ☐ transfers (such as moving from bed to chair, from bed to commode)
(3) ☐ gait (walking)
(a) ☐ on level   (c) ☐ on ramps
(b) ☐ on stairs (d) ☐ on uneven terrain

b ☐ Difficulty with self-care (such as bathing, dressing, eating, toileting)

c ☐ Difficulty with home management (such as household chores, shopping, driving/transportation, care of dependents)

d ☐ Difficulty with community and work activities/integration
(1) ☐ work/school
(2) ☐ recreation or play activity

25 MEDICATIONS

a Do you take any prescription medications?   (1) ☐ Yes (2) ☐ No
If yes, please list:_____

b Do you take any nonprescription medications? (Check all that apply.)

(1) ☐ Advil/Aleve		(6) ☐	Decongestants
(2) ☐ Antacids		(7) ☐	Herbal supplements
(3) ☐ Ibuprofen/ Naproxen		(8) ☐	Tylenol
(4) ☐ Antihistamines		(9) ☐	Other:_____
(5) ☐ Aspirin			

c Have you taken any medications previously for the condition for which you are seeing the physical therapist?
(1) ☐ Yes   (2) ☐ No   If yes, please list:
_____

26 OTHER CLINICAL TESTS—Within the past year, have you had any of the following tests? (Check all that apply.)

a ☐ Angiogram		m ☐	Mammogram
b ☐ Arthroscopy		n ☐	MRI
c ☐ Biopsy		o ☐	Myelogram
d ☐ Blood tests		p ☐	NCV (nerve conduction velocity)
e ☐ Bone scan		q ☐	Pap smear
f ☐ Bronchoscopy		r ☐	Pulmonary function test
g ☐ CT scan		s ☐	Spinal tap
h ☐ Doppler ultrasound		t ☐	Stool tests
i ☐ Echocardiogram		u ☐	Stress test (eg, treadmill, bicycle)
j ☐ EEG (electroencephalogram)		v ☐	Urine tests
k ☐ EKG (electrocardiogram)		w ☐	X-rays
l ☐ EMG (electromyogram)		x ☐	Other:_____

© American Physical Therapy Association 1999; revised September 2000

■ **Figure 2–8** (continued)

**DOCUMENTATION TEMPLATE FOR
PHYSICAL THERAPIST PATIENT/CLIENT MANAGEMENT**
Systems Review

	Not Impaired	Impaired
CARDIOVASCULAR/PULMONARY SYSTEM	☐	☐

Heart rate:_____

Respiratory rate: _____

Blood pressure: _____

Edema: _____

INTEGUMENTARY SYSTEM	☐	☐

Integrity
Integumentary disruption:_____
Continuity of skin color:_____
Pliability (texture):_____

	Not Impaired	Impaired
MUSCULOSKELETAL SYSTEM		
Gross Symmetry	☐	☐

Standing:_____
Sitting: _____
Activity specific: _____

Gross Range of Motion	☐	☐
Gross Strength	☐	☐

Other: _____

Height _____

Weight _____

NEUROMUSCULAR SYSTEM

Gait	☐	☐
Locomotion (includes transfers, sit-to-stand transitions, bed mobility)	☐	☐
Balance	☐	☐
Motor function (motor control, motor learning)	☐	☐

	Not Impaired	Impaired
COMMUNICATION, AFFECT, COGNITION, LEARNING STYLE		
Communication (eg, age-appropriate)	☐	☐
Orientation × 3 (person/place/time)	☐	☐
Emotional/behavioral responses	☐	☐

Learning barriers:
☐ None
☐ Vision
☐ Hearing
☐ Unable to read
☐ Unable to understand what is read
☐ Language/needs interpreter
☐ Other:_____

Education needs:
☐ Disease process
☐ Safety
☐ Use of devices/equipment
☐ Activities of daily living
☐ Exercise program
☐ Other:_____

How does patient/client best learn? ☐ Pictures ☐ Reading ☐ Listening ☐ Demonstration ☐ Other:_____

© American Physical Therapy Association 1999; revised September 2000

Guide to Physical Therapist Practice   Appendix 6: Documentation Template 713/**S705**

Systems Review

American Physical Therapy Association

■ **Figure 2–9** Documentation Template for Physical Therapist Patient/Client Management: Systems Review. Reprinted with permission from the American Physical Therapy Association.

**DOCUMENTATION TEMPLATE FOR
PHYSICAL THERAPIST PATIENT/CLIENT MANAGEMENT
Tests and Measures**

KEY TO TESTS AND MEASURES:

1 Aerobic Capacity/Endurance
2 Anthropometric Characteristics
3 Arousal, Attention, and Cognition
4 Assistive and Adaptive Devices
5 Circulation (Arterial, Venous, Lymphatic)
6 Cranial and Peripheral Nerve Integrity
7 Environmental, Home, and Work (Job/School/Play) Barriers
8 Ergonomics and Body Mechanics
9 Gait, Locomotion, and Balance
10 Integumentary Integrity
11 Joint Integrity and Mobility
12 Motor Function (Motor Control and Motor Learning)
13 Muscle Performance (Including Strength, Power, and Endurance)

14 Neuromotor Development and Sensory Integration
15 Orthotic, Protective, and Supportive Devices
16 Pain
17 Posture
18 Prosthetic Requirements
19 Range of Motion (Including Muscle Length)
20 Reflex Integrity
21 Self-Care and Home Management (Including Activities of Daily Living and Instrumental Activities of Daily Living)
22 Sensory Integrity
23 Ventilation and Respiration/Gas Exchange
24 Work (Job/School/Play), Community, and Leisure Integration or Reintegration (Including Instrumental Activities of Daily Living)

NOTES:

_____

© American Physical Therapy Association 1999; revised September 2000

Guide to Physical Therapist Practice

Appendix 6: Documentation Template 715/**S707**

Tests and Measures

■ **Figure 2–10** Documentation Template for Physical Therapist Patient/Client Management: Tests and Measures. Reprinted with permission from the American Physical Therapy Association.

DOCUMENTATION TEMPLATE FOR PHYSICAL THERAPIST PATIENT/CLIENT MANAGEMENT
Evaluation

DIAGNOSIS:

Musculoskeletal Patterns

- ☐ A: Primary Prevention/Risk Reduction for Skeletal Demineralization
- ☐ B: Impaired Posture
- ☐ C: Impaired Muscle Performance
- ☐ D: Impaired Joint Mobility, Motor Function, Muscle Performance, and Range of Motion Associated With Connective Tissue Dysfunction
- ☐ E: Impaired Joint Mobility, Motor Function, Muscle Performance, and Range of Motion Associated With Localized Inflammation
- ☐ F: Impaired Joint Mobility, Motor Function, Muscle Performance, Range of Motion, and Reflex Integrity Associated With Spinal Disorders
- ☐ G: Impaired Joint Mobility, Muscle Performance, and Range of Motion Associated With Fracture
- ☐ H: Impaired Joint Mobility, Motor Function, Muscle Performance, and Range of Motion Associated With Joint Arthroplasty
- ☐ I: Impaired Joint Mobility, Motor Function, Muscle Performance, and Range of Motion Associated With Bony or Soft Tissue Surgery
- ☐ J: Impaired Motor Function, Muscle Performance, Range of Motion, Gait, Locomotion, and Balance Associated With Amputation

Neuromuscular Patterns

- ☐ A: Primary Prevention/Risk Reduction for Loss of Balance and Falling
- ☐ B: Impaired Neuromotor Development
- ☐ C: Impaired Motor Function and Sensory Integrity Associated With Nonprogressive Disorders of the Central Nervous System—Congenital Origin or Acquired in Infancy or Childhood
- ☐ D: Impaired Motor Function and Sensory Integrity Associated With Nonprogressive Disorders of the Central Nervous System—Acquired in Adolescence or Adulthood
- ☐ E: Impaired Motor Function and Sensory Integrity Associated With Progressive Disorders of the Central Nervous System
- ☐ F: Impaired Peripheral Nerve Integrity and Muscle Performance Associated With Peripheral Nerve Injury
- ☐ G: Impaired Motor Function and Sensory Integrity Associated With Acute or Chronic Polyneuropathies
- ☐ H: Impaired Motor Function, Peripheral Nerve Integrity, and Sensory Integrity Associated With Nonprogressive Disorders of the Spinal Cord
- ☐ I: Impaired Arousal, Range of Motion, and Motor Control Associated With Coma, Near Coma, or Vegetative State

Cardiovascular/Pulmonary Patterns

- ☐ A: Primary Prevention/Risk Reduction for Cardiovascular/Pulmonary Disorders
- ☐ B: Impaired Aerobic Capacity/Endurance Associated With Deconditioning
- ☐ C: Impaired Ventilation, Respiration/Gas Exchange, and Aerobic Capacity/Endurance Associated With Airway Clearance Dysfunction
- ☐ D: Impaired Aerobic Capacity/Endurance Associated With Cardiovascular Pump Dysfunction or Failure
- ☐ E: Impaired Ventilation and Respiration/Gas Exchange Associated With Ventilatory Pump Dysfunction or Failure
- ☐ F: Impaired Ventilation and Respiration/Gas Exchange Associated With Respiratory Failure
- ☐ G: Impaired Ventilation, Respiration/Gas Exchange, and Aerobic Capacity/Endurance Associated With Respiratory Failure in the Neonate
- ☐ H: Impaired Circulation and Anthropometric Dimensions Associated With Lymphatic System Disorders

Integumentary Patterns

- ☐ A: Primary Prevention/Risk Reduction for Integumentary Disorders
- ☐ B: Impaired Integumentary Integrity Associated With Superficial Skin Involvement
- ☐ C: Impaired Integumentary Integrity Associated With Partial-Thickness Skin Involvement and Scar Formation
- ☐ D: Impaired Integumentary Integrity Associated With Full-Thickness Skin Involvement and Scar Formation
- ☐ E: Impaired Integumentary Integrity Associated With Skin Involvement Extending Into Fascia, Muscle, or Bone and Scar Formation

PROGNOSIS: _____
_____
_____
_____
_____
_____
_____
_____
_____
_____
_____
_____

© American Physical Therapy Association 1999; revised September 2000

Guide to Physical Therapist Practice

Appendix 6: Documentation Template 717/**S709**

Evaluation

American Physical Therapy Association

■ **Figure 2–11** Documentation Template for Physical Therapist Patient/Client Management: Evaluation. Reprinted with permission from the American Physical Therapy Association.

Diagnosis

Diagnosis is the orderly categorization and labeling of the impact of conditions on function and the assignment of conditions to a specific practice pattern presented in the *Guide*. The assigned diagnostic label provides a basis for prognosis and directs the plan of care. An example of a diagnosis is impaired joint mobility associated with localized inflammation. This diagnosis is within the musculoskeletal practice pattern and may arise in a patient who has a diagnosis by a physician of osteoarthritis. Assignment of a diagnosis, and conveying the diagnosis to the patient, is the responsibility of a physical therapist.

■ **Take Note**

Based on physical therapy practice patterns.

Prognosis

Prognosis is the determination of a predicted optimal level of improvement in function and the time needed to achieve the predicted optimal level of improvement. A prognosis also may include predictions of intermediate levels of improvement and time needed to attain these intermediate outcomes necessary to reach the predicted optimal level of improvement. Establishing a prognosis, and conveying the prognosis to the patient, is the responsibility of a physical therapist.

Plan of Care

A plan of care (■ **Figure 2–12**) specifies (1) goals, (2) outcomes, (3) interventions, (4) education, (5) informed consent, and (6) discharge planning. Designing a plan of care is the responsibility of physical therapists. Physical therapists may delegate implementation of appropriate interventions within the plan of care to physical therapist assistants.

Goals

Establishment of a diagnosis and prognosis permits clarification and description of expected patient outcomes. Physical therapists and patients both contribute to setting goals. Goals are statements of expected patient outcomes based on the results of the evaluation. Goal statements are written using terms describing specific, objective, and measurable patient behaviors related to patient function. Descriptions of what physical therapists will do, or interventions to be provided, are *not* goal statements. **Long-term goals (LTGs)** are statements describing functional capabilities a patient will have upon discharge. **Short-term goals (STGs)** are individual activities a patient will achieve to perform functional activities stated as long-term goals. A clear progression of short-term goals provides the basis for successful attainment of long-term goals.

The mnemonic ABCDFT[12,13] can be used to ensure the inclusion of all components of a goal:

- **A**udience: To whom the goal applies. Examples of audience are the patient, patient's family, and patient's caregivers.
- **B**ehavior: What the patient is expected to perform described in observable and measurable terms. Examples of behaviors for short-term goals are strength, range of motion, gait speed, or distance of ambulation. Behaviors for long-term goals are functional abilities, such as transfers, community participation, and work tasks.
- **C**onditions: Variables that describe how behaviors are performed. Examples of conditions include type of assistive device used, speed of performance, or type or amount of assistance required.
- **D**egree: How often the patient is expected to perform the behavior under the conditions described. An example of degree is "walking to the bathroom five times each day." When no specific degree is stated, a patient is expected to perform the behavior at 100 percent each time the behavior is required.

**DOCUMENTATION TEMPLATE FOR
PHYSICAL THERAPIST PATIENT/CLIENT MANAGEMENT**
Plan of Care

_____

Anticipated Goals: _____
_____
_____
_____
_____
_____

Expected Outcomes: _____
_____
_____
_____

Interventions: _____

Frequency of Visits/Duration of Episode of Care:
_____
_____
_____
_____

Education (including safety, exercise, and disease information): _____
_____
_____

Who was educated?   ☐ Patient/Client   ☐ Family (name and relationship): _____
How did patient/family demonstrate learning:
☐ Patient/client verbalizes understanding
☐ Family/significant other verbalizes understanding
☐ Patient/client demonstrates correctly
☐ Demonstration is unsuccessful (describe): _____
_____
_____

Informed Consent:

Does patient/legal guardian agree with plan of care?   ☐ Yes ☐ No

_____
Signature of patient/client or legal guardian

Discharge Plan: _____
_____
_____
_____
_____
_____
_____
_____
_____
_____
_____

Guide to Physical Therapist Practice

Appendix 6: Documentation Template 719/**S711**

Plan of Care

American Physical Therapy Association

■ **Figure 2–12**   Documentation Template for Physical Therapist Patient/Client Management: Plan of Care. Reprinted with permission from the American Physical Therapy Association.

- **F**unction: Behaviors must be related to specified functional abilities. For example, the behavior in a short-term goal is increasing strength as a requirement for the long-term goal's behavior of ambulation, a functional ability. Connecting behaviors of short-term goals to functional abilities of long-term goals assists patients, physicians, and third-party payers, among others, in understanding patient management progression.
- **T**ime: How long it will take a patient to achieve a short-term or long-term goal. Time can be stated by number of treatments or number of days.

It should be noted that in *Writing SOAP Notes* (3rd ed.),[13] Kettenbach uses only ABCD of the mnemonic. Function and Time are incorporated within Degree.

Intervention

"Intervention is the purposeful interaction of physical therapists with the patient/client and, when appropriate, other individuals involved in patient/client care."[6] Diagnosis, prognosis, and goals direct the selection of specific physical therapy procedures designed to achieve stated goals. Interventions include (1) type, (2) amount, (3) duration, and (4) frequency of physical therapy interventions. Examples of interventions include exercise, modalities, education, selection of patient care equipment, and discharge planning.

Documentation

There are many aspects of patient care and a large number of professionals involved in the care of each patient. Coordination of these aspects and professionals requires a high level of communication among all concerned. A patient's chart serves as the single repository of pertinent facts concerning the patient's history, illness(es), and treatment. Events and actions must be documented and are deemed to have occurred only if documented in the patient's chart. Charts can be physical or computer files.

Documentation is the medico-legal record of patient care provided by all practitioners for a given patient. Documentation that is precise and concise is required for providing appropriate communication and is an essential function of health-care professionals. The most important rationale for appropriate documentation is to provide the highest possible level of patient care at all times. With proper documentation, those involved with providing care for the patient and support for the patient's family will know many pieces of information:

1. What has been determined about the patient's condition based upon interviews and tests;
2. Specific problems identified;
3. Goals of treatment;
4. Intervention strategies employed;
5. Patient's response to treatment;
6. Rationale upon which goals and interventions are based.

Formats of Medical Records

There are several major formats of medical records. The **source-oriented method** and the **problem-oriented medical record (POMR)**[7–11] **method** are two popular formats. Ideally, all departments within a facility will use the same method of documentation. Formats of documentation used must provide appropriate information in a "user-friendly" manner, both for the person providing documentation and for those reviewing documentation.

In the source-oriented method, charts are divided into sections for each health profession providing service for a patient (e.g., clinical lab results, physical therapy notes, physician notes, nursing notes, etc.). The source-oriented system segregates patient information by discipline, which may limit the ability to identify patient problems and focus treatment resources on the specific needs of a patient. Documentation of the flow of patient care among professions and the interaction of professional interventions for the benefit of the patient may be lost when using the source-oriented format in medical charts. A narrative format is usually used for writing notes in source-oriented charts.

The Problem-Oriented Medical Record (POMR) system, introduced by Lawrence Weed,[7] was designed to facilitate care provided to patients by organizing each medical record in a format based upon identified patient problems rather than by professional discipline. The POMR is composed of (1) database, (2) problem list, and (3) notes—initial, daily, progress or interim, and discharge. In the POMR system, the Subjective–Objective–Analysis–Plan (SOAP) format is used for note writing.

A database contains subjective and objective information, including medical, family, and social history, and medical examination and test results. A problem list is a list of the patient's problems identified from information contained in the database. Problems may be identified by any professional in a discipline providing patient care and may be listed as an abnormal test result, chief complaint, diagnosis, physical finding, physiological finding, or symptom. Notes are sequential records of decisions, actions, and events describing the course of a patient's treatment by all involved professionals relevant to a specified problem. Initial notes present initial findings and the plan of care. Daily notes briefly present a description of treatment and patient responses for each day. Progress (interim) notes present the progression of treatment, patient responses to treatment, and changes in the plan of care over intervals. Discharge notes present the status of patient problems, and the current course of treatment, at the time of patient discharge.

Formats of Notes

The purpose of a note format is to organize and facilitate the flow of information. When there is a lack of uniformity of note formats within a single chart, difficulty in identifying where or how specific information is contained within the medical record may occur. Each note format may appear in a chart sequentially, separated by discipline, or not separated by discipline. The major formats for writing notes by physical therapists include the (1) narrative note, (2) SOAP note, and (3) patient/client management note formats.

In the narrative format, patient information is entered in narrative form. Headings and subheadings may or may not be used in narrative notes to organize information. Physical therapists may use a narrative format for daily notes, which are usually brief descriptions of daily treatments and patient responses. The complexity and detail required in initial, evaluation, progress, and discharge notes may be difficult to achieve when using the narrative format. For this reason, the narrative format is rarely used by physical therapists other than for daily notes.

The SOAP note format originated with the POMR system and now is used more widely for medical chart notes. The SOAP acronym denotes the note section headings: (1) Subjective, (2) Objective, (3) Analysis, and (4) Plan. Physical therapist assistants may document in the SOAP note format but do not document evaluation and planning in the analysis and plan sections, as these sections are within the scope of practice of only the physical therapist.

Each section of the SOAP note need not be included in every note. Initial notes, however, should include all sections. Only relevant sections are needed for any specific note. Progress notes should include only those sections necessary for indicating changes in patient status (i.e., progress or regression). Discharge notes summarize interventions, progress achieved, and patient profile upon discharge. In this way, initial status, final status, and the effectiveness of therapeutic intervention are presented in an organized manner.

■ Take Note

SOAP = subjective, objective, analysis, plan.

In a SOAP note, a section identifying the patient often precedes the first "S" section. This section contains information such as name, gender, age and date of birth, primary and secondary diagnoses, and physicians. Others, however, may place this information in the "Subjective" section even though this information is not truly subjective. "S" denotes subjective data. Relevant data concerning the patient's history that are not verifiable in medical records are considered subjective data. The patient's description of functional problems, pain, and the date of onset also are included as subjective data. Symptoms are the patient's subjective perceptions that may be indicative of disease. Complaints reported by patients or significant others also are considered to be subjective data. A patient's goals of treatment are considered to be subjective data.

"O" denotes objective data. Objective data are verifiable. These data include examination results, observations by health-care providers, interventions, and patient response to interventions. Signs are objective evidence of disease perceptible by a health-care provider and reported in the objective data. Subheadings are helpful in organizing the content of this section.

"A" denotes analysis by physical therapists of data included in the subjective and objective sections. A list of patient problems is included in this section. This section also includes professional opinions concerning a patient's problems and reasoning used as the basis for the plan of care. Diagnosis and prognosis related to physical therapy care are included in this section.

One limitation of the SOAP note format is the lack of coherent timelines. Interventions and patient responses to interventions for a given date are documented in the objective section before analysis of data appears in the analysis section for the same date.

"P" denotes a plan developed by the physical therapist for providing patient treatment. Each plan has a number of components for the care of a specific patient. While the plan must be developed by a physical therapist, some components of the plan may be delegated to physical therapist assistants. In some facilities, goals of treatment are included in the plan section, whereas other facilities include goals in the analysis section of the note.

■ Figure 2–13 shows an example of a SOAP note for a patient with a recently healed fracture.

The patient/client management note format of documentation is developing in response to the implementation of the Physical Therapy Patient/Client Management Process.[6,13] This approach has components of both the narrative and SOAP note formats. The elements of the Patient/Client Management process provide major divisions (see Figure 2–4) of the note. Subheadings are used to enhance the ease of locating specific information. Not all subheadings are appropriate for each patient.

Using the Documentation Template for Physical Therapist Patient/Client Management for either inpatient or outpatient treatment (Figures 2–7 and 2–8) provides a systematic and organized way to conduct the interview and systems review. Based upon these data, and any other existing data in records, physical therapists implement the patient/client management process. Templates for physical therapy patient/client management to assist in developing the plan of care are found in Figure 2–12.

■ Figure 2–14 presents the organization, including headings and subheadings, used in the Patient/Client Management note format. Subheadings are selected and inserted as deemed necessary to convey patient information in a precise and concise manner. There are three levels of organization in Figure 2–14. Main headings (EXAMINATION, EVALUATION, PLAN OF CARE) present the order of major components within the patient/client management process. Subheadings (History, Systems Review, Tests and Measures within EXAMINATION) are the usual sections necessary for complete information within each component. Other subheadings may be added as necessary for complete patient presentation. Each cell (Social Information within History within EXAMINATION) provides indicators of specific information that may be included.

■ Figure 2–15 offers a sample Patient/Client Management note.

02/01/2010

Mrs. Rita Jones is a 43-year-old automotive assembly-line worker, referred by Dr. Parker. She is 8 weeks post fracture L olecranon process and 10 days post cast removal.

First visit today, 02/01/2010.

S. *Mrs. Jones' chief complaint is inability to use her left arm for activities of daily living and for work. Patient's goal is to return to previous job.*

O. *Active ROM: L elbow ext – flex 15–110 degree*

Passive ROM: L elbow ext – flex 10–115 degree

Strength:		
	L elbow ext	3/5
	L elbow flex	3+/5
	L supination	3+/5
	L pronation	3+/5
	L wrist (all)	4/5
	L hand (all)	4/5
	L shoulder (all)	5/5

Pain:	
	L elbow 2/10 in dependent position with no motion.
	L elbow 4/10 during passive ROM.
	L elbow 5/10 during active flexion, supination, pronation.
	L elbow 7/10 during active extension.

A. *Problem 1 – Decreased ROM L elbow*

Problem 2 – Decreased strength L elbow and wrist

Problem 3 – Pain L elbow

Problems 1 through 3 result of recent fracture L olecranon process and casting of L upper extremity.

LTG: The patient is able to use L arm for washing, dressing, and combing hair.

Patient will be able to perform pervious job as automotive assembly-line worker.

STG: The patient has 5–110 degrees ROM in L elbow to perform job skills in 2 weeks.

The patient has 4/5 muscle strength in all major muscle groups of the L upper extremity to perform job skills in 2 weeks.

The patient is free of pain in L elbow while performing job skills in 5 weeks.

P. *Priorities: Increase ROM L elbow.*

Increase strength L elbow and wrist muscles.

Decrease in pain expected as ROM and strength return to normal.

Treatment: Cryotherapy prior to and following each exercise session to decrease swelling and pain.

Passive and active stretching of left elbow and forearm to increase ROM.

Progressive resistance exercises for all planes of motion starting with 3 sets of 10 repetitions with five pound weight.

Home exercise program of stretching and strengthening.

Schedule: Clinic visits 45 min 3×/wk for 2 weeks followed by

45 min 2×/wk for 2 weeks.

Independent ADL using L arm in 2 weeks.

Return to work in 5 weeks.

Mary Minor, PT

02/01/2010

■ **Figure 2–13**   Sample SOAP note.

PATIENT/CLIENT MANAGEMENT NOTE FORMAT

EXAMINATION		
History		
General Demographics	Social History	Employment/Work (Job/School/Play)
Growth and Development	Living Environment	General Health Status
Social/Health Habits	Family History	Medical/Surgical History
Current Conditions	Functional Status and Activity Level	Medications
Other Clinical Tests		
Systems Review		
Cardiovascular/Pulmonary	Integumentary	Musculoskeletal
Neuromuscular	Communication	Affect
Cognition	Language	Learning Style
Tests and Measures		
Aerobic Capacity/Endurance	Anthropometric Characteristics	Arousal, Attention/Cognition
Assistive and Adaptive Devices	Circulation	Cranial/Peripheral Nerve Integrity
Environmental/Home/Work Barriers	Ergonomics and Body Mechanics	Gait/Locomotion and Balance
Integumentary Integrity	Joint Integrity	Motor Function
Muscle Performance	Neuromotor Development and Sensory Integration	Orthotic/Protective Devices
Pain	Posture	Prosthetics
ROM/Muscle Length	Reflex Integrity	Self-Care/Home Management
Sensory Integrity	Ventilation/Respiration	Work/Community, Leisure Integration

EVALUATION		
Diagnosis	Prognosis (Timeframe and Outcomes/Goals)	Preferred Practice Pattern (Cardiovascular/pulmonary, integumentary, musculoskeletal, and neuromuscular)

PLAN OF CARE		
Interventions and Parameters (Specifics of interventions)	Frequency (Number of times/week)	Duration (Number of weeks or treatment sessions for plan of care)
Equipment and Devices (Assistive/Adaptive)	Coordination of Services	Re-examination Timeline

■ **Figure 2–14** Patient/Client Management Note Format Headings and Subheadings.

02/01/2010

HISTORY

John Jones is a 57-year-old white male self-employed carpenter who sustained a fracture of the right distal humerus 8 weeks ago when a beam fell on his arm. Right handed. Lives with his wife and three children in a ranch-style home. Does not smoke and drinks alcohol only occasionally. General health has been good. Takes no prescription medications and only occasionally takes OTC medications for pain. Prior to the fracture he was independent in all ADLs and work situations. Cast removed RUE just prior to physical therapy.

SYSTEMS REVIEW

Mr. Jones is alert, oriented, with no cardiovascular/pulmonary/neuromuscular problems. Integumentary and musculoskeletal problems are only noted in right UE. Affect and communication skills are appropriate. He prefers to learn by being told and given material to read.

TEST and MEASURES

Only the right UE was examined.

ROM: Shoulder normal, Elbow: 15 to 100 degrees of flexion. Forearm supination and pronation 0-10 degrees. Wrist and hand normal

Strength: Shoulder: all motions 4/5. Elbow and forearm: 3/5 within available ROM. Brachial and radial pulses present and strong.

Integumentary: Skin over right UE is pale, dry and has large areas of dry skin from being casted for 8 weeks.

Pain: 3/10 with movement on 10-point scale.

Sensation: intact

EVALUATION

Practice Pattern G: Impaired Joint Mobility, Muscle Performance, and Range of Motion Associated with Fracture.

Diagnosis: Impaired ROM and strength due to fracture

Prognosis: ROM to permit independence in ADLs within 4 weeks, strength to 5/5 in 10 weeks; return to prior level of function 8 weeks.

LTG: Mr. Jones will return to independent ADLs and resume work within 8 weeks.

STG: Mr. Jones will have increased elbow and forearm ROM by 10 degrees in all planes to permit him to perform ADLs independently within 10 days.

Mr. Jones will have increased strength in available ROM to 3+/5 in all planes to permit him to perform ADLs independently within 10 days.

INTERVENTIONS

Treatment twice a week for 2 weeks, then once a week for 3 weeks. Each treatment session will be approximately 45 minutes.

Interventions will include:

Stretching for all planes of motion for right elbow and forearm—2 sets of 5 repetitions, held 20 seconds each.

Progressive strengthening exercises for all planes of motion of right elbow and forearm—3 sets of 10 repetitions with manual resistance.

Re-examine at each session.

Mary Minor, PT

02/01/2010

■ **Figure 2–15** Sample Patient/Client Management Note Format.

Requirements for Adequate Documentation

The role of documentation is to enhance communication for medical and legal purposes. The rules of proper grammatical usage should be followed. Documentation must be precise, concise, complete, legible, and timely.

Precise documentation requires measurements and test results be recorded accurately using appropriate terminology. Abbreviations (see Glossary of Abbreviations) may be used *only* if they are generally accepted abbreviations. *Concise* documentation requires information be organized effectively, conveying important information in a brief, clear, and unfettered fashion. Only relevant information is to be included. *Complete* documentation requires all necessary information be included. *Legible* documentation requires easily and accurately read chart entries. Entries may be in either handwritten or electronic format as long as it can be read by others. *Timely* documentation requires notes be entered into the medical record as required by rule or regulation.

An important aspect of medical documentation is the presentation of information in a manner that can be read and interpreted quickly and efficiently. Outline format may be significantly more concise than prose. Flow charts and tables can be used to report individual and serial test results, enabling communication of large amounts of information in formats that can be read quickly and interpreted easily.

Medicare Guidelines

Medicare guidelines are issued by the Center for Medicare and Medicaid Services (CMS).[14] These guidelines must be followed if reimbursement for services rendered under Medicare is expected. CMS guidelines change relatively frequently, requiring updates, which can be obtained online from the federal government website http://www.cms.hhs.gov/manuals/. Of specific interest may be section 220, Coverage of Outpatient Rehabilitation Therapy Services (Physical Therapy, Occupational Therapy, and Speech-Language Pathology) Under Medical Insurance. This section appears in Chapter 15, Covered Medical and Other Health Services, within the Medicare Benefit Policy Manual. In a significant number of cases, Medicare guidelines are adopted by nonfederal government agencies and third-party payers, necessitating an understanding of CMS rules and regulations for more than just services rendered under Medicare.

Highlights of Medicare documentation guidelines include a variety of topics:

- Conditions of coverage for patients requiring physical therapy services
  - Services are required because patient requires therapy.
  - Plans for services developed by physical therapists must be certified by a physician.
  - Physician recertification of plans of care for therapy services must occur every 30 days.
  - Physical therapy services must be of a complexity that requires the clinical decision-making skills of a physical therapist and the intervention skills of either physical therapists or physical therapist assistants.
  - Physical therapy services may only be rendered by physical therapists, or physical therapist assistants under the supervision of a physical therapist.
- Contents of Physical Therapy Plans of Care
  - Each patient's Plan of Care must be consistent with evaluation results.
  - Diagnosis
  - Long-term treatment goals
  - Type, amount, duration, and frequency of therapy services
- Documentation requirements
  - Consistently and accurately reported
  - Legible, relevant, and sufficient to justify services
  - Evaluation and Plan of Care
  - Certification

■ Take Note
Documentation: precise, concise, complete, legible, timely.

- Indication of active participation by a physical therapist during each progress report period
- Progress reports shall be at least once every 10 treatment days, or within one certification cycle.
- Complete progress reports shall be written by physical therapists.
- Physical therapist assistants may write certain elements of progress reports.
- Treatment/Daily notes for each treatment day
- Treatment/Daily notes may be written by either a physical therapist or physical therapist assistant.

Audit of Patient Care

Periodic and consistent evaluation of patient-care activities is necessary to measure and analyze the quality of patient care. **Audits** are systematic reviews of documentation that examine the efficacy and efficiency of patient-care outcomes with respect to interventions used. Only through the availability of properly completed records can useful audits be performed appropriately.

When appropriate and significant data are reported in a consistent format, peer review and quality assurance are facilitated. One question that an audit can answer is to determine if actual patient-care outcomes are dependent upon the type of interventions employed. Potential benefits to be gained from performing audits include improved patient care and patient outcomes. A partial list of information that an audit may yield is whether

- Individual physical therapists are including pertinent and required information in medical chart notes;
- Department or individual physical therapist interventions are appropriate for the patients to which the interventions are applied;
- Changes in department policy or protocols are necessary to improve patient care and patient outcomes;
- Continuing education is necessary to improve patient care skills.

Chapter Review

Review Questions

1. State the purpose of HIPAA rules and regulations.

2. List the eighteen specific HIPAA identifiers.

3. Describe why patient identifiers are protected under HIPAA rules and regulations.

4. Describe the elements of the Patient/Client Management process.

5. Describe the purposes of an initial patient interview.

6. Define the two styles of questions used in an interview.

7. When are the two styles of questions best used in an interview?

8. List and provide examples of the content of the information to be elicited during an initial patient interview.

9. List the purposes of documentation.

10. Describe the two formats of medical records.

11. Describe the components of the SOAP note format of documentation.

12. Describe the Patient/Client Management note format, using examples of the note content of each component.

13. State where Medicare requirements for documentation are located.

14. Write an example of a long-term goal and two short-term goals appropriate for the long-term goal in proper format.

15. Discuss the requirements of adequate documentation.

16. List the information provided by a medical records audit.

Suggested Activities

1. Indicate in which component of the SOAP note each of the following statements should be by placing the appropriate letter, S, O, A, or P, before the statement.

   _____ ROM: R shoulder flexion: 0–85.
   _____ The family reports that the patient frequently falls at night.
   _____ TX 2/wk for 3 wks.
   _____ The patient will ambulate with a straight cane on all surfaces for functional distances without fatigue within 4 weeks.
   _____ Pain 5/10 after treatment.
   _____ Patient's pain level ↓ following treatment.
   _____ Patient ↑↓ 12 stairs step over step using the hand rail 4 times.
   _____ The patient's ability to assume standing from sitting is impaired because of weakness of both quadricep muscles.

2. Identify the components of the following goal statement by writing the word or phrase in the appropriate space:

Goal statement: The patient will have full left knee extension ROM for ambulation, dressing, and getting in and out of a chair within 2 weeks of daily treatment.

A: _____

B: _____

C: _____

D: _____

F: _____

T: _____

Case Study

Eduardo Jiminez

415 Main Street

Any City, USA

(555) 212-2222

SSN: 123-45-6789

DOB: 05/08/37

Record: 444-3-45-897

Mr. Jiminez is a 67-year-old male 2 days post left total knee replacement. Mr. Jiminez is to be discharged to a skilled nursing care facility in 2 days where he will receive additional therapy. The goal is for Mr. Jiminez to ambulate independently without an assistive device as a community ambulatory. The physician has indicated that when Mr. Jiminez has 90 degrees of left knee flexion, good strength of knee flexors and extensors, and can ambulate 200 ft $\times$ 4, he can be discharged to his home. Mr. Jiminez reports pain of 4/10 about the incision. The incision is anterior over the left knee in a proximal distal direction. Some clear discharge is noted at the distal end of the incision. The circumference of the left knee at 2 inches above the tibial tuberosity is ¾ inch larger than the right.

a. Using the Case Study information, identify and write information that would be covered by HIPAA regulations.

b. Organize the preceding narrative note into the Patient/Client Management note format.

References

1. http://www.cms.hhs.gov/home/regsguidance.asp
2. Nagi S. Some conceptual issues in disability and rehabilitation. In: Sussman M (ed). *Sociology and Rehabilitation.* Washington, DC: American Sociological Association, 1965, 100–113.
3. Nagi S. *Disability and Rehabilitation.* Columbus: Ohio State University Press, 1969.
4. Nagi S. Disability concepts revisited: Implications for prevention. In: Pope A, Tarlov A (eds). *Disability in America: Toward a National Agenda for Prevention.* Washington, DC: Institute of Medicine, National Academy Press, 1991.
5. http://www.who.int/classifications/icf/site/beginners/bg.pdf
6. *Guide to Physical Therapist Practice,* 2nd ed. In *Physical Therapy.* 2001; 81; 1.
7. Weed LL. *Medical Record, Medical Education, and Patient Care.* Chicago: Yearbook Medical Publishers, 1970.
8. Feitelberg SB. *The Problem-Oriented Medical Record System in Physical Therapy.* Self-published. Copyright 1975, revised 1984, 1999.
9. Dunsdale SM, Mossman PL, Guleckson G, Jr. et al. The problem-oriented medical record in rehabilitation. *Arch Phys Med Rehabil.* 1970; 51; 488–492.
10. Milhous R. The problem-oriented medical record in rehabilitation management and training. *Arch Phys Med Rehabil.* 1972; 53; 182–185.
11. Editorial. Ten reasons why Weed is right. *N Engl J Med.* 1971; 51; 284.
12. Kettenback G. *Writing SOAP Notes,* 2nd ed. Philadelphia: F.A. Davis, 1995.
13. Kettenback G. *Writing SOAP Notes,* 3rd ed. Philadelphia: F.A. Davis, 2004.
14. http://www.cms.hhs.gov

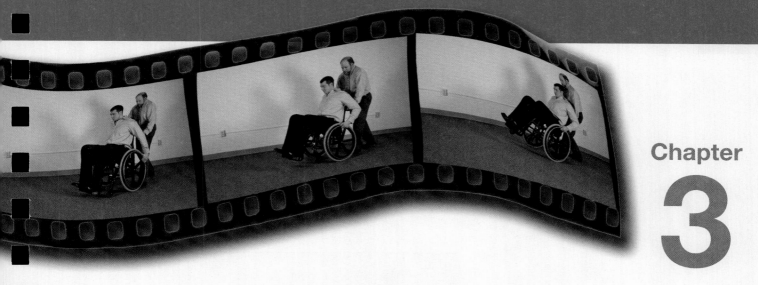

Preparation
for Patient Care

Learning Objectives

Upon completion of this chapter, you will be able to:

1. State who is responsible for properly managing the patient care environment.
2. Describe general guidelines for properly managing the patient care environment.
3. Describe correct body mechanics for safety of both patients and physical therapists/assistants.
4. Describe the physical therapist's/assistant's position when guarding a patient during ambulation and transporting in a gurney or wheelchair.
5. Discuss the decision-making tree used to incorporate proper body mechanics when treating patients/clients.
6. Describe the characteristics of instructions and verbal commands.
7. Describe the purposes of proper draping.
8. Describe proper draping techniques.
9. Describe how to transport patients safely via gurney and wheelchair.

Key Terms

Base of support
Body mechanics
Center of gravity
Draping
Instructions

Isometric muscle
   contractions
Proper posture
Valsalva maneuver
Verbal commands

Introduction

Fundamental to all patient care are skills of management of the treatment environment, body mechanics, and communication. Safe implementation of interventions is best achieved when all components of an intervention are given proper attention. By planning and preparing prior to treatment sessions, physical therapists/assistants increase the likelihood of safe, efficient, and effective treatment sessions. Safety of all involved in patient care, both patients and providers, must be of paramount consideration at all times.

Management of the Environment

The patient care environment must be organized for protection of patients and clinicians, as well as for efficient use (■ Figure 3–1). Managing the patient care environment to achieve these goals is a serious responsibility of all clinicians. Physical therapists have the responsibility to ensure that all clinicians are trained properly in patient care environment management. Although some tasks may be delegated to certain clinicians, the user always retains final responsibility for maintaining a safe and efficient environment for patients and clinicians.

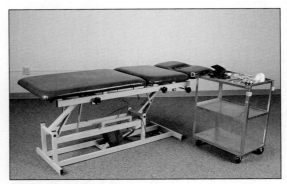

■ **Figure 3–1**   Preparing a clear patient care environment.

Preparation for the next treatment to be given in a patient care area begins at the end of the previous treatment session. Following use, equipment is cleaned and returned to the proper storage area in a safe, functioning condition. Equipment that is not functioning correctly, or is unsafe, must be tagged, removed from the treatment area, and reported immediately. Used supplies must be disposed of properly. Unused supplies must be returned to the proper storage area. The person responsible for ordering supplies should be notified in the appropriate manner when consumable supplies are low.

Risk management dictates that all equipment must be inspected to ensure safe function. Annual inspection of all electrical, thermal, and mechanical equipment by a biomedical engineer is required. Nonfunctioning or unsafe equipment must be removed from use. A simple inspection of equipment, including checking for frayed wiring, worn mechanical parts, and proper function, before each treatment session promotes patient safety. Equipment that malfunctions, or is determined to be unsafe, during a pretreatment inspection must not be used for that treatment session and must be tagged and reported.

Maintaining clean and orderly environments is part of managing treatment sessions. Some, but not all, tasks to be considered are cleaning of floors, mats, and treatment tables. Proper cleaning of equipment prolongs its life of safe and effective use. Guidelines for safe and clean environments are developed by Centers for Disease Control and Prevention (CDC) and are incorporated into facility policies and procedures. Specifics of some of these procedures are covered in Chapter 4.

All facility personnel, not just Housekeeping/Environmental Services personnel, are responsible for following and implementing policies and procedures correctly. These personnel include physical therapists, physical therapist assistants, and physical therapy aides. Ensuring that the treatment environment is safe and clean is ultimately the responsibility of the supervising physical therapist.

Prior to initiating any physical therapy patient interaction, the surrounding area must be readied. For transport, transfer, or intervention, the bed, chair, and surrounding areas must be prepared. Treatment tables, mats, chairs, stools, or beds should be prepared before patients arrive in treatment areas. Supplies necessary for treatment areas include linens and pillows. Additional sheets are used as pull sheets for transfers or for draping. Pillows for patient positioning, comfort, and safety must be within easy reach. Supporting a patient's head while reaching for a misplaced pillow, or leaving a patient in an uncomfortable or unsafe position while equipment is retrieved, is not acceptable patient care. Call bells or patient call buttons must be placed within a patient's reach when patients will be left unattended. Timers, when necessary, must also be available and set properly.

Specific equipment required for a treatment session should be prepared and placed properly prior to escorting a patient into a treatment environment (■ Figure 3–2). Having equipment and supplies required in the area avoids leaving a patient unguarded or interrupting treatment.

■ **Take Note**
Ready treatment areas prior to bringing patient into the area.

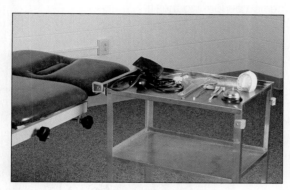

■ **Figure 3–2**   Equipment and supplies for interventions.

Adequate room in a treatment environment is necessary for unimpeded movement. Clinicians and patients must be able to maneuver in the area without bumping into, or tripping over, equipment. Equipment and furniture not needed during a transport or transfer, such as a mobile stool, should be moved away from the area prior to arrival of patients in treatment areas. Besides getting in the way, many of these pieces of equipment are not stable and become dangerous when patients try to use them as support. When equipment is used in the treatment of a patient/client, physical therapists/assistants should position the equipment and patient/client to allow easy access to the patient. Improperly positioned equipment may hamper the ability of clinicians to provide patient assistance quickly.

PROCEDURE 3–1   Body Mechanics

MEDIALINK Watch the video on the CD under the heading of Body Mechanics.

When lifting, lowering, pushing, or pulling, stresses and strains upon the musculoskeletal system are increased. Proper posture and body mechanics are required to limit stress and strain on musculoskeletal structures of both patients and physical therapy clinicians. **Proper posture** is appropriate alignment of the musculoskeletal system such that the stresses and strains placed on bones, muscles, ligaments, and cartilage are as few as possible. **Body mechanics**

(continued)

requires strength, range of motion (ROM), and motor control. Proper body mechanics uses these elements to maintain proper skeletal alignment during standing and proper skeletal movement during activity by maintaining the **center of gravity** within the **base of support**. Although the five cardinal rules of correct body mechanics for lifting are titled for lifting only, they apply to any activity in which a person must lift, lower, push, pull, or carry any object or person. By following these rules, as presented in the following photos, a person can maintain balance and decrease the potential for injury. The five cardinal rules are

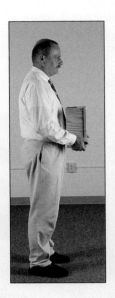

1. Keep the load close: Keep the center of gravity of the person or object being lifted/lowered should be kept as close as possible to the body of the person performing the lifting/lowering. In this way the center of gravity remains within the base of support provided by physical therapy clinicians.

2. Create an appropriate base of support: The base of support of the person performing the lifting/lowering should be as wide (side to side) and long (front to back) as necessary to maintain balance throughout the lifting/lowering activity. If movement beyond the original base of support is required, an appropriately changing base of support must be maintained. While changing a base of support, avoid awkward positions. When feet must be moved, move in a manner that avoids crossing of the extremities. Use of these strategies decreases the potential for tripping or falling by maintaining an appropriately sized base of support.

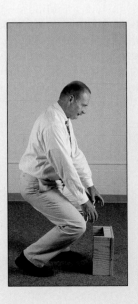

3. Use **isometric muscle contractions** of the trunk (extensor and abdominal muscles): Maintain the trunk in a constant position, preferably erect, during the lifting/lowering activity. Prior to performing the actual lifting/lowering movement, move into position and set trunk position. Use isometric contractions to the trunk and abdominal muscles. Creating isometric contractions in the muscles of the trunk prior to lifting can reduce the potential for injury. Although isometric contractions of trunk musculature are used, avoid performing a Valsalva maneuver. A **Valsalva maneuver** is closing of the glottis during heavy exertion resulting in increased intrathoracic and intra-abdominal pressure, which can cause a rapid increase in blood pressure.

4. Lift with the legs: Use the large and strong muscles of the legs to perform lifting/lowering activities, avoiding active flexion or extension of the trunk.

5. Do not twist: Avoid rotation of the spine as the lifting/lowering activity is performed. When a change of direction is required, move the feet to achieve the change of direction. Avoid twisting or crossing of the lower extremities, which can decrease the available base of support and interfere with balance while moving.

The initial stance for lifting/lowering requires placing the feet in stride and slightly apart. This stance widens the base of support in both the lateral (side to side) and anterior/posterior (front and back) directions, mitigating the effects of shifts in the center of gravity during lifting/lowering activities. Centering a load within the base of support and keeping it close to the base of support aids stability. In this way, a balanced position can be maintained.

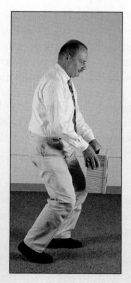

■ **Take Note**
Keep the load close; large base of support, "set" trunk muscles, use leg muscles, do not twist.

Initiate lifting a person or object from the floor from a squatting position (rule 4). This is the lowest level from which a person or object will need to be lifted. Modifications of these instructions pertaining to lifting from different heights, such as a chair or treatment table, are included in Chapter 7.

The depth of the squat should be sufficient to permit reaching the person or object to be lifted but, if possible, not so deep that the leg muscles are at a disadvantage in regaining the upright position. The person or object is reached by squatting, achieved by flexing the hips and knees, rather than by flexing the trunk. Trunk position should be set (rule 3). Maintain the load as close as possible (rule 1) and an appropriate base of support (rule 2). When the center of gravity is centered within the base of support and near the body's midline, both balance and correct postural alignment are easier to maintain. Lowering a person or object uses the same concepts of posture and alignment as lifting, but with the steps in the reverse order.

Transfers require movements that move the center of gravity away from the center of the base of support. These movements have the potential of causing loss of balance as the combined center of gravity moves toward the boundaries of the base of support. Increasing the size of the base of support by setting the feet in stride and slightly apart provides a larger base of support. Proper arrangement of patient and chair, bed, or treatment table can reduce the distance that must be moved during a transfer. Proper environmental management means that the area is free of unnecessary equipment, allowing room for movement and avoiding interference with free movement of the feet. Avoid crossing the legs (rule 5) because it decreases the size of the base of support and constrains freedom of foot movement. Specific examples are illustrated in Chapter 7.

When moving large pieces of equipment, such as treadmills or parallel bars, or when guarding a patient during ambulation, a physical therapist/assistant should be positioned behind the equipment or patient, facing in the direction of movement. Positioned this way the clinician does not obstruct the patient's view and path of movement, and the clinicians assisting the patient then can determine a path free from obstruction.

When guarding a patient during ambulation training, a physical therapist/assistant should be positioned with feet in stride and the body at a 45-degree angle slightly to the side and behind the patient. If a patient starts to fall forward, backward, or to either side, this position of the physical therapist/assistant allows a patient's center of gravity to be pulled toward the physical therapist/assistant and the combined center of gravity to be maintained within the base of support with a relatively small shift of a physical therapist's/assistant's weight. In this way, large foot movements are usually not required. The base of support must be large enough to support such shifts in the center of gravity should a patient start to fall. To permit unencumbered weight shifting or foot movements, a physical therapist/assistant should not cross feet during ambulation or become entangled with the patient's feet or ambulatory equipment.

In all cases, plan movements and prepare areas to be used prior to implementing any portion of a treatment session. Use of proper decision making and selection of appropriate body mechanics provides safety for patients and clinicians. When in doubt about your ability to lift, transfer, or guard a patient or object safely, always obtain appropriate assistance.

There are many examples of how proper body mechanics is related to physical therapy. Ambulation guarding, as follows, is one example. Selection of methods of guarding patients requires a physical therapist to determine the activity to be performed, the capabilities of the patient, and the status of the patient's injury or illness. One example is that there may be differences in where physical therapists/assistants stand when guarding ambulating patients who have a unilateral non-weight-bearing status of a lower extremity and are progressing to partial weight-bearing status and then to full weight-bearing status. When initiating ambulation training with an assistive device during the non–weight-bearing stage, a physical therapist determines the optimal position on either the involved or uninvolved side. A decision-tree thinking process of where to stand must occur.

The decision to be positioned on the side of the uninvolved lower extremity is based on the non–weight-bearing status and the first cardinal rule of body mechanics: Keep the load close. A patient who should be non–weight-bearing on one lower extremity will shift weight away from the involved lower extremity. This moves the center of gravity into the base of support of the physical therapist/assistant and avoids weight-bearing on the involved lower extremity. If this patient falls, the physical therapist/assistant should be able to move the patient away from weight-bearing on the involved extremity by pulling the patient into the physical therapist's/assistant's base of support. This occurs only when the physical therapist/assistant is guarding a patient on the side of the uninvolved lower extremity. When a physical therapist/assistant is guarding a patient on the side of the involved lower extremity, and the patient starts to fall, the physical therapist/assistant is required to push the patient away from the physical therapist's/assistant's base of support to ensure that the patient's weight-bearing occurs on the uninvolved extremity. If a physical therapist/assistant pulls the patient into the base of support, weight-bearing on the involved lower extremity is likely to occur. Guarding a patient on the side of the involved lower extremity thus requires a choice of pulling the patient into the physical therapist's/assistant's base of support while creating weight-bearing on the involved lower extremity or avoiding weight-bearing on the involved extremity by pushing the patient away from the therapist's or assistant's base of support. Either choice in this example violates one aspect of proper patient care and safety: maintaining non–weight-bearing status or keeping the load within the base of support.

As this patient moves from non–weight-bearing to partial weight-bearing, the situation changes and the physical therapist must return to the decision-tree thinking process. For partial weight-bearing status, there is no one right way of guarding a

■ **Take Note**

The rules for body mechanics apply to gait training.

■ **Take Note**

When patient's goal is non–weight-bearing/partial weight-bearing on one lower extremity, and to protect the involved lower extremity, guard from the side of the uninvolved side. When patient's goal is to increase weight-bearing, guard from the side of the involved lower extremity.

patient. A physical therapist must consider how much weight will be appropriate to bear on the involved extremity, how good a patient's balance and coordination are, and how well the physical therapist believes the patient's ambulation can be controlled from one side or the other. In this case, the better guarding position might be on the side of the uninvolved or involved lower extremity. This is the physical therapist's choice based on clinical expertise.

If a patient's balance and coordination are good, and a physical therapist believes ambulation can be well controlled, guarding on the side of the involved lower extremity can be safe. With a physical therapist/assistant on the side of the involved extremity, the patient will feel more comfortable shifting to that side, thus creating partial weight-bearing. If a patient begins to fall, the patient's coordination and the physical therapist's/assistant's capability to control ambulation can allow controlled weight-bearing onto the involved extremity as the patient moves into the physical therapist's base of support. If the patient's balance and coordination are not good, then maintaining guarding position on the side of the uninvolved lower extremity promotes safety. There is no one best answer, and decisions must be based on the physical therapist's clinical decision making.

As a patient moves to full weight-bearing, guarding can be performed by a physical therapist/assistant being positioned on the side of either the involved or uninvolved lower extremity.

■ **Take Note**

When a patient is partial weight-bearing, guarding from either side may be appropriate. Safety is the basis of this decision.

Instructions and Verbal Commands

To participate effectively during interventions, patients must know what they are to do and when they are to do it. Patients must be able to hear instructions and commands if oral instructions or commands are to be used. When a patient cannot hear, or does not understand, spoken words, gestures, and demonstrations may convey necessary meanings. **Instructions** inform patients of what is to be done and provide information as part of the teaching process. Instructions may include oral description, visual demonstration, and written description. **Verbal commands** are auditory cues to patients and are provided during activity performance. Prior to activity performance, patients should be instructed about the verbal commands that will be provided during activity performance.

■ **Take Note**

Instructions are given before, and verbal commands during, activity performance.

Instructions must be simple, informative, and in a language and terms a patient can understand. Lay language should be used unless patients readily understand medical terminology. When a patient's inability to understand English interferes with safe and effective intervention, instructions need to be provided in a language the patient understands. When a physical therapist/assistant cannot communicate fluently in the required language, the physical therapist/assistant is responsible for securing the services of an interpreter. Many facilities maintain lists of clinicians who speak specific languages in addition to English.

Physical therapists and physical therapist assistants should describe to a patient the general sequence of events that will occur during a treatment session. Safety and learning are enhanced when patients understand what they are expected to do. Physical therapists/assistants must determine that patients understand instructions provided before activity performance. Asking a patient, "Do you understand the instruction?" does not ensure understanding. Having patients repeat instructions in proper sequence indicates an appropriate level of understanding and provides an opportunity for mental rehearsal of the task. Verbal commands focus a patient's attention on specifically desired actions. A command is a cue for a specific action during activity performance.

■ Take Note
Verbal commands are clear, brief, specific, and require proper timing, tone, and volume.

Verbal commands must be clear, brief, specific, properly timed, and spoken in appropriate tone and volume. Tone and volume must vary as a situation requires. Generally, commands spoken in a sharp or loud manner receive quick responses, and commands spoken in a soft or low manner elicit slower responses.

Patients may become confused when provided a long series of actions to implement with only one cue provided. In such situation, each specific action may require a specific verbal command. Verbal commands must be specific to the action desired. For example, counting to three does not direct a patient to perform a specific action. When a patient is to look up, the instruction may be "I will count to three and then say 'look up.' When I say 'look up,' you should look up." The verbal command is "look up," which is a specific command and does not require translating the word "three" into "look up." In this example, a patient has been provided an instruction that includes the verbal command to be used and the expected response. Commands must be timed for each action to occur in the proper sequence, and at the appropriate time, so an entire activity is completed safely and effectively.

Patient Preparation

■ Take Note
The purposes of draping are to protect a patient's modesty and expose only necessary body area, keep a patient warm, and protect wounds.

For efficient use of treatment time, preparation of treatment areas should be completed prior to bringing patients into treatment environments. When patients are transported to a physical therapy department for treatment, scheduling involves nursing and transport personnel and preparation of treatment environments to limit patient waiting times. When treating patients at the bedside or in private homes, physical therapists/assistants must ensure that environments are safe and ready for activity performance. In all cases, part of patient preparation is ensuring that patients are properly dressed to ensure modesty, safety, and effective treatment before activities are performed.

Appropriate draping for modesty, safety, and effective treatment is the right of every patient and the responsibility of all clinicians. **Draping** is covering a patient appropriately in a manner that maintains patient modesty and comfort. Draping uses a patient's clothing, as well as sheets and towels, to (1) protect patient modesty, (2) provide warmth, (3) protect wounds, scars, and residual limbs, and (4) expose specific body segments for treatment. Edges of sheets and towels should be secured to avoid shifting of draping material and exposing a patient. Planning is necessary to maintain appropriate draping throughout all aspects of treatment sessions.

Hospital gowns are designed for ease in dressing and access during nursing care. They may not provide effective draping during movements required for transfers or treatment. Properly securing the ties of a hospital gown may provide some coverage. Mid-length robes, or two hospital gowns with one opening in front and one opening in back, can be used. Long robes may interfere with movement, and their use as draping should be avoided.

Whenever possible, patients should be dressed in slacks or shorts to provide ease of movement without loss of modesty. Shorts are especially useful if a lower extremity must be observed. If slacks or shorts are loose-fitting at the waist, a belt should be worn to prevent slacks or shorts from falling, which restricts movement and poses a safety hazard. A halter top or bra is appropriate when the upper trunk is treated for female patients. Shoes that offer support are required when a patient is to stand, ambulate, or practice transfers. When shoes are worn, socks should be worn for protection, comfort, and sanitation. For patients who are not ambulatory, slippers may be acceptable as they are easier to put on and take off. In all situations, decisions concerning dress must be tempered by a patient's needs, a patient's ability to manipulate clothing, and the requirements of treatment.

Gait belts are a piece of safety equipment that should be considered for use for each movement of a patient, whether it is a transfer or guarding during ambulation. When used properly, and under appropriate conditions, gait belts provide a significant margin of safety for patients. Physical therapists use clinical decision making to determine if gait belts should be used for safe and effective performance of specific activities.

During gait training, gait belts provide a sturdy and significant measure of control. However, they must not impede patient movement, interfere with patient equipment such as lines and leads, and be used as the only means of controlling an upright patient. Exercise diligence in fastening gait belts, for security of the fastening device, and for how tightly or loosely gait belts are applied. If security of the fastening device is not complete, gait belts can release unexpectedly. When secured too tightly, gait belts may impede patient breathing, cause pain about the torso, or be difficult for the physical therapist/assistant to grasp effectively. When secured too loosely, gait belts may slip along the patient's torso, causing pain and abrasions, or may not provide the physical therapist/assistant with proper control.

Physical therapist/assistant control of patient movements during transfers is achieved by using manual contacts to guide patients during movement and to provide support when necessary. Consider how gait belts will affect patient safety and comfort. When a physical therapist's clinical decision making indicates that gait belts will increase patient and physical therapist/assistant safety and proper performance of the transfer, then use of gait belts is indicated. Pulling on gait belts to lift and move patients is improper use of gait belts during transfers. Pulling on gait belts may interfere with patients participating actively during activity and applies both compression and shear forces to a patient's body. In some environments, application of gait belts to patients for transfers is required, and gait belts are considered safety devices to be used when transfers start to fail. When a physical therapist/assistant uses manual contacts on a patient for guiding movements, the gait belt is available should it be necessary to support a patient who starts to fall. Whenever a physical therapist/assistant determines a patient cannot be transferred safely by one person, alternative methods of transfer or additional trained clinicians are required to assist.

Physical therapists treat patients in a variety of settings. In many settings, primarily hospitals but also in nursing homes and some personal homes, patients may present with intravenous (IV) lines, chest tubes, catheters, respirators, cardiac monitors, or any combination of these. When positioning, transferring, or treating patients, take care not to disrupt lines, tubes, or electrodes, as these are vital to patient well-being. A dislodged chest tube or respirator can be life threatening. When a line, tube, or electrode is disrupted, a physical therapist/assistant must initiate emergency measures properly, which includes notification of appropriate clinicians.

Lines, tubes, and electrodes limit the amount of movement available to a patient. Before moving patients, or having patients move, physical therapists/assistants must check that the desired movement can occur without disrupting patient equipment, lines, and tubes, or the clinician should consider repositioning IV containers, catheter bags, oxygen masks, chest tubes, etc. for unimpeded patient movement. Repositioning of containers, tubes, lines, and other equipment may require additional equipment or clinicians. Do not allow tubes or lines to become tangled, pinched, kinked, stretched, or pulled out from their insertion or attachment site. Any of these occurrences will interrupt proper function, perhaps even be life threatening. IV drip rates and oxygen flow rates must not be changed without a physician's order. IV fluid containers must remain above the level of the patient's heart. Urinary drainage collection bags must remain below the level of the patient's bladder. Proper placement of IV fluid containers and urinary drainage collection bags is necessary to maintain the correct direction of fluid flow. Dislodging chest tubes requires replacement of tubes by qualified clinicians. Closing off chest tubes or the chest opening for chest tubes is the immediate action to take when chest tubes are dislodged.

■ **Take Note**
Gait belts must be secured properly.

■ **Take Note**
Checking for tubes, lines, and monitor electrodes is part of examining the patient and preparing the treatment area at the initiation of each intervention session.

All facilities have policies and procedures for dealing with occurrences of a variety of emergencies. Physical therapists/assistants are responsible for knowing the policies and procedures and for implementing them properly. Many times these situations may be ones concerning a patient with whom a physical therapist/assistant is providing or supervising treatment. At other times, physical therapists/assistants may be designated responders for emergencies not associated with a patient for whom they are providing treatment. Physical therapists/assistants must maintain certification in cardiopulmonary resuscitation and be capable of providing basic first aid.

Transporting

Transporting patients from one area to another is frequently necessary. A gurney (cart) or wheelchair may be required because of patient condition or facility regulations. Patients should be transferred onto/into the required transport device in an appropriate manner while proper draping is maintained throughout transfer and transport. Appropriate transfers in preparation for transporting patients are covered in Chapter 7.

Make sure wheel locks on wheelchairs or gurneys are locked before initiating transfers. Adjust patient clothing, draping, and medical equipment (IVs, etc.) to avoid problems discussed previously under *Patient Preparation*, becoming tangled in wheels, or dragged on the floor, during transport. A patient's arms and legs must be within the boundaries of a gurney or wheelchair to avoid injury during transport. Gurneys may have straps or side rails to keep patients within the confines of a gurney, and wheelchairs may have seat belts to keep patients from sliding or falling out of the chair. Use safety devices routinely for patient safety during transport.

Mattresses on gurneys and cushions on wheelchairs are used for patient comfort and protection. Pillows and padding are positioned for patient comfort and protection as necessary. Appropriate patient positioning is covered in Chapter 8.

MEDIALINK Watch the video on the CD under the heading of Body Mechanics.

Gurneys have four swivel wheels, making it easier to maneuver them from either end. Locks are located on each wheel. Generally, there are three positions in which a lock can be set. The three positions allow the lock to be used to stop swivel, stop rolling, or both.

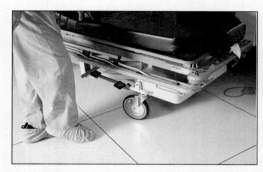

① With the locking lever in the horizontal position, both swivel and rolling movements are permitted.

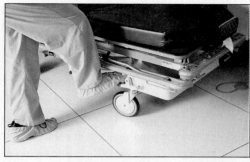

② When locking levers are tilted in one direction, swivel movements are not possible and rolling motions are permitted. Tilting locking levers in the other direction locks wheels completely, prohibiting both swivel and rolling movements. To engage locking levers, hold the gurney in a stable position and activate locking levers with your foot.

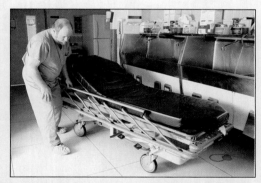

③ Gurney side rails raise or swing up to prevent patients from falling off gurneys. Rails are lowered or swung down for easier transfers.

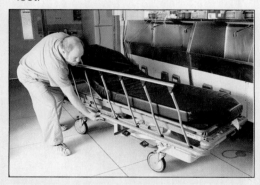

④ Gurney rails have locking mechanisms to secure them in the up position.

⑤ Push gurneys from the end at which a patient's head is placed so patients are moving feet first. The pace of transport should be slow and steady. Quick, jerky movements may upset or nauseate patients. Maintain control of gurneys at all times. Turn corners cautiously because of the potential for limited visibility and maneuvering space. Additional clinicians may be needed to maneuver on and off elevators, through doorways, and at blind corners. When necessary, medical equipment, such as IVs, can be attached to gurneys at an appropriate height.

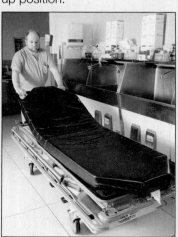

PROCEDURE 3–3   Transporting Via Wheelchair

Proper patient positioning in a wheelchair includes having a patient seated well back on the seat, lower extremities placed on the footrests or leg rests, arms resting on armrests or in laps, and available safety straps or seat belts secured. Push wheelchairs at a slow and steady pace without quick or jerky movements. Maintain control of wheelchairs at all times. When necessary, medical equipment, such as IVs, can be attached to the wheelchair at the appropriate height.

The method chosen to ascend and descend curbs depends on the (1) height of the curb, (2) size and weight of the patient and wheelchair, and (3) height and strength of the person transporting the patient. Use proper body mechanics to prevent potential injury. When descending an average height curb, the backward method places less stress on a physical therapist/assistant. When ascending an average height curb, the forward method places less stress on a physical therapist/assistant.

Descending Curb—Backward Method

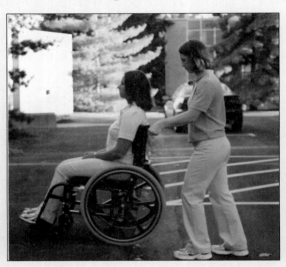

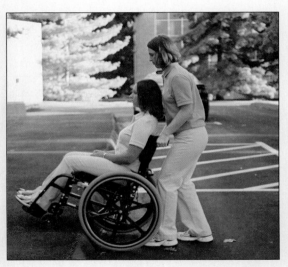

1 To lower a patient in a wheelchair down a curb, position the wheelchair with the patient facing away from the curb. The larger rear wheels are now at the edge of the curb to be descended.

2 Facing the wheelchair from behind, the physical therapist/assistant steps off the curb backward. Holding onto the wheelchair's push handles, the physical therapist/assistant slowly and smoothly rolls the rear wheels of the wheelchair to street level.

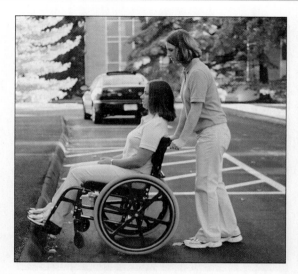

■ **Take Note**
The easier methods are to descend a curb backward and ascend a curb forward.

③ Securely holding a wheelchair's push handles and maintaining the wheelchair in a tilted position, the physical therapist/assistant continues to roll the wheelchair backward until the front wheels are clear of the curb. The physical therapist/assistant slowly lowers the front wheels until all four wheels are securely on the street level.

Descending Curb—Forward Method

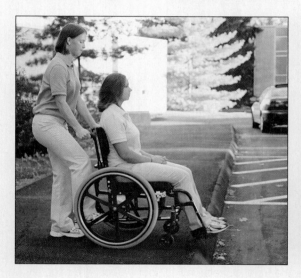

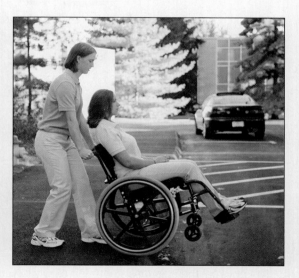

① This method places stress on a physical therapist/assistant, who must maintain backward tilt of the wheelchair while controlling the roll of the wheelchair's rear wheels over the edge of the curb. There is danger of losing control of the wheelchair when using this method. This method is recommended for use only with low curbs.

② When using the forward method, a wheelchair is positioned with the front of the wheelchair facing the curb. Facing the wheelchair from behind, the physical therapist/assistant tilts the wheelchair backward so the front wheels are approximately 8 inches above the ground. The wheelchair is rolled on its rear wheels to the edge of the curb.

(continued)

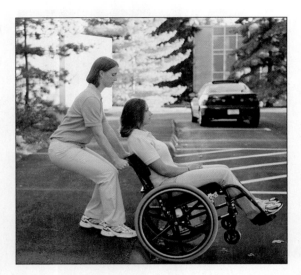

③ The rear wheels of the wheelchair are rolled slowly and smoothly off the curb onto the street level. As the wheelchair rolls over the curb, the physical therapist/assistant must step forward and bend at the hips and knees to control descent.

■ **Take Note**
Check traffic before descending curbs. Go slowly.

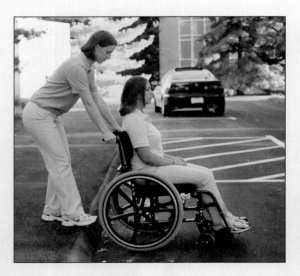

④ The physical therapist/assistant then slowly lowers the front wheels until all four wheels are securely on the lower level. Control of the lowering motion may be increased by placing one foot on one of the anti-tipping bars.

When a curb is high, a physical therapist/assistant may step off the curb while maintaining the wheel-chair in a tilted position.

Ascending Curb—Backward Method

This method places stress on the physical therapist/assistant while controlling the roll of the wheelchair over the edge of the curb. This method is recommended only for use with low curbs.

1 To raise a patient in a wheelchair up onto a curb, position the wheelchair with the patient facing away from the curb. Position the larger rear wheels of the wheelchair at the edge of the curb to be ascended. Facing the wheelchair from behind, the physical therapist/assistant tilts the chair backward and steps onto the curb backward. The physical therapist/assistant is positioned on the curb with feet in stride, hips and knees flexed, and trunk erect.

Holding onto a wheelchair's push handles, the physical therapist/assistant slowly and smoothly pulls the wheelchair in a tilted orientation up the curb on its rear wheels to sidewalk level.

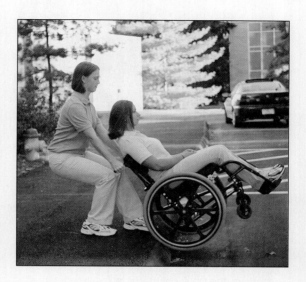

2 The wheelchair is rolled backward until the front wheels are clearly past the curb and over the sidewalk. The physical therapist/assistant then slowly lowers the front wheels until all four wheels are securely on the sidewalk. The physical therapist/assistant may place one foot on one of the antitipping bars to control the rate of lowering the wheelchair onto all four wheels.

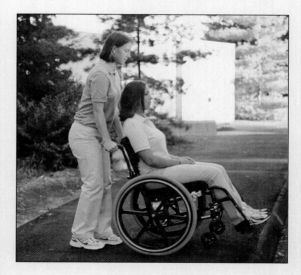

(continued)

Ascending Curb—Forward Method

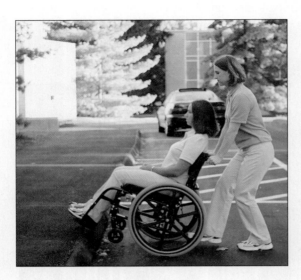

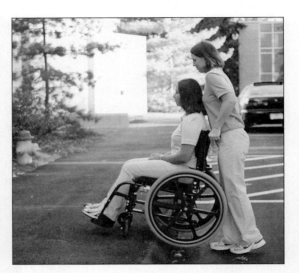

1 To raise a wheelchair and patient up onto a curb, position the wheelchair with the patient facing the curb. Facing the wheelchair from behind, the physical therapist/assistant tilts the wheelchair backward so the front wheels are higher than the curb. The physical therapist/assistant can use the antitip bars, and appropriate biomechanics, to assist in tilting the wheelchair safely.

2 Holding onto a wheelchair's push handles, the physical therapist/assistant slowly and smoothly pushes the wheelchair forward until the front wheels are clearly over the sidewalk. The wheelchair is lowered slowly, placing the front wheels on the sidewalk.

3 The physical therapist/assistant continues to wheel the wheelchair until the rear wheels contact the curb. Then the wheelchair is pushed and lifted so the rear wheels roll up and over the curb. Good body mechanics requires that the arms be held in a steady position and that the legs be straightened during the lifting motion.

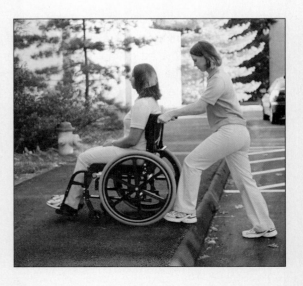

Doorways

Most public buildings have automatic doors, both opening and closing, to allow independent access for individuals using ambulation aides. The time an automatic door takes to open or close may vary. Doors with automatic closers may have varying degrees of door-closing force. Patients should be instructed to be aware of how automatic doors react and to learn details about the specific doors they use frequently.

Assisted Progression Through Doorways

Door Opening Away From Patient

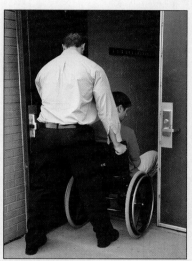 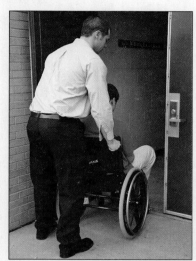

① To assist a patient in a wheelchair to progress through doors opening away from the patient, the physical therapist/assistant positions a patient facing away from the door. Using the door handles, the physical therapist/assistant releases the latch. The physical therapist/assistant walks backward through the doorway pulling the wheelchair backward through the doorway, using his or her back, shoulder, or foot to open and block the door.

② As a wheelchair passes the doorjamb, the physical therapist/assistant uses his or her body to keep the door open while steering the wheelchair with his or her hands, turning the wheelchair so the patient is facing the direction of progression.

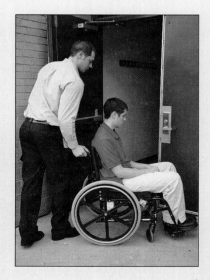

③ As the physical therapist/assistant, patient, and wheelchair progress through a doorway, the physical therapist/assistant may also use his or her shoulder, hip, or foot to continue blocking the door. Doors should not be allowed to close and hit either the patient or the wheelchair.

(continued)

Door Opening Toward Patient

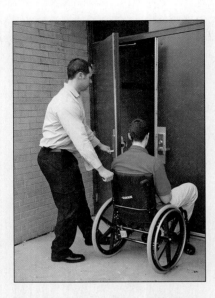

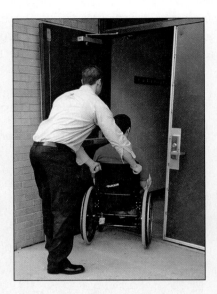

① To assist a patient in a wheelchair to progress through a doorway opening toward the patient, a physical therapist/assistant positions the patient and wheelchair parallel to the door at the latch side of the door. The physical therapist/assistant uses one hand to unlatch and pull the door open.

② The physical therapist/assistant opens the door sufficiently for passage of the wheelchair. Blocking the door open, the physical therapist/assistant aligns the patient and wheelchair while the door is open.

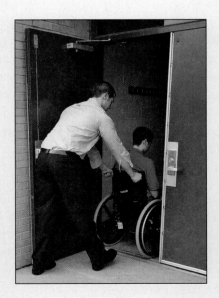

③ Walking forward through the doorway, the physical therapist/assistant pushes the wheelchair forward through a doorway, using his or her shoulder, hip, or foot to continue blocking the door. Doors should not be allowed to close and hit either the patient or the wheelchair.

Independent Progression Through Doorways

Techniques for independent wheelchair ambulation through doorways are determined by the (1) abilities of the patient, (2) direction in which doors open, (3) side of door jamb from which the patient can approach (hinge or latch), and (4) whether doors are automatic opening/closing doors.

Door Opening Toward Patient (With Automatic Door Closer)

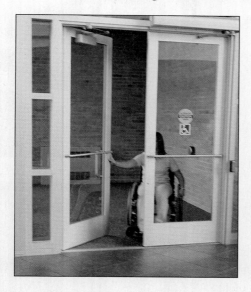

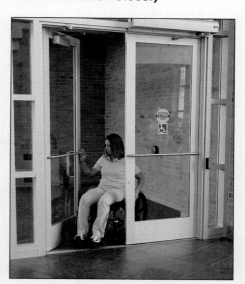

① The patient wheels to the latch side of the door and grasps the door handle with the hand toward the hinge side of the door. The patient pulls the door open wider than necessary for progression through the doorway, because the door will begin to close prior to the patient completing progression through the doorway.

② The patient may use the front rigging of the wheelchair or a hand to block open the door. The patient must progress into the doorway quickly to block the closing door. Take care that the closing door does not strike the patient or hit the wheelchair hard enough to cause a loss of control of the wheelchair.

③ Patients may pull on the doorjamb to assist propulsion through the doorway. Take care to avoid crushing a patient's fingers between a door and the propulsion wheels as the door is blocked.

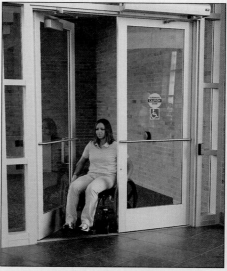

(continued)

Door Opens Away From Patient
(With Automatic Door Closer)

1. The patient approaches the door and grasps the door handle.

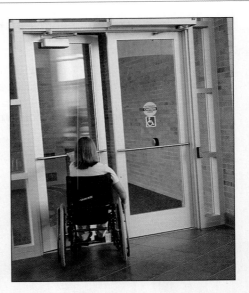

2. Pushing hard to open the door wide, a patient must enter the doorway before the door can close. Take care that the closing door does not strike a patient or hit the wheelchair hard enough to cause a patient to lose control of the wheelchair. Some patients may pull on the doorjamb to assist progression through the doorway, while blocking the closing door with the other hand. Other patients propel their wheelchair in the usual manner or use a combination of pulling on the doorjamb and normal propulsion.

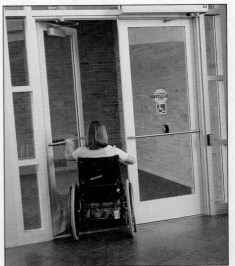

3. When a patient is nearly through a doorway, the door may be given one more opening push. The patient then propels the wheelchair quickly out of the arc of the closing door. Then the door is allowed to close behind the patient's wheelchair. Some patients turn wheelchairs around the latch side of the doorjamb and away from the closing door to move quickly out of the arc of closing door.

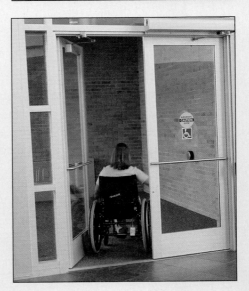

Doors With Automatic Door Openers
(Opening Away/Toward Patient)

Several types of activators are available for automatic door openers. Most commonly, push-plate activators are located along the path to the door at an appropriate height. A pressure activator may be located in the floor in front of the door, or a motion sensor may be used. When doors open toward patients, patients must make sure to be clear of the arc of the opening doors to avoid being struck. Doors usually stay open until patients have progressed completely through doorways. Patients, however, should not hesitate while progressing through doorways, because automatic door openers release after a set amount of time.

Wheelchair Wheelies

Wheelchair wheelies are performed by balancing on the rear wheels of a wheelchair with the (front) caster wheels in the air. Patients must be able to perform wheelies to ascend and descend curbs independently when no curb ramps/cuts are available. It is critical to guard a patient while a patient learns to perform a wheelie to prevent injury.

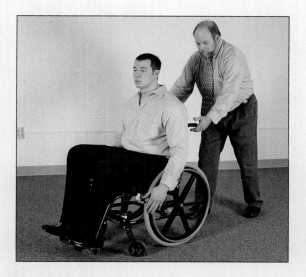

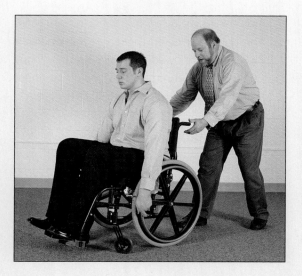

❶ A physical therapist/assistant must be positioned behind, and move with, the wheelchair to guard as patients practice. The physical therapist's/assistant's hands must be beneath or on a wheelchair's push handles, ready to catch a wheelchair if it tilts too far backward.

❷ The patient begins a wheelie by grasping the anterior portion of the push rims.

(continued)

3 A quick backward movement of the wheels places the patient's hands in position for the forward thrust that achieves the wheelie position.

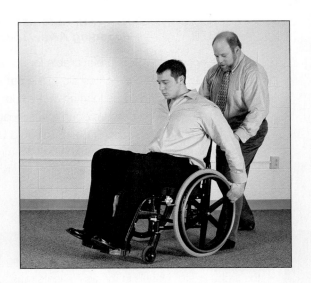

4 The quick backward motion of the wheels is immediately followed by a quick forward thrust on both wheel rims. The result of these maneuvers causes the wheelchair to tilt backward, rising onto the rear wheels only.

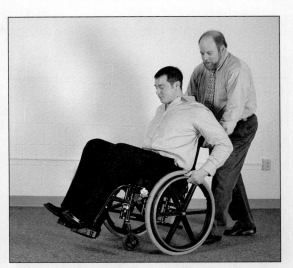

5 Patients control balancing and moving on the rear wheels by forward and backward movements of the rear wheels.

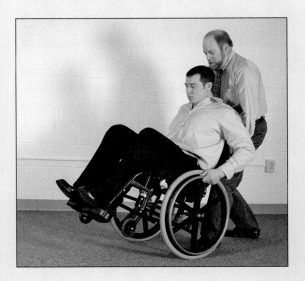

Elevators

When riding in an elevator, patients should be positioned facing an elevator door, the position most commonly assumed when riding an elevator. When space is sufficient, a patient may enter an elevator forward, and then turn around. When space is limited, patients should enter an elevator backward. Facing forward allows patients to monitor floor displays and have access to control panels. Exiting facing forward is usually safer.

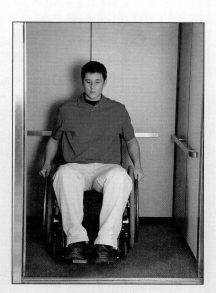

Chapter Review

Review Questions

1. Who is responsible for ensuring that patient care environments are safe and efficient?

2. Describe the general guidelines for properly managing the patient care environment.

3. List the five rules of proper body mechanics.

4. Describe how to apply rules of proper body mechanics in each of the following situations:
   a. When transporting a patient on a gurney.
   b. When guarding a patient who is ambulating.
   c. When moving large equipment.

5. Distinguish between instructions and commands, giving examples of each.

6. List the purposes of draping a patient.

7. Describe how to transport a patient safely in a wheelchair.

Suggested Activities

1. Demonstrate how to correctly adjust locking mechanisms on the wheels of a gurney, railings on a gurney, and wheel locks on a wheelchair.

2. Demonstrate how to maneuver gurneys and wheelchairs through doorways, around corners, and along hallways properly and safely.

3. Demonstrate how to ascend and descend curbs.

4. Demonstrate how to guard a person performing wheelchair wheelies.

5. Perform wheelchair wheelies.

6. Discuss experiences in activities 1–5, including:
   a. Perceptions of self when being transported compared to being the person doing the transporting.
   b. Realization of the challenge of moving about the environment while in a wheelchair or on a gurney.

7. Rotate through several stations related to body mechanics. Suggestions for stations include:

   a. Foot placement.

   Place foot marks on the floor indicating foot placement. Make some foot placements correct and some incorrect. Students should perform tasks such as lifting boxes from a wheelchair to a mat table, from a wheelchair to a treatment table, and from a table in front to a table behind. Discuss which foot placements are appropriate and why.

   b. Center of Gravity (CoG) centered.

   Carry books in a book bag from the front of a classroom to the rear of a classroom, with the book bag on one shoulder, properly positioned on both shoulders, held in one hand at the side, and held in one hand out in front. Discuss experiences to determine which positions are easier and why.

8. Document experiences such as ascending and descending curbs in SOAP note format.

Case Study

You are working in a rehabilitation facility with a patient who has a recent complete cervical spinal cord injury. A power wheelchair has been ordered but has not yet been delivered, so transport requires family members to maneuver a manual wheelchair. The patient's family wishes to take her to a restaurant in an older section of town. The family has determined that the restaurant is wheelchair accessible. The parking lot, however, is across the street from the restaurant and there are no curb ramps on either side of the street. List and describe the transport activities that might be required. Indicate what you would review with the patient and family prior to their departure for the restaurant.

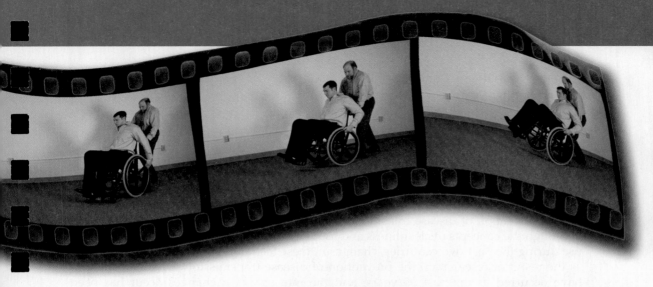

Aseptic Techniques

Learning Objectives

Upon completion of this chapter, you will be able to:

1. Describe Standard Precautions, including who is responsible for implementation, when to implement, and methods of implementation.
2. Recognize when the guidelines for a sterile field are violated, and act appropriately.
3. Demonstrate proper procedure for donning a sterile gown.
4. Demonstrate proper procedure for donning sterile gloves.
5. Demonstrate proper procedure for removal of contaminated gloves.
6. Describe the requirements and components of a sterile field.
7. Describe the purposes, types, materials, and methods of wound dressings.
8. List the five major areas of recommendations for isolation precautions.
9. Describe the five modes of transmission of infectious microorganisms.
10. Describe the implementation of selected procedures of isolation precautions.

Key Terms

Airborne precautions	Hand antisepsis
Airborne transmission	Hand hygiene
Alcohol-based hand rub	Hand-washing
Antimicrobial soap	Hospital Infection Control
Antiseptic agent	Practices Advisory
Antiseptic hand rub	Committee (HICPAC)
Antiseptic hand wash	Indirect-contact
Aseptic technique	transmission
Bacterial barrier	Isolation
Centers for Disease	Mask
Control and	Noncritical items
Prevention (CDC)	Nosocomial infection
Cleaning	Occlusive dressing
Cleanliness	Patient-care equipment
Common vehicle	categories
transmission	Plain soap
Compression wrap	Recommendations
Contact precautions	ranking scheme
Contact transmission	Respirator
Contaminated	Rigid dressing
Critical items	Semicritical items
Damp-to-damp dressing	Shelf life
Damp-to-dry dressing	Spiral wrap
Decontaminate hands	Standard precautions
Detergent	Sterile
Direct-contact	Sterile field
transmission	Sterilization
Disinfection	Surgical hand antisepsis
Droplet precautions	Transmission-based
Droplet transmission	precautions
Dry-to-dry dressing	Unsterile (nonsterile)
Figure-of-eight wrap	Vectorborne transmission
Gauze wrap	Waterless antiseptic agent

Introduction

Much of the material in this chapter is from publications in the public domain produced by the CDC,[1, 2, 3, 4] which is continually updating recommendations for cleaning, disinfecting, and sterile technique based on an increasing body of scientific knowledge. While the information in this chapter provides a starting point for understanding disease-transmission prevention and practices in aseptic techniques, individuals are strongly advised to become familiar with the specific practices of the institution in which they work and to obtain updated information directly from the CDC. Information can be found at the CDC website by entering a key term such as "Isolation Precautions" in the search box, and then downloading the desired information.

Centers for Disease Control and Prevention

1600 Clifton Rd, Atlanta, GA 30333

(404) 639–3311

(404) 639–3534 / (800) 311–3435 (public inquiries)

www.cdc.gov

Each institution will use information and protocols specific to that institution. Institution-specific information and protocols can be obtained from the appropriate department within the institution.

The prevention of disease transmission in health-care settings is of major concern.[2, 3] Although the concepts of cleanliness and aseptic technique in patient care have been in use during the past two centuries, changes in these techniques occur from time to time as the result of research on the prevention of disease transmission. Dramatic changes have occurred in the past 35 years, and the rate at which changes occur has been increasing. For this reason, a brief history of isolation protocols is presented.

In 1970, the **Centers for Disease Control and Prevention** (CDC) recommended isolation procedures based on seven categories: Strict Isolation, Respiratory Isolation, Protective Isolation, Enteric Precautions, Wound and Skin Precautions, Discharge Precautions, and Blood Precautions. The precautions recommended for each category were based primarily on the epidemiologic features of the diseases grouped in the category. The diseases were grouped primarily by routes of transmission, and recommended precautions were the minimum believed necessary to prevent transmission of all diseases in a specific category. In 1983, the CDC published guidelines, which included revision of the original categories, and permitted facilities to use either category-specific guidelines or disease-specific guidelines. CDC guidelines published in 1997 required guidelines to (1) have a basis that is epidemiologically sound; (2) emphasize the importance of all body fluids, secretions, and excretions in the transmission of nosocomial pathogens; (3) contain adequate precautions for infections transmitted by the airborne, droplet, and contact routes of transmission; (4) be simple to understand and use; and (5) use new terms to avoid confusion with existing systems. CDC guidelines published in 2007 encompass updated recommendations and emphasize that these guidelines cover all health-care settings and not just hospitals. Current specific infection-control recommendations are contained in *Guidelines for Isolation Precautions: Preventing Transmission of Infectious Agents in Healthcare Settings 2007.*

Recent increased emphasis on the importance of prevention of disease transmission and the spread of infection through proper patient-care techniques has occurred in part because of the increasing incidence of catastrophic diseases, such as acquired immunodeficiency syndrome (AIDS). The CDC and its **Hospital Infection Control Practices Advisory Committee (HICPAC)**, operating within the Department of Health and Human Services, are responsible for issuing guidelines related to prevention of disease transmission. These guidelines are updated periodically, and personnel should obtain the most updated information from the infection control officer at their specific institution or directly from the CDC. The Occupational Safety and Health Agency (OSHA), an agency of the federal government, establishes rules and regulations to protect workers in a variety of work environments, including workers in health-care facilities.

One means of preventing disease transmission is placing patients in isolation. **Isolation** is the separation and placement of patients in environments that reduce the potential for transmission of infectious microorganisms. The principles followed and the techniques used to prevent disease transmission as part of isolation precautions are generally appropriate for the prevention of disease transmission as part of patient care in general.

■ **Take Note**

Isolation precautions are aimed at preventing disease transmission.

When a patient is placed in isolation, signage is posted outside the patient's room indicating specifically required isolation practices or a request for visitors to see the patient's nurse prior to entering the patient's room. There are two methods indicating which isolation precautions are to be used. Hospitals choose which method is most appropriate for their facility.

Definitions

Definitions are used by the medical community to standardize terminology. Several terms used in this chapter are defined below. Not all definitions related to *Aseptic Techniques* are included.

Alcohol-based hand rub: An alcohol-containing preparation designed for application to the hands for reducing the number of viable microorganisms on the hands. In the United States, such preparations usually contain 60 percent to 95 percent ethanol or isopropanol.

Antimicrobial soap: Soap (i.e., detergent) containing an antiseptic agent.

Antiseptic agent: Antimicrobial substances that are applied to the skin to reduce the number of microbial flora. Examples include alcohols, chlorhexidine, chlorine, hexachlorophene, iodine, chloroxylenol (PCMX), quaternary ammonium compounds, and triclosan.

Antiseptic hand rub: Applied to all surfaces of the hands to reduce the number of microorganisms present.

Antiseptic hand wash: Washing hands with water and soap or other detergents containing an antiseptic agent.

Aseptic technique: The methods and procedures used to create and maintain a sterile field.

Bacterial barrier: A barrier that keeps microorganisms from coming in contact with sterile items.

Cleanliness: Three levels of cleanliness—cleaning, disinfection, and sterilization— have been established for equipment use in patient care.

   Cleaning: The physical removal of organic material or soil from objects. The process of cleaning is usually performed with water, with or without detergents. Cleaning is the least rigorous of the three levels and is designed to remove microorganisms rather than kill them. Cleaning usually precedes either of the next two levels, disinfection or sterilization.

   Disinfection: An intermediate level between cleaning and sterilization. Three levels of disinfection—high, intermediate, and low—have been defined. Disinfection is usually performed using pasteurization or chemical germicides.

   Sterilization: The highest level of cleanliness. Sterilization is the destruction of all forms of microbial life by steam under pressure, liquid or gaseous chemicals, or dry heat.

Contaminated: An item, surface, or field that comes in contact with anything that is not sterile.

Decontaminate hands: To reduce bacterial counts on hands by performing antiseptic hand rub or antiseptic hand wash.

Detergent: Compounds that possess a cleaning action. Detergents (i.e., surfactants) are composed of both hydrophilic and lipophilic parts and can be divided into four groups: anionic, cationic, amphoteric, and nonionic detergents. Although products used for hand-washing or antiseptic hand wash in health-care settings represent various types of detergents, the term "soap" is used to refer to such detergents in this guideline.

Hand antisepsis: Either antiseptic hand wash or antiseptic hand rub.

Hand hygiene: A general term that applies to hand-washing, antiseptic hand wash, antiseptic hand rub, or surgical hand antisepsis.

Hand-washing: Washing hands with plain (i.e., nonantimicrobial) soap and water.

Mask: A nonactive device that filters environmental air.

Nosocomial infection: Infection acquired while hospitalized for treatment of other conditions.

Patient-care equipment categories: Three categories of patient care equipment— critical, noncritical, and semicritical,[2,3]—provide a basis for the level of cleanliness deemed necessary.

Critical items: Introduced directly into the circulatory system or other normally sterile areas of the body. Surgical instruments, implants, and the blood compartment of a hemodialyzer are examples of critical items.

Noncritical items: Do not touch the patient or touch the patient in areas that are normally not sterile, such as intact areas of skin. Blood pressure cuffs and crutches are examples of noncritical items.

Semicritical items: Introduced into body cavities not usually considered sterile, and include, but are not limited to, endotracheal tubes and fiberoptic endoscopes. There is a lower degree of risk of infection associated with semicritical items.

Plain soap: Detergents that do not contain antimicrobial agents or that contain low concentrations of antimicrobial agents that are effective solely as preservatives.

Recommendations ranking scheme: The CDC's Center for Infectious Diseases has established four categories to indicate the scientific support for their recommendations.[3]

Category IA: Strongly recommended for all hospitals and strongly supported by well-designed experimental or epidemiologic studies.[3]

Category IB: Strongly recommended for all hospitals and reviewed as effective by experts and a consensus of HICPAC, based on strong rationale and suggestive evidence, although definitive scientific studies have not been done.[3]

Category II: Suggested for implementation in many hospitals. Recommendations may be supported or suggested by clinical or epidemiologic studies, a strong theoretical rationale, or definitive studies applicable to some, but not all, hospitals.[3]

No recommendation/unresolved issues: Practices for which insufficient evidence or consensus regarding efficacy exists.[3]

Respirator: A mechanical device that provides a source of air not associated with the immediate environment.

Shelf life: The length of time an unopened sterilized package is considered to remain sterile.

Standard precautions: Precautions designed for the care of all patients, particularly hospitalized patients, regardless of their diagnosis or presumed infection status. This is new terminology to replace the term universal precautions.

Sterile: An item or environment free from living microorganisms.

Sterile field: An area considered free from living microorganisms.

Surgical hand antisepsis: Antiseptic hand wash or antiseptic hand rub performed preoperatively by surgical personnel to eliminate transient, and reduce resident, hand flora. Antiseptic detergent preparations often have persistent antimicrobial activity.

Unsterile (nonsterile): Any item or environment that has not been sterilized, has come into contact with an item that is no longer considered sterile, has entered a field that is not sterile, or has exceeded its shelf life.

Waterless antiseptic agent: An antiseptic agent that does not require use of exogenous water. After applying such an agent, the hands are rubbed together until the agent has dried.

Guidelines for Isolation Precautions in Health Care Settings

Rationale

Transmission of infection requires three elements: (1) a source of infecting microorganisms, (2) a susceptible host, and (3) a means of transmission for the microorganism. Human sources of infecting microorganisms in hospitals may be patients, personnel, or visitors. Included may be persons with acute disease, or persons in the incubation period of a disease, persons who are colonized by an infectious agent but have no apparent disease, or persons who are chronic carriers of an infectious agent. Other sources of infecting microorganisms can be the patient's own endogenous flora, which may be difficult to control, and inanimate environmental objects that have become contaminated, including equipment and medications.

Resistance among persons to pathogenic microorganisms varies greatly. Some may be immune to infection or may be able to resist colonization by an infectious agent. Others exposed to the same agent may establish a commensal relationship with the infecting microorganism and become asymptomatic carriers. Still others may develop clinical disease. Host factors may include, but are not limited to, (1) age; (2) underlying diseases; (3) certain treatments with antimicrobials, corticosteroids, or other immunosuppressive agents; (4) irradiation; and (5) breaks in the first line of defense mechanisms caused by surgical operations, anesthesia, and indwelling catheters, which may render patients more susceptible to infection.

Microorganisms are transmitted in hospitals by several routes, and the same microorganism may be transmitted by more than one route. There are five main routes of transmission: contact, droplet, airborne, common vehicle, and vectorborne. Isolation precautions are designed to prevent transmission of microorganisms by these routes in hospitals. Because agent and host factors are more difficult to control, interruption of transfer of microorganisms is directed primarily at transmission. CDC recommendations are based on this concept.

There are two tiers of isolation precautions. The first, and most important, tier of isolation precautions is standard precautions, as described previously. The second tier of precautions is **transmission-based precautions**, based on the concept of avoiding infection by limiting the potential for transmission of microorganisms. Transmission-based precautions are designed for the care of only specified patients: patients known, or suspected, to be infected by epidemiologically important pathogens, highly transmissible pathogens for which additional precautions, beyond standard precautions, are needed to interrupt transmission in health-care settings. There are three types of transmission-based precautions: contact, droplet, and airborne. Combinations of these precautions may be used for diseases that have multiple routes of transmission. Whether used singularly or in combination, they are to be used in addition to standard precautions.

Modes of Transmission

Contact transmission, the most important and frequent mode of nosocomial infection transmission, is divided into two subgroups—direct-contact transmission and indirect-contact transmission. **Direct-contact transmission** involves direct body-surface-to-body-surface contact and physical transfer of microorganisms between a susceptible host and an infected or colonized person, such as when turning or transferring a patient or when performing other patient-care activities that require direct personal contact. Direct-contact transmission can also occur when one patient serves as a source of the infectious microorganisms and the other as a susceptible host. **Indirect-contact transmission** involves contact of a susceptible host with a contaminated intermediate object, usually inanimate, such as whirlpool water that is not changed between patient treatments, reuse of self-adhesive electrodes on more than one patient, contaminated hands that are not washed, and gloves that are not changed between patients.

Droplet transmission, theoretically, is a form of contact transmission. The mechanism of transfer of the pathogen, however, is quite distinct from either direct- or indirect-contact transmission. Therefore, droplet transmission is considered a separate route of transmission. Droplets are generated from a source person, primarily during coughing, sneezing, and talking, and during the performance of certain procedures such as suctioning or wound care. Transmission occurs when droplets containing microorganisms generated from the infected person are propelled a short distance through the air and deposited on a host's conjunctivae, nasal mucosa, or mouth.

■ **Take Note**

Modes of transmission include contact, droplet, airborne, common vehicle, and vectorborne.

Droplets do not remain suspended in the air, and droplet transmission must not be confused with airborne transmission.

Airborne transmission occurs by two modes of dissemination, the first mode of which is airborne droplet nuclei, which are particle residue 5 μm or smaller in size. These nuclei are evaporated droplets containing microorganisms that remain suspended in the air for long periods of time. The second mode of dissemination is in dust particles containing the infectious agent that are dispersed widely by air currents and inhaled by a susceptible host. The distance over which such dissemination may occur is dependent upon environmental factors, thus special air handling and ventilation are required to prevent airborne transmission.

Common vehicle transmission applies to microorganisms transmitted by contaminated items such as food, water, medications, devices, and equipment.

Vectorborne transmission occurs when vectors such as mosquitoes, flies, rats, and other vermin transmit microorganisms; this route of transmission is of less significance in hospitals in the United States than in other regions of the world.

Precautions

When outlining the precautions to be used in isolation, the CDC deemed five areas crucial to maintaining isolation precautions in health-care settings: (1) administrative controls, (2) standard precautions, (3) contact precautions, (4) droplet precautions, and (5) airborne precautions. Current CDC recommendations for all five areas are at the Category IB level. The recommendations are limited to the topic of isolation. Therefore, they must be supplemented by hospital policies and procedures for other aspects of infection and environment control, occupational health, and administrative and legal issues.

Following are selected isolation precaution recommendations from the CDC.[3]

Administrative Controls

Education.   Develop a system to ensure that hospital patients, personnel, and visitors are educated about use of precautions and their responsibility for adherence to them.

Adherence to Precautions.   Periodically evaluate adherence to precautions and use findings to direct improvements.

Standard Precautions

Standard precautions combine the major features of universal precautions (UP) and body substance isolation (BSI) and are based on the principle that all body fluids (blood and secretions, excretions except sweat), nonintact skin, and mucous membranes may contain transmissible infectious agents. Standard precautions include a group of infection-prevention practices that apply to all patients, regardless of suspected or confirmed infection status, in any setting in which health care is delivered. These include hand hygiene; use of gloves, gown, mask, eye protection, or face shield, depending on the anticipated exposure; and safe injection practices. Also, equipment or items in the patient environment likely to have been contaminated with infectious body fluids must be handled in a manner to prevent transmission of infectious agents (e.g., wear gloves for direct contact, contain heavily soiled equipment, properly clean and disinfect or sterilize reusable equipment before use on another patient). The application of standard precautions during patient care is determined by the nature of the health-care-worker (HCW)–patient interaction and the extent of anticipated blood, body fluid, or pathogen exposure. For some interactions (e.g., performing venipuncture), only gloves may be needed; during other interactions (e.g., intubation), use of gloves, gown, face shield or mask, and goggles is necessary. Education and training on the principles and rationale for recommended

■ **Take Note**

IB recommendations are strongly indicated based on rationale and suggested evidence.

■ **Take Note**

Standard precautions are to be used with all patients.

practices are critical elements of standard precautions because they facilitate appropriate decision making and promote adherence when HCWs are faced with new circumstances. An example of the importance of the use of standard precautions is intubation, especially under emergency circumstances when infectious agents may not be suspected, but later are identified (e.g., SARS-CoV, *Neisseria meningitides*). Standard precautions are also intended to protect patients by ensuring that health-care personnel do not carry infectious agents to patients on their hands or via equipment used during patient care.

New Elements of Standard Precautions

Infection-control problems that are identified in the course of outbreak investigations often indicate the need for new recommendations or reinforcement of existing infection-control recommendations to protect patients. Because such recommendations are considered a standard of care and may not be included in other guidelines, they have been added to standard precautions. Three such areas of practice that have been added are respiratory hygiene/cough etiquette, safe injection practices, and the use of masks for insertion of catheters or injection of material into spinal or epidural spaces via lumbar puncture procedures (e.g., myelogram, spinal or epidural anesthesia). While most elements of standard precautions evolved from universal precautions that were developed for protection of health-care personnel, these new elements of standard precautions focus on protection of patients.

Respiratory Hygiene/Cough Etiquette

The transmission of SARS-CoV in emergency departments by patients and their family members during the widespread SARS outbreaks in 2003 highlighted the need for vigilance and prompt implementation of infection-control measures at the first point of encounter within a health-care setting (e.g., reception and triage areas in emergency departments, outpatient clinics, and physician offices). The strategy proposed has been termed respiratory hygiene/cough etiquette and is intended to be incorporated into infection-control practices as a new component of standard precautions. The strategy is targeted at patients and accompanying family members and friends with undiagnosed transmissible respiratory infections and applies to any person with signs of illness, including cough, congestion, rhinorrhea, or increased production of respiratory secretions when entering a health-care facility. The term *cough etiquette* is derived from recommended source control measures for *Mycobacteria tuberculosis*. The elements of respiratory hygiene/cough etiquette include (1) education of health-care facility staff, patients, and visitors; (2) posted signs, in language(s) appropriate to the population served, with instructions to patients and accompanying family members or friends; (3) source control measures (e.g., covering the mouth/nose with a tissue when coughing and prompt disposal of used tissues, use of a surgical mask on the coughing person when tolerated and appropriate); (4) hand hygiene after contact with respiratory secretions; and (5) spatial separation, ideally greater than 3 feet, of persons with respiratory infections in common waiting areas when possible. Covering sneezes and coughs and placing masks on coughing patients are proven means of source containment that prevent infected persons from dispersing respiratory secretions into the air. Masking may be difficult in some settings (e.g., pediatrics, in which case the emphasis by necessity may be on cough etiquette). Physical proximity of less than 3 feet has been associated with an increased risk for transmission of infections via the droplet route (e.g., *N. meningitidis* and group A streptococcus) and, therefore, supports the practice of distancing infected persons from others who are not infected. The effectiveness of good hygiene practices, especially hand hygiene, in preventing transmission of viruses and reducing the incidence of respiratory infections both within and outside health-care settings is summarized in several reviews.

■ **Take Note**
Respiratory hygiene/cough etiquette is just like mom says—cover your mouth and nose with a tissue when sneezing/coughing.

Respiratory hygiene and cough etiquette should be effective in decreasing the risk of transmission of pathogens contained in large respiratory droplets (e.g., influenza virus, adenovirus, *Bordetella pertussis*, and *Mycoplasma pneumonia*). Although fever will be present in many respiratory infections, patients with pertussis and mild upper respiratory tract infections are often afebrile. The absence of fever, however, does not always exclude a respiratory infection. Patients who have asthma, allergic rhinitis, or chronic obstructive lung disease also may be coughing and sneezing. While these patients often are not infectious, cough etiquette measures are prudent.

Health-care personnel are advised to observe droplet precautions (i.e., wear a mask) and practice hand hygiene when examining and caring for patients with signs and symptoms of a respiratory infection. Health-care personnel who have a respiratory infection are advised to avoid direct patient contact, especially with high-risk patients. If this is not possible, then a mask should be worn while providing patient care.

Standard Precaution Guidelines

Assume that every person is potentially infected or colonized with an organism that could be transmitted in the health-care setting, and apply the following infection-control practices during the delivery of health care.

A. Hand hygiene
   1. During the delivery of health care, avoid unnecessary touching of surfaces in close proximity to the patient to prevent both contamination of clean hands from environmental surfaces and transmission of pathogens from contaminated hands to surfaces.
   2. When hands are visibly dirty, contaminated with proteinaceous material, or visibly soiled with blood or body fluids, wash hands with a nonantimicrobial or antimicrobial soap and water.
   3. If hands are not visibly soiled, or after removing visible material with nonantimicrobial soap and water, decontaminate hands in clinical situations. The preferred method of hand decontamination is with an alcohol-based hand rub. Alternatively, hands may be washed with an antimicrobial soap and water. Frequent use of alcohol-based hand rub immediately following handwashing with nonantimicrobial soap may increase the frequency of dermatitis. Perform hand hygiene:
      a. Before having direct contact with patients.
      b. After contact with blood, body fluids or excretions, mucous membranes, nonintact skin, or wound dressings.
      c. After contact with a patient's intact skin (e.g., when taking a pulse or blood pressure or lifting a patient).
      d. If hands will be moving from a contaminated body site to a clean body site during patient care.
      e. After contact with inanimate objects (including medical equipment) in the immediate vicinity of the patient.
      f. After removing gloves.
   4. Wash hands with nonantimicrobial or antimicrobial soap and water if contact with spores (e.g., *C. difficile* or *Bacillus anthracis*) is likely to have occurred. The physical action of washing and rinsing hands under such circumstances is recommended because alcohols, chlorhexidine, iodophors, and other antiseptic agents have poor activity against spores. Steps to proper hand-washing:
      a. Hands should be washed using soap and warm, running water.
      b. Hands should be rubbed vigorously during washing for at least 20 seconds with special attention paid to the backs of the hands, wrists, between the fingers, and under fingernails.
      c. Hands should be rinsed well while leaving the water running.

      d. With the water running, hands should be dried with a single-use towel.

      e. Turn off the water using a paper towel, covering washed hands to prevent recontamination.

  5. Do not wear artificial fingernails or extenders if duties include direct contact with patients at high risk for infection and associated adverse outcomes (e.g., those in ICUs or operating rooms). As an administrative control, an institution should develop an organizational policy on the wearing of nonnatural nails by health-care personnel who have direct contact with patients outside the groups specified above.

B. Personal protective equipment (PPE)

  1. Observe the following principles of use:

      a. Wear PPE when the nature of the anticipated patient interaction indicates that contact with blood or body fluids may occur.

      b. Prevent contamination of clothing and skin during the process of removing PPE.

      c. Before leaving the patient's room or cubicle, remove and discard PPE.

  2. Gloves

      a. Wear gloves when it can be reasonably anticipated that contact with blood or other potentially infectious materials, mucous membranes, nonintact skin, or potentially contaminated intact skin (e.g., of a patient incontinent of stool or urine) could occur.

      b. Wear gloves with fit and durability appropriate to the task.

        i. Wear disposable medical examination gloves for providing direct patient care.

        ii. Wear disposable medical examination gloves or reusable utility gloves for cleaning the environment or medical equipment.

      c. Remove gloves after contact with a patient and/or the surrounding environment (including medical equipment) using proper technique to prevent hand contamination. Do not wear the same pair of gloves for the care of more than one patient. Do not wash gloves for the purpose of reuse, since this practice has been associated with transmission of pathogens.

      d. Change gloves during patient care if the hands will move from a contaminated body site (e.g., perineal area) to a clean body site (e.g., face).

  3. Gowns

      a. Wear a gown that is appropriate to the task to protect skin and prevent soiling or contamination of clothing during procedures and patient-care activities when contact with blood, body fluids, secretions, or excretions is anticipated.

        i. Wear a gown for direct patient contact if the patient has uncontained secretions or excretions.

        ii. Remove gown and perform hand hygiene before leaving the patient's environment.

      b. Do not reuse gowns, even for repeated contacts with the same patient.

      c. Routine donning of gowns upon entrance into a high-risk unit (e.g., ICU, NICU, HSCT unit) is not indicated.

  4. Mouth, nose, eye protection

      a. Use PPE to protect the mucous membranes of the eyes, nose, and mouth during procedures and patient-care activities that are likely to generate splashes or sprays of blood, body fluids, secretions, and excretions. Select masks, goggles, face shields, and combinations of these according to the need anticipated by the task to be performed.

      b. During aerosol-generating procedures (e.g., suctioning of the respiratory tract [if not using inline suction catheters], endotracheal intubation) in patients who are not suspected of being infected with an agent for which

■ **Take Note**

Nonsterile examination gloves can be used for most routine patient-care activities.

respiratory protection is otherwise recommended (e.g., *M. tuberculosis,* SARS, or hemorrhagic fever viruses), wear one of the following: a face shield that fully covers the front and sides of the face, a mask with attached shield, or a mask and goggles (in addition to gloves and gown).

C. Respiratory hygiene/cough etiquette
    1. Educate health-care personnel on the importance of source control measures to contain respiratory secretions to prevent droplet and fomite transmission of respiratory pathogens, especially during seasonal outbreaks of viral respiratory tract infections (e.g., influenza, RSV, adenovirus, parainfluenza virus) in communities.
    2. Implement the following measures to contain respiratory secretions in patients and accompanying individuals who have signs and symptoms of a respiratory infection, beginning at the point of initial encounter in a health-care setting (e.g., triage, reception, and waiting areas in emergency departments, outpatient clinics, physical therapy clinics/offices, and physician offices).
        a. Post signs at entrances and in strategic places (e.g., elevators, cafeterias) within ambulatory and inpatient settings with instructions to patients and other persons with symptoms of a respiratory infection to cover their mouths/noses when coughing or sneezing, to use and dispose of tissues, and to perform hand hygiene after hands have been in contact with respiratory secretions.
        b. Provide tissues and no-touch receptacles (e.g., foot-pedal-operated lid or open, plastic-lined waste basket) for disposal of tissues.
        c. Provide resources and instructions for performing hand hygiene in or near waiting areas in ambulatory and inpatient settings; provide conveniently located dispensers of alcohol-based hand rubs and, where sinks are available, supplies for hand-washing.
        d. During periods of increased prevalence of respiratory infections in the community (e.g., as indicated by increased school absenteeism, increased number of patients seeking care for a respiratory infection), offer masks to coughing patients and other symptomatic persons (e.g., persons who accompany ill patients) upon entry into the facility or medical office and encourage them to maintain special separation, ideally a distance of at least 3 feet, from others in common waiting areas. Some facilities may find it logistically easier to institute this recommendation year-round as a standard of practice.

D. Patient-care equipment and instruments/devices
    1. Establish policies and procedures for containing, transporting, and handling patient-care equipment and instruments/devices that may be contaminated with blood or body fluids.
    2. Remove organic material from critical and semicritical instrument/devices using recommended cleaning agents before high-level disinfection and sterilization to enable effective disinfection and sterilization processes.
    3. Wear PPE (e.g., gloves, gown) according to the level of anticipated contamination when handling patient-care equipment and instruments/devices that are visibly soiled or may have been in contact with blood or body fluids.

E. Care of the environment
    1. Establish policies and procedures for routine and targeted cleaning of environmental surfaces as indicated by the level of patient contact and degree of soiling.
    2. Clean and disinfect surfaces that are likely to be contaminated with pathogens, including those that are in close proximity to the patient (e.g., bed rails, over bed tables) and frequently touched surfaces in the patient-care

environment (e.g., door knobs, surfaces in and surrounding toilets in patients' rooms) on a more frequent schedule compared to that for other surfaces (e.g., horizontal surfaces in waiting rooms).

3. Use EPA-registered disinfectants that have microbiocidal (i.e., killing) activity against the pathogens most likely to contaminate the patient-care environment. Use in accordance with manufacturer's instructions.

4. In facilities that provide health care to pediatric patients or have waiting areas with child play toys, establish policies and procedures for cleaning and disinfecting toys at regular intervals. *Category IA recommendation.* Use the following principles in developing this policy and procedures:

   a. Select play toys that can be easily cleaned and disinfected.

   b. Do not permit use of stuffed furry toys if they will be shared.

   c. Clean and disinfect large stationary toys (e.g., climbing equipment) at least weekly and whenever visibly soiled.

   d. If toys are likely to be mouthed, rinse with water after disinfection; alternatively, wash in a dishwasher.

   e. When a toy requires cleaning and disinfection, do so immediately or store in a designated labeled container separate from toys that are clean and ready for use.

5. Include multiuse electronic equipment in policies and procedures for preventing contamination and for cleaning and disinfection, especially those items that are used by patients, those used during delivery of patient care, and mobile devices that are moved in and out of patient rooms frequently (e.g., daily).

F. Textiles and laundry

1. Handle used textiles and fabrics with minimum agitation to avoid contamination of air, surfaces, and persons.

2. If laundry chutes are used, ensure that they are properly designed, maintained, and used in a manner to minimize dispersion of aerosols from contaminated laundry.

Contact Precautions

Contact precautions are intended to prevent transmission of infectious agents, including epidemiologically important microorganisms, that are spread by direct or indirect contact with the patient or the patient's environment. Contact precautions also apply where the presence of excessive wound drainage, fecal incontinence, or other discharges from the body suggest an increased potential for extensive environmental contamination and risk of transmission. A single-patient room is preferred for patients who require contact precautions. When a single-patient room is not available, consultation with infection-control personnel is recommended to assess the various risks associated with other patient placement options (e.g., cohorting, keeping the patient with an existing roommate). In multipatient rooms, greater than 3 feet spatial separation between beds is advised to reduce the opportunities for inadvertent sharing of items between the infected/colonized patient and other patients. Health-care personnel caring for patients on contact precautions should wear a gown and gloves for all interactions that may involve contact with the patient or potentially contaminated areas in the patient's environment. Don PPE before room entry and discard before exiting the patient room to contain pathogens, especially those that have been implicated in transmission through environmental contamination

Contact Precaution Guidelines

Use contact precautions for patients with known or suspected infections or evidence of syndromes that represent an increased risk for contact transmission.

■ **Take Note**

Select toys that are washable.

■ **Take Note**

Contact precautions use gowns and gloves, which should be donned before entering the patient's room and removed before exiting the patient's room.

A. Use of personal protective equipment

    1. Wear gloves whenever touching the patient's intact skin or surfaces and articles in close proximity to the patient (e.g., medical equipment, bed rails). Don gloves upon entry into the room or cubicle.

    2. Gowns

        a. Don gown upon entry into the room or cubicle. Remove gown and observe hand hygiene before leaving the patient-care environment.

        b. After gown removal, ensure that clothing and skin do not contact potentially contaminated environmental surfaces that could result in possible transfer of microorganism to other patients or environmental surfaces.

B. Patient transport

    1. In *acute-care hospitals and long-term care and other residential settings*, limit transport and movement of patients outside the room to medically necessary purposes.

    2. When transport or movement in any health-care setting is necessary, ensure that infected or colonized areas of the patient's body are contained and covered.

    3. Remove and dispose of contaminated PPE and perform hand hygiene following transport of patients on contact precautions.

    4. Don clean PPE to handle the patient at the transport destination. *Category II recommendation.*

C. Patient-care equipment and instruments/devices

    1. Handle patient-care equipment and instruments/devices according to standard precautions.

    2. In *acute-care hospitals and long-term care and other residential settings*, use disposable noncritical patient-care equipment or implement patient-dedicated use of such equipment. If common use of equipment for multiple patients is unavoidable, clean and disinfect such equipment before use on another patient.

    3. In *home-care settings*

        a. Limit the amount of nondisposable patient-care equipment brought into the home of patients on contact precautions. Whenever possible, leave patient-care equipment in the home until discharge from home-care services.

        b. If noncritical patient-care equipment (e.g., stethoscope) cannot remain in the home, clean and disinfect items before taking them from the home using a low- to intermediate-level disinfectant. Alternatively, place contaminated reusable items in a plastic bag for transport and subsequent cleaning and disinfection.

    4. In *ambulatory settings*, place contaminated reusable noncritical patient-care equipment in a plastic bag for transport to a soiled utility area for reprocessing.

D. Environmental measures

    1. Ensure that rooms of patients on contact precautions are prioritized for frequent cleaning and disinfection (e.g., at least daily) with a focus on frequently touched surfaces (e.g., bed rails, overbed table, bedside commode, lavatory surfaces in patient bathrooms, doorknobs) and equipment in the immediate vicinity of the patient.

Droplet Precautions

Droplet precautions are intended to prevent transmission of pathogens spread through close respiratory or mucous-membrane contact with respiratory secretions. Because these pathogens do not remain infectious over long distances, special air handling and ventilation are not required to prevent droplet transmission. A single-patient room is preferred for patients who require droplet precautions. When a single-patient room is not available, consultation with infection-control personnel is recommended to assess the various risks associated with other patient placement options (e.g., keeping the patient with an existing roommate). Spatial separation of patients by at least 3 feet and drawing the curtain between patient beds is especially important for patients in multibed rooms with infections transmitted by the droplet route. Health-care personnel wear a mask for close contact with infectious patients; the mask is generally donned upon room entry. Patients on droplet precautions who must be transported outside the room should wear a mask if tolerated and follow respiratory hygiene/cough etiquette.

Droplet Precaution Guidelines

In addition to standard precautions, use transmission-based precautions for patients with documented or suspected infection or colonization with highly transmissible or epidemiologically important pathogens for which additional precautions are needed to prevent transmission.

A. Use droplet precautions as recommended for patients known or suspected to be infected with pathogens transmitted by respiratory droplets (i.e., large-particle droplets greater than 5 μm in size) that are generated when a patient is coughing, sneezing, or talking.

B. In *ambulatory settings,* place patients who require droplet precautions in an examination room or cubicle as soon as possible. Instruct patients to follow recommendations for respiratory hygiene/cough etiquette.

C. Use of personal protective equipment
   1. Don a mask upon entry into the patient room or cubicle.
   2. No recommendation for routinely wearing eye protection (e.g., goggle or face shield), in addition to a mask, for close contact with patients who require droplet precautions.

D. Patient transport
   1. In *acute-care hospitals and long-term care and other residential settings,* limit transport and movement of patients outside the room to only medically necessary purposes.
   2. If transport or movement in any health-care setting is necessary, instruct the patient to wear a mask and follow respiratory hygiene/cough etiquette.
   3. No mask is required for persons transporting patients on droplet precautions.

Airborne Precautions and Guidelines

Airborne precautions prevent transmission of infectious agents that remain infectious over long distances when suspended in the air (e.g., rubeola virus [measles], varicella virus [chickenpox], *Mycobacterium tuberculosis,* and possibly SARS-CoV). The preferred placement for patients who require airborne precautions is in an airborne infection isolation room (AIIR). An AIIR is a single-patient room that is equipped with special air handling and ventilation capacity that meet the American Institute of Architects/Facility Guidelines Institute (AIA/FGI) standards for AIIRs (i.e., monitored negative pressure relative to the surrounding area, twelve air exchanges per hour for new construction and renovation and six air exchanges per hour for existing facilities, air exhausted directly to the outside or recirculated through HEPA filtration before return). Some states require the availability of such rooms in hospitals, emergency departments, and nursing homes that care for patients with *M. tuberculosis.* A respiratory-protection program that includes education about use of respirators, fit-testing, and user seal checks is required in any facility with AIIRs. In settings where airborne precautions cannot be implemented due to limited engineering resources (e.g., physician offices), masking the patient, placing the patient in a private room (e.g., office examination room) with the door closed, and providing N95 or higher level respirators or masks if respirators are not available for health-care personnel will reduce the likelihood of airborne transmission until the patient is either transferred to a facility with an AIIR or returned to the home environment as deemed medically appropriate. Health-care personnel caring for patients on airborne precautions should wear a mask or respirator, depending on the disease-specific recommendations for respiratory protection, which is to be donned prior to entering the patient's room. Whenever possible, nonimmune health-care workers should not care for patients with vaccine-preventable airborne diseases (e.g., measles, chickenpox, and smallpox).

Transmission-Based Precautions and Guidelines

In addition to standard precautions, use transmission-based precautions for patients with documented or suspected infection or colonization with highly transmissible or epidemiologically important pathogens for which additional precautions are needed to prevent transmission.

    A. In *ambulatory settings:*

        1. Develop systems upon entry into ambulatory settings (e.g., triage, signage) to identify patients with known or suspected infections that require airborne precautions.

        2. Place the patient in an AIIR as soon as possible. If an AIIR is not available, place a surgical mask on the patient, and place him/her in an examination room. Once the patient leaves, the room should remain vacant for the appropriate time, generally one hour, to allow for a full exchange of air.

        3. Instruct patients with a known or suspected airborne infection to wear a surgical mask and observe respiratory hygiene/cough etiquette. Once in an AIIR, the mask may be removed; the mask should remain on if the patient is not in an AIIR.

    B. An administrative control is to restrict susceptible health-care personnel from entering the rooms of patients known or suspected to have measles (rubeola), varicella (chickenpox), disseminated zoster, or smallpox if other immune health-care personnel are available.

    C. Use of PPE

        1. Wear a fit-tested National Institute of Occupational Safety and Health (NIOSH)–approved N95 or higher-level respirator for respiratory protection when entering the room or home of a patient when the following diseases are suspected or confirmed:

            a. Infectious pulmonary or laryngeal tuberculosis or when infectious tuberculosis skin lesions are present and procedures that would aerosolize viable organisms (e.g., irrigation, incision and drainage, whirlpool treatments) are performed.

            b. Respiratory protection is recommended for all health-care personnel, including those with a documented "take" after smallpox vaccination due to the risk of a genetically engineered virus against which the vaccine may not provide protection or of exposure to a very large viral load (e.g., from high-risk aerosol-generating procedures, immunocompromised patients, or hemorrhagic or flat smallpox).

Apparel

The purposes of apparel have been covered earlier in this chapter. Specific points regarding apparel are presented in this section.

Scrub suits are not sterile. Gowns, whether paper or cloth, should be worn only once, removed properly, and discarded in an appropriate receptacle.

When the use of a mask is indicated, it should be used only once and discarded in an appropriate receptacle. Lowering a mask around the neck and then placing it over the nose and mouth again is the same as reusing a mask and should not be done. Masks should cover both the nose and the mouth.

In most cases, glasses only provide a barrier in front of the eyes. Glasses with side shields provide an additional barrier. When prescription glasses are necessary, shields or goggles should be worn over prescription glasses, providing the best degree of protection. Shields and goggles are usually constructed of clear plastic, providing a barrier in front and on the sides of the eyes.

Nonsterile gloves are worn as a standard precaution. Whether using sterile or non-sterile gloves, hand-washing is required after gloves are removed. Used gloves should be removed properly and discarded into an appropriate receptacle.

Additional apparel, including caps, beard covers, and shoe covers, must be worn as necessary to maintain clean or sterile fields.

Sterile Field

The primary goal of using aseptic techniques is to prevent infection. One aseptic technique is to provide and maintain a sterile field. A sterile field is most commonly required in an operating room; however, there also may be a necessity for a sterile field in patient-care areas other than the operating room for the performance of minor procedures.

There are eight requirements for providing and maintaining a sterile field. The first four requirements concern creation of a sterile field. The remaining four requirements concern maintenance of the sterile field.

■ **Take Note**
Sterile field: There are four requirements for establishment and four requirements for maintenance.

Requirement 1

All items used within the boundaries of a sterile field must be sterile. The items must have been properly sterilized and maintained to preserve their sterile state. Once items have been sterilized, they must be used within the allowable shelf life of the item and sterilization process. The expiration date, or end of shelf life, is marked on each sterile package. Certain types of equipment and different types of packaging may affect the shelf life of a sterile package.

Whenever possible, single-use items are preferred. Because single-use items are discarded after use, there is no concern about contamination because of reuse. This does not mean, however, that single-use items cannot become contaminated before the initial use through improper technique or carelessness.

The shelf-life date of a sterile package is not a guarantee that the package is sterile. Packages are only considered to remain sterile when the

1. Initial packaging was performed properly;
2. Package was stored in a proper manner;
3. Package was not mishandled during distribution; and
4. Shelf-life date has not been exceeded.

Requirement 2

Once a sterile package has been opened, the edges are not considered sterile. Care in opening sterile packages is required to avoid having the edges touch the contents of the package or having the edges touch the gloved hands or sterile gown. Most sterile packages have enough packaging material around the edges to keep the unsterile edges away from the sterile contents.

Requirement 3

Once donned properly, sterile gowns are considered to be sterile in the front from shoulder level to tabletop level, including the sleeves. For this reason, the hands must be held above tabletop level and in front of the body during and after scrubbing, gowning, and gloving.

Requirement 4

In all cases, only the top surface of a table is considered sterile. Sterile drapes cover the top of a surface and descend on all sides of the surface. Such draping may be covering a patient or on an instrument table. Demarcation of sterile surfaces is fairly easy on tables but more difficult on patients. A guideline to use for demarcation on a patient that is draped is to consider that a surface above the level of the instrument table, or above waist level, whichever is higher, is a sterile surface as long as it is draped properly. Undraped or improperly draped surfaces, or surfaces below the top level of the instrument table or waist, are considered unsterile.

When a sterile field is created using only a sterile towel, a perimeter of 1 inch inside the edges of the towel is not considered sterile.

Requirement 5

Only sterile items and personnel in sterile attire may enter the sterile field or touch items in a sterile area. Personnel considered nonsterile may not touch any item in a sterile area or any item to be placed in a sterile area. Usually, sterile packages are opened by nonsterile personnel, and the contents are released into the sterile area without actually being touched by nonsterile personnel. Transfer of sterile items into a sterile area may also be accomplished by using sterile forceps to hold the item as it is passed into the sterile area. The set of forceps is considered contaminated after a single use and may not be used again until sterilized properly. Nonsterile personnel may not reach across or into a sterile area.

Requirement 6

Activity in a sterile area cannot be allowed to render the area unsterile. Personnel in sterile attire should not sit on or lean against unsterile surfaces. Movement within the sterile area must be measured and careful to avoid contact between sterile and unsterile surfaces.

All personnel, sterile or nonsterile, in or around a sterile area must be aware of the boundaries of a sterile area. Any contamination of a sterile area must be pointed out immediately by any personnel present for protection of the patient.

Requirement 7

Penetration of a sterile covering or barrier is considered to cause contamination of a sterile field. Liquids are the most likely cause of penetration of a sterile barrier. Liquids spilled within a sterile field may cause penetration of a sterile barrier.

A less noticeable but highly potential cause of penetration is air flow. Design of climate control for sterile areas provides for the most purified air possible and a slightly higher gradient of air pressure in the sterile area. Higher air-pressure gradient in the sterile area will cause air flow away from the site of potential infection. Climate-control systems should also be physically separated from other areas of the institution so that airborne microorganisms picked up in sterile areas do not permeate the atmosphere of the entire institution.

Requirement 8

Sterile areas and fields should be prepared as close to the time of use as feasible. They should not be left unattended. Sterile fields should not be prepared and then covered for later use. A delay in using equipment or supplies laid out in a sterile field necessitates the preparation of a new sterile field with new sterile equipment and supplies.

When there is doubt about the sterile quality of an area, a field, or an item, it should be considered unsterile. Improper packaging, sterilization processing, storage, or handling can occur without overt signs. Appropriate use of all items in a sterile environment is the responsibility of the user. Only proper judgement, rigid discipline, and appropriate use provide protection for a patient.

Scrubbing vs. Hand-Washing

Hand-washing techniques have been presented previously under Infection Control Guidelines. Hand-washing procedures are used prior to donning sterile gloves for procedures other than surgery. Scrubbing is a series of specific steps of hand cleaning using nail cleaners and soap or antimicrobial products prior to donning sterile gloves for surgery. Specific scrubbing procedures are beyond the scope of this text.

■ Take Note
Everyone is responsible for maintaining a sterile field and ensuring that the sterile field remains uncontaminated.

PROCEDURE 4–1   Gowning

When necessary for maintaining a sterile environment, don a freshly laundered scrub suit (pants and shirt or gown), scrub cap, and a new mask. Fasten the scrub suit completely and properly. All hair must be covered by a scrub cap. Facial hair, when present, must be covered by a mask and beard cover when necessary. The mask is formed to fit tightly but comfortably over the nose and mouth. Wear eye shields to protect the eyes.

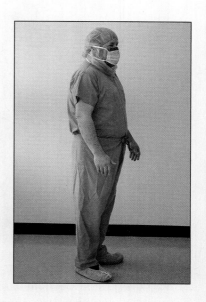

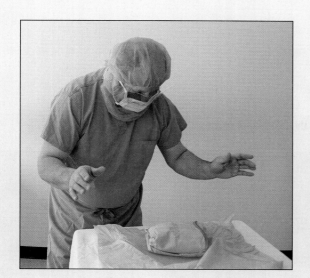

① Open the sterile pack containing the gown. The part of the gown facing you as you look at an open sterile pack is the inside of the gown.

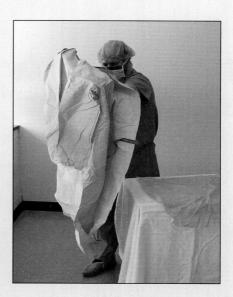

② Grasp the gown firmly, and lift it up and away from the sterile field. Move away from the table on which the sterile pack rests, keeping hands above waist height at all times. Shake open the gown so it unfolds. Holding the inside of the gown only, locate the neck and armholes of the gown.

(continued)

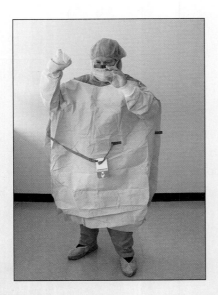

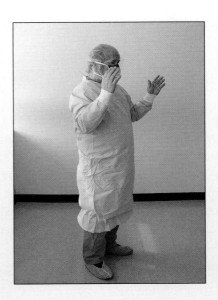

③ Without touching the outside, or sterile side, of the gown, work both arms into the sleeves at the same time. Stop when the hands reach the stockinette cuffs.

④ The gown is tied using back and neck closures by personnel who are not in the sterile field.

PROCEDURE 4–2 Gloving

MEDIALINK Watch the video on the CD under the heading of gloving.

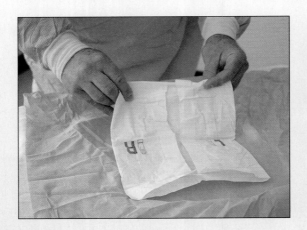

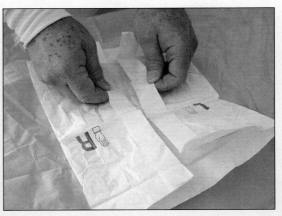

① Open a glove pack and place the sterile paper enclosure that contains the gloves on a sterile surface with the cuffs toward the person who will be gloving.

② Open the sterile portion of a glove pack by grasping the folds of the paper enclosing the gloves.

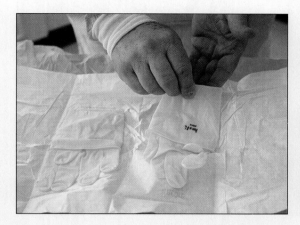

3 The wrist end of each glove has been turned back on itself, creating a cuff where the inside, or unsterile side, is now outward.

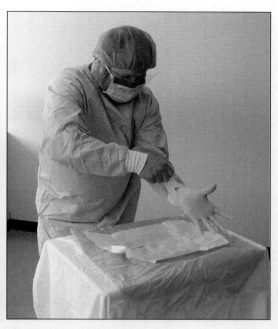

4 Grasping the left glove by its cuff on the non-sterile portion with a bare right hand, work the left hand into the left glove.

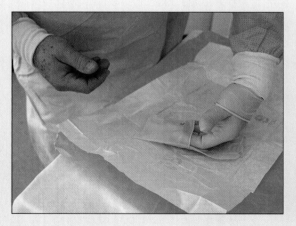

5 Once the left glove is in place, it is now a sterile surface. Slip the first two or three fingers of the gloved left hand down inside the sterile side of the cuff of the right glove, starting at the palm of the right glove and pointing toward the crease of the cuff at the wrist.

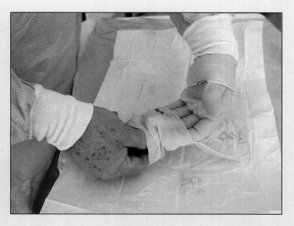

6 Then lift the right glove using the fingers inside the cuff only. The thumb of the gloved left hand cannot be used to grasp the right-hand glove. As the right glove is held by the first two or three fingers on the inside (sterile side) of the cuff, work the right hand into the right glove.

(continued)

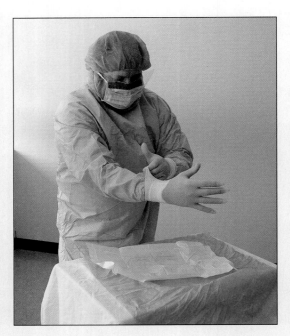

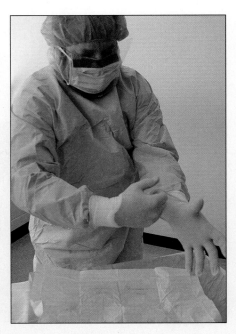

7 Once the right hand is gloved, unfold the cuff by pulling the cuff up over the sleeve of the gown and letting the wrist portion of the glove snap into place.

8 Now the fingers of the right hand, now sterile, can be placed on the inside (sterile side) of the left glove cuff. Unfold the left cuff in the same manner as was done for the right glove. If necessary, the gloves can be adjusted on the fingers once both glove cuffs have been properly placed.

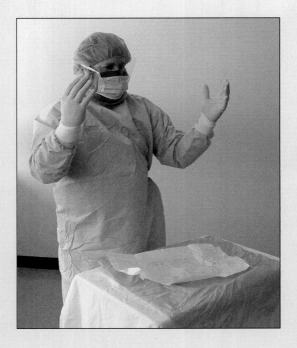

9 Once gloved, both hands must remain above waist level or the level of draping that defines the sterile field, whichever is appropriate.

Removal of Contaminated Gloves

When a glove becomes torn or punctured during a sterile procedure, it no longer provides proper protection and must be removed and discarded as soon as is feasible, and another sterile glove must be donned. This may require interruption of a procedure provided that the interruption does not threaten the patient's welfare.

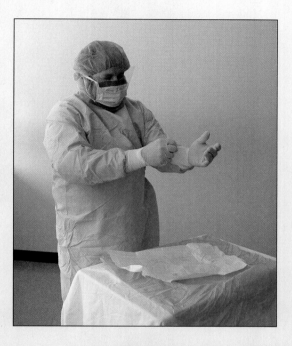

1 Remove contaminated gloves in a manner that prevents the spread of contaminants. One hand grasps the cuff of the other glove.

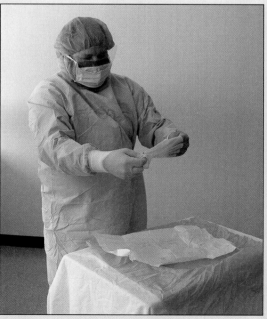

2 The glove that has been grasped at the cuff is turned inside out as it is removed.

(continued)

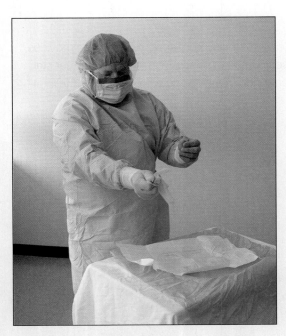

3 Compact the glove that has been removed into the palm of the hand that still is gloved.

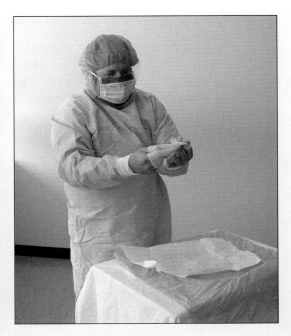

4 Hook the thumb of the ungloved hand inside the remaining glove and pull the remaining glove toward the fingers, turning it inside out over the compacted glove.

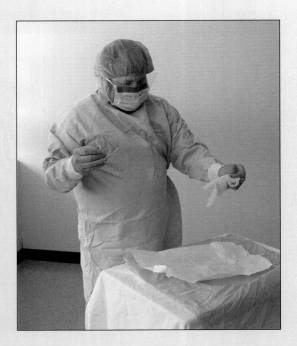

5 Remove both gloves with the contaminated sides inward. When removing gloves, the material should not be permitted to snap in order to avoid dislodging material that has accumulated on the gloves. Dispose of the gloves in an appropriate container, and wash the hands.

Wounds and Wound Dressings

There are specific classifications for pressure wounds and burns. Pressure wounds are described by the depth of the wound. Burns are classified by the cause of burn (thermal, electrical, chemical, radiation), depth of burn (superficial or epidermal, superficial partial-thickness burn, deep partial-thickness burn, full-thickness burn), and extent of burn (rule of nines). Other types of wounds are abrasions, lacerations, and surgical incisions.

The location of a wound can dictate the type of dressing applied or the method of application. Wounds over joints may require rigid dressings to prevent joint motion from disrupting the wound, or the dressings may have to be applied in a way that accommodates joint motion. Wounds can require extensive modification of bedding and seating arrangements so sleeping and sitting activities do not disrupt a dressing or put pressure on a wound.

Underlying pathological conditions may have an impact on the dressings chosen and the application of dressings. No dressing should ever be applied in a manner that impedes circulation. The existence of peripheral vascular disease is a condition that requires special attention to avoid further impairment of circulation.

When long-term care of a wound is required, care may be provided outside an institutional setting. When noninstitutional care is appropriate, a patient or patient's family must be instructed carefully in proper wound care. Whenever possible, use simple procedures. Give careful evaluation and consideration to the patient's, or family's, ability to understand and carry out specific instructions. A wound site that cannot be seen easily by the patient may not be well cared for by a patient. A physical impairment, such as a stroke, or mental impairment, such as Alzheimer's disease, may prohibit a patient from providing wound care. Provide supervision to ensure that proper techniques are followed.

Purpose

The purposes of wound dressings are to

1. Physically protect the site of injury
2. Prevent contamination of a wound
3. Prevent transmission of infection from a wound
4. Promote healing

Many institutions and health-care professionals have preferred methods of caring for specific types of wounds, and there is increasing evidence to support several methods. This section presents basic information concerning wound dressings. Information for a specific institution should be sought from the appropriate departments or practitioners within the institution.

Evaluation

Examination of wound characteristics is necessary for appropriate selection of dressing materials and protective agents. A physical therapist performs the initial examination and evaluates the results using the clinical decision-making process to determine a plan of care. A plan of care may be implemented by a physical therapist assistant where permitted by state law. Documentation of wound characteristics and management must be explicit and precise.

Evaluation of the wound is necessary to determine

1. The cause of the wound
2. The location, area, and depth of the wound
3. Whether the wound is wet or dry
4. Whether the wound is infected; and if infected, the source, mechanism, and microorganism of infection

Measurement of a wound can be performed using a ruler (■ Figure 4–1). In addition to regular rulers, there are specialized clear plastic circular rulers. The ruler should not make contact with the wound itself and should be limited to single-patient use. Measurements should include width, length, and depth. Another method of documenting the extent of a wound is by photographing the wound.

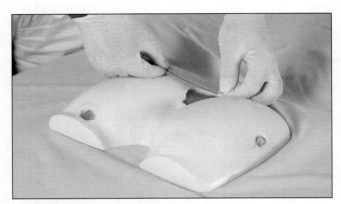

■ **Figure 4–1**   Measuring a wound using a ruler.

Types of Dressings

Five methods of dressing applications generally used for wound management are

1. Dry to dry
2. Damp to damp
3. Damp to dry
4. Occlusive
5. Rigid

A **dry-to-dry dressing** is the application of a dry absorbent or nonabsorbent dressing to cover the wound. A **damp-to-damp dressing** is the application of a gauze pad moistened with normal saline solution or another similar solution before application. Remoistening a damp dressing is performed while the dressing remains in place. This prevents the dressing from drying out and becoming embedded in the eschar. The damp-to-damp dressing assists in softening the eschar in preparation for removal. A **damp-to-dry** dressing is the application of a moistened dressing that is allowed to dry before removal. The dressing dries embedded in the eschar and debrides the wound when the dried, embedded dressing is removed. **Occlusive dressings** are applied to provide a semipermeable barrier to air and moisture penetration. **Rigid dressings** provide physical protection to a wound and the adjacent area.

Choice of materials for, and method of, application of dressings may depend on

1. The cause of the wound
2. Whether the wound is clean or infected; and if infected, the microorganism causing the infection
3. The type of dressing (damp, dry)
4. The type, if any, of antimicrobial agent to be applied
5. The site, area, and depth of the wound
6. Whether a trained professional, the patient, or the patient's family will be responsible for monitoring and changing the dressing

Identification of the specific microorganism responsible for infection is beneficial in treating any wound. Specific antimicrobial agents may require specific types of dressing materials to ensure that the antimicrobial agent is applied properly to the wound.

When a wound is draining, absorption of exudate can be a consideration requiring a dry dressing. When a wound tends to be dry and the dryness impedes healing, a damp dressing would be required. Limiting exposure to air or maintaining a moist environment within the wound can require an occlusive dressing.

■ **Take Note**

Wet wound—dry dressing.

Dry wound—moist dressing.

Materials

The size of dressings, whether prepackaged or constructed, should cover a wound site, plus some portion of healthy tissue on all sides of the wound. In no case should the adhesive portion of a dressing come in contact with a wound.

The most basic dressing is an adhesive strip with a small gauze center, commonly known by the brand name Band-Aid®. These dressings are available from a number of companies in various shapes and sizes. Topical antimicrobial agents may be applied under the gauze portion of this dressing. The adhesive portion of the dressing may be plastic or paper, with a hypoallergenic adhesive that limits skin reaction to the adhesive.

Dressings with nonadhering pads that do not stick to wounds or the exudate from wounds are also available. These dressings, commonly known by the brand name Telfa® pads, are available from a number of companies in various shapes and sizes. These basic dressings are usually best for small wounds, although self-made dressings of the same nature can be constructed in any size when the necessary material is available.

Gauze is the most common material used for dressings and is available in pads and rolls. Sterile and nonsterile gauze is available in several sizes. If sterile gauze is to be used, perform proper aseptic handling techniques during opening and application. Dressings constructed from gauze can be used with topical antimicrobial agents under the dressing when required.

Compression wraps are applied to control edema in a limb segment or to provide some support for a joint. Compression wraps are constructed of an elastic material and are commonly known by the brand name Ace® wrap. Common sizes are 2-, 3-, 4-, 5-, and 6-inch widths.

Edges of lacerations can be approximated using thin adhesive strips, commonly known by the brand name Steri-Strips™. The edges of a wound are placed together, and the adhesive strips are placed across the wound. The number of strips required is determined by the open length of the wound.

Tape used to secure a dressing can be cloth adhesive tape or paper tape that has a hypoallergenic adhesive. Tape can be cut to the required length with scissors or torn from the roll. Tear tape by unrolling the desired amount and firmly grasping the tape between the pad of the thumb and the side of the index finger of each hand, with the hands approximately 1 inch apart. Take care not to roll the edges of the tape over, because this makes the tape harder to tear. A quick movement of one hand away from the body and the other hand toward the body will cause the tape to tear between the two hands. Even cloth adhesive tape can be torn in this manner as long as the edges have not been rolled.

Preparation

Necessary supplies, such as gauze pads, roll gauze, tape, and topical agents, must be easily accessible during the procedure. Sterile fields, when required, must be prepared appropriately. Protection of the wound from contamination requires the appropriate application of aseptic techniques. Proper preparation for personnel includes handwashing or scrubbing, and masking, gowning, and gloving, when required.

Tape for securing dressings may need to be prepared before starting the application of a dressing because tearing or cutting tape usually takes two hands. The pieces can be hung from the edge of a table, cabinet, or bed frame by sticking only a small portion of one end to the object and letting the remainder of the piece hang free. The pieces should be hung in an accessible place, since one hand is usually required to secure the dressing or wrap while tape is applied. When tape is applied circumferentially on a limb segment, the ends should not overlap. Adhesive and paper tape do not have enough elasticity to avoid impairment of circulation if the ends overlap in this situation.

PROCEDURE 4–3 Application of Dressings and Wraps

Packing a Wound

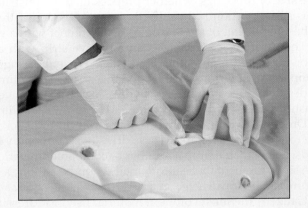

1 Depending on the depth of a wound, it may be packed with gauze to ensure that deeper layers of a wound heal before surface layers, avoiding development of an unhealed cavity.

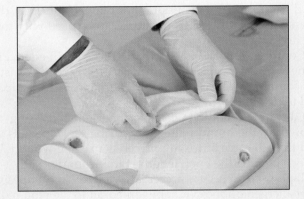

2 Once packed, the wound and packing are covered with additional dressing that is secured with roll gauze or tape.

Applying a Gauze Wrap

Gauze pads are secured by tape or a gauze roll. Gauze rolls are applied in a spiral wrap or in a "figure-of-eight" wrap. To avoid impairing circulation, the amount of pressure applied when using gauze wraps should not be excessive.

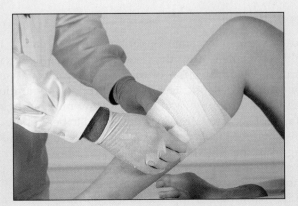

1 To apply a **gauze wrap**, lay the portion of the gauze roll that is unwrapping against the limb segment, with the still-rolled gauze away from the limb.

2 A **spiral wrap** is applied by wrapping gauze in a continuous manner around the limb segment. The roll of gauze is angled slightly to accommodate for the sloping contour of the limb segment to be wrapped and to avoid creating a tourniquet. The roll of gauze is unrolled around the limb segment, with each successive wrap overlapping the previous wrap by half. When the wrap is completed, secure the gauze with tape.

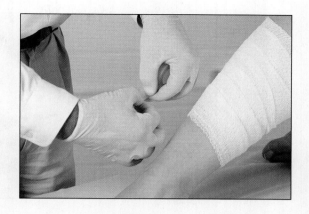

3 Removal of a gauze wrap secured with tape requires careful cutting to avoid injuring patients; use bandage scissors (scissors with one flat arm). The flat arm slides under the wrap and next to the skin, permitting the wrap and tape to be cut without cutting the skin.

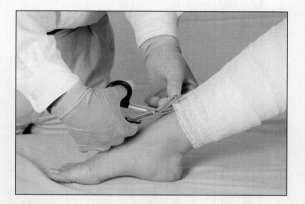

Applying a Compression Wrap

Compression wraps may be applied in spiral or figure-of-eight wraps. When applying compression wraps to control edema, use a spiral wrap, with more pressure applied distally than proximally. This provides for compression on edematous segments without constricting the flow of fluid toward the core of the body for subsequent elimination. When controlling edema, use the wrap with approximately graded pressure to cover the entire limb segment distal to the proximal edge of the wrap. When applying compression wraps for joint support, a figure-of-eight or spiral wrap may be used. When providing support, apply a compression wrap with even pressure from distal to proximal. Applying a compression wrap for support does not require the entire limb segment distal to the proximal edge of the wrap to be covered. In no case should a wrap be applied with the proximal pressure greater than the distal pressure.

The technique for applying a compression wrap is the same as for applying a gauze wrap. Frequent examination of compression wraps is necessary to ensure that the amount of compression applied is appropriate and that the wrap remains in place.

Start a **figure-of-eight wrap** in the same manner as a spiral wrap. Rather than a continuous wrap in the same direction, however, change the direction of wrapping each time the wrap completes one loop of the figure-of-eight. The illustrations for this section demonstrate application of a compression wrap of the ankle.

(continued)

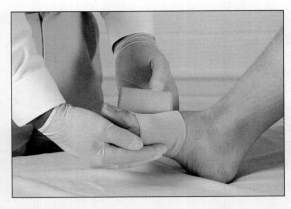

1 Start with a circumferential anchoring loop around the foot.

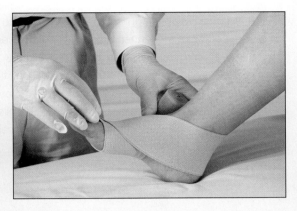

2 Wrap from lateral to medial around the ankle.

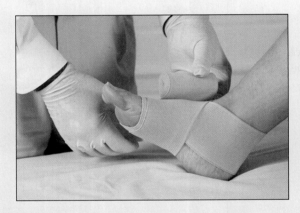

3 Wrap from lateral to medial around the foot.

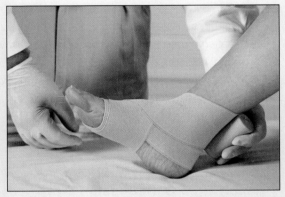

4 Wrap from lateral to medial around the ankle (second time) with an angle that will permit continuing a spiral wrap up the ankle from distal to proximal. Secure the end of the compression wrap with adhesive tape.

Chapter Review

Review Questions

1. Which federal agency is responsible for developing and issuing guidelines for aseptic techniques and isolation systems?

2. Describe the eight guidelines for providing and maintaining a sterile field.

3. What apparel is necessary for aseptic techniques?

4. What is the most important procedure for preventing transmission of nosocomial infections?

5. List and describe the steps performed during
   a. Gowning
   b. Gloving
   c. Removal of contaminated gloves

6. List the four purposes of wound dressing.

7. Describe five methods of dressing applications.

8. List five factors affecting selection of wound-dressing materials.

9. What are the five main routes of microorganism transmission?

10. Who is responsible for implementing and monitoring isolation procedures?

11. What is the usual level of infection control practiced for contact with all patients?

12. What is the difference between standard precautions and transmission-based precautions?

Suggested Activities

1. Practice the skills of hand-washing, gowning, gloving, wound assessment, and application of wound dressings.

2. Observe other students performing wound dressings using a sterile field, and make note of any violation of the guidelines for maintaining a sterile field.

3. Role-play wound assessment and application of dressings.

4. Document wound-dressing procedures.

■■■

Case Study

Mrs. Shimizu is an 80-year-old female 16 days status post left transtibial amputation as a result of peripheral vascular disease secondary to Type II diabetes. She also has Stage I ulcerations over her sacrum and right greater trochanter. The medial border of her surgical incision has not closed completely and may be infected.

1. What characteristics of the wounds should be examined and described in documentation?
2. What infection-control guidelines, including apparel, are applicable for daily care and management of the wounds?
3. What wound dressings might be best for each of the wounds?

■■■

References

1. Boyce JM, Pittet D. *Guideline for Hand Hygiene in Health Care Settings.* Recommendations of the Centers for Disease Control and Prevention, Healthcare Infection Control Practices Advisory Committee and the HICPAC/SHEA/APIC/IDSA Hand Hygiene Task Force, 2002.
2. Department of Health and Human Services. *Part I: Evolution of Isolation Practices.* Centers for Disease Control and Prevention, Hospital Infection Control Practices Advisory Committee, 1997.
3. Department of Health and Human Services. *Part II: Recommendations for Isolation Precautions in Hospitals.* Centers for Disease Control and Prevention, Hospital Infection Control Practices Advisory Committee, 1997.
4. Schulster L, Chinn RYW. *Guidelines for Environmental Infection Control in Health Care Facilities.* Recommendations of the Centers for Disease Control and Prevention, Healthcare Infection Control Practices Advisory Committee, 2003.

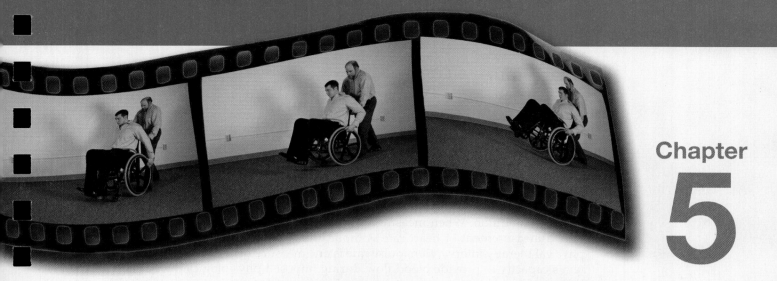

Vital Signs

Learning Objectives

Upon completion of this chapter, you will be able to:

1. Describe the purposes, methods, and norms for the measurement of vital signs of pulse, blood pressure, respiration, temperature, and pain.
2. Describe the purposes and methods for the subjective measurement of pain levels perceived by a patient.
3. Indicate the sites at which measurements of vital signs of pulse, blood pressure, respiration, and temperature are usually taken.
4. Correctly and accurately measure pulse, blood pressure, respiration, and temperature.
5. Correctly and accurately measure patient pain levels.
6. Use terms that correctly describe vital-sign measurements outside normal ranges.
7. Identify vital-sign measurements that are below, within, or above normal ranges.
8. Correctly and accurately document vital-sign measurements.
9. Correctly and accurately document pain measurements.
10. Describe the use of the anthropometric measures of height and weight and how they relate to body mass index.

Key Terms

Afebrile
Anthropometric measures
Auscultation
Basal heart rate
Blanching
Blood pressure
Body mass index (BMI)
Bradycardia
Diastolic pressure
Doppler
Febrile
Hyperthermia
Hypothermia
Maximal heart rate

Pain
Patency
Pulse
Red flag
Regularity
Respiratory rate
Resting heart rate
Systolic pressure
Tachycardia
Target heart rate
Temperature
Trophic
Visual analog scale

Introduction

Physical therapists/assistants should be aware of, and able to perform, objective measurements of physiological functions known as vital signs. Vital signs are used to monitor a patient's status prior to, and at any given time during, patient care. Changes in vital-sign measurements may indicate physiological responses to treatment. Vital signs consist of heart rate (HR) or pulse (P), blood pressure (BP), respiration (R), and temperature (T). Although historically not considered a vital sign, indications of pain are now considered a vital sign and determined when vital signs are measured. Pain levels are subjective measurements. Also historically not considered a vital sign, anthropometric measures of height and weight are used in assessing patient health. They are often monitored in conjunction with vital signs.

■ Take Note
Vital signs: heart rate, blood pressure, respiration rate, temperature, pain.

117

Heart Rate

Purpose

Pulse (in beats per minute) is a measurement of heart rate. **Basal heart rate** is the pulse rate measured after an extended period of rest and is one indication of cardiovascular function in the absence of physical stress.

Pulse rates are measured before, during, or following an imposed physiological or physical stress arising from physical therapy intervention. Determination of when pulse rate is measured during physical therapy interventions is contingent upon a patient's condition. When measured during rest, pulse rate is called the **resting heart rate**, a measurement of heart rate without imposed stresses. When measured during physical therapy intervention, pulse rate is one measurement of the cardiovascular system's capacity to provide blood flow during imposed physiological or physical stress. When measured after treatment or other exercise, pulse rate is one measure of the cardiovascular system's recovery capability following the imposition of physiological or physical stress.

Measurements of pulse are also used to determine **patency**, which is the openness of the peripheral portion of the cardiovascular system. When used for this purpose, the important measurement is the presence or absence of a pulse at a chosen site. Such measurements of pulse can provide a preliminary indication of arterial occlusion resulting from physical blockage or peripheral vascular insufficiency secondary to disease states, such as diabetes. Lack of patency must be documented accurately, and precautions and contraindications must be reviewed with the physical therapist assistant when interventions are delegated. When a lack of patency is noted that does not fit with a known medical diagnosis for a specific patient, this is a **"red flag"** that physical therapists must document and refer patients to an appropriate health-care provider immediately. When such a condition is observed by a physical therapist assistant, he or she should notify the supervising physical therapist immediately. Physical therapy interventions should not be implemented with such patients until the medical condition is evaluated and the patient is cleared by medical personnel.

Examination for patency of peripheral vessels should be accompanied by observation for **trophic** changes, which are physiological sequels to decreased circulation, such as loss of hair, dry or flaky skin, and muscle atrophy. Skin temperature changes are often noted in areas of decreased patency. **Blanching** is a noted loss of color of the skin resulting from decreased circulation. Blanching of an extremity is more pronounced and occurs more rapidly when the extremity has decreased circulation. Blanching may be produced by two methods. One method is to raise the extremity above the level of the heart, artificially increasing the difficulty of supplying circulation to the extremity. A second method is to press firmly and briefly on a patient's skin to occlude circulation in the area of pressure. The rate of capillary refill indicates circulatory status in that area. The presence of edema makes the determination of patency difficult.

In addition to patency and rate, pulse regularity and amplitude can provide information concerning cardiovascular status. Measuring pulse rate allows examination of the regularity of heartbeat. **Regularity** refers to the evenness of heart rate. This measure of regularity is subjective. Amplitude of a pulse is rated on a subjective scale of 0–4+. This scale includes the measures of

    0 = absent
 1+ = thready, weak
 2+ = normal
 3+ = strong
 4+ = full bounding

A pulse that varies from normal in rate, regularity, or amplitude may be indicative of disease or injury.

Methods

The most common clinical method of measuring pulse is manual palpation. In addition to manual measures of pulse, there are mechanical devices that may be used. **Auscultation** of the heart, which is monitoring of the heart using a stethoscope, is also used to obtain heart rate. **Doppler** measurements, which use frequency changes during blood flow, are used to examine patency (■ Figure 5–1).

An oximeter is a device that measures pulse rate and blood oxygen concentrations (■ Figure 5–2). Results are provided by digital display. This is an easy method of monitoring pulse rate and blood oxygen concentration during activities. These devices are used more and more to measure important vital signs during activity, allowing patient response to activity to be monitored in real-time.

To palpate a pulse manually, place the pads of the index and middle fingers of one hand over the site where the pulse is to be measured. Do not use the pad of the thumb for palpation when measuring pulse because there is an artery in the pad of the thumb. If a thumb is used for palpation, one's own pulse may be mistaken for the patient's pulse. Take care not to press too hard while palpating pulses. Excessive pressure during palpation can obliterate the pulse, impede blood flow, or cause arterial spasm. Obliterating a pulse prevents measurement, and impeding blood flow or causing arterial spasm can be dangerous to a patient. This is especially true when examining distal pulses, most commonly palpated when measuring peripheral vascular patency.

Heart rate is measured in beats per minute (bpm). The use of units is advocated to ensure conveying complete information. To obtain a heart rate, use a watch or clock that displays time in seconds. Once a pulse is palpated, count beats within a specified interval of time. The most accurate method is to count beats for a period of 60 seconds. The count is reported without additional calculation.

Alternative methods require less time to monitor the pulse but require additional calculation. Counting beats for a 10-second time period and multiplying by six or using a 15-second time period and multiplying by four are the most common shortcuts used. Using a shorter sampling period may result in a measurement that is less precise. Many times, a whole number of beats does not occur within a shorter period of time. An estimate of a fractional heart rate is not as accurate as an exact count. Irregularities in heart rate are not detected as readily when a shorter sampling period is used. The necessity of additional calculation provides a potential source of error. Sometimes one beat in a time period is missed. In either of these cases, using a shortcut will increase the error, either six-fold or four-fold, respectively.

As an example, an error of one beat during measurements taken over a 60-second period of time and over a 10-second period will provide two very different results. For a patient with an actual heart rate of 72 bpm, missing one beat during the 60-second count produces an error of 1/72 or 1.4 percent. Using a 10-second count, the same heart

■ **Take Note**
Means of measuring pulse: palpation, auscultation, EKG, doppler.

■ **Take Note**
Use index and middle fingers to palpate pulses.

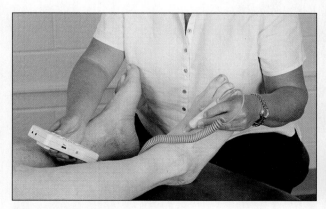

■ **Figure 5–1**   Doppler sonography.

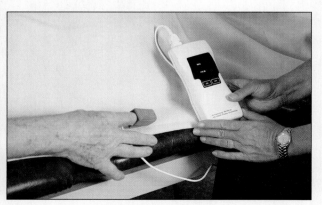

■ **Figure 5–2**   Pulse oximeter.

■ **Take Note**
It is most accurate to count a pulse for 60 seconds.

■ **Take Note**
Calculating pulse:
• Count for 60 seconds.
• Count for 30 seconds and double (multiply by 2).
• Count for 15 seconds and quadruple (multiple by 4).

rate should yield 12 beats. If one beat is missed during the 10-second count, only 11 beats will be counted. This is multiplied by six, resulting in a calculation of 66 bpm for the same patient, an error of 6/72, or 8.3 percent. Although shortcut methods are used routinely, and their results are recorded without question, take care to provide an accurate and valid measurement.

There are two methods of timing when counting heart rate. The key factor in counting heart rate is that the number of heartbeats within a given time period is counted. The first, or traditional, method starts the time period of counting at a specific time on a clock or watch, and the first heartbeat felt after the time period has started is considered beat 1. This is beat 1 because it is the first heartbeat within the specified time period. The second method starts the time period of counting when a heartbeat is felt; that heartbeat is beat 0. This is beat 0 because it does not occur within the specified time period but marks the beginning of the specified time period. Whichever method is used will provide an accurate count when attention is paid to the basis for when the interval begins and the number of counts that fall *within* the specified interval.

Norms

The normal range of heart rate for adults is 60–100 bpm. Resting heart rate in adults can vary greatly, depending on the state of physical conditioning of each individual. Individuals who maintain a high level of physical training may have a resting heart rate between 40 and 60 bpm. Individuals who maintain a moderately sedentary lifestyle may have a resting heart rate between 60 and 85 bpm. A resting heart rate greater than 85 bpm is usually indicative of a state of deconditioning or a medical condition.

PROCEDURE 5–1   Measuring Heart Rate

The radial and carotid arteries are the most commonly used sites for measuring pulse, an indicator of heart rate.

The radial pulse is most easily palpated on the distal volar surface of the wrist, just lateral to the tendons of the finger flexors.

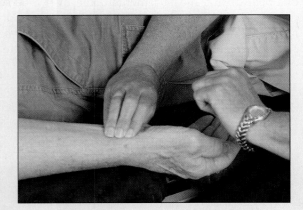

The carotid pulse is most easily palpated on the lateral aspect of the neck, inferior to the angle of the mandible.

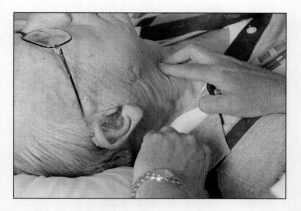

Take care to palpate the carotid pulse without reaching across the patient's throat. Placing a hand across the patient's throat creates the potential for compromising a patient's airway. Baroreceptor reflexes produce decreased heart rate and strength of heart contractions. "Massage" to the carotid artery can elicit this reflex, so take care to be accurate in placement and type of palpation when measuring carotid artery pulses.

The site used to obtain a pulse via auscultation is medial to the mid-clavicular line at the level of the fifth intercostal space.

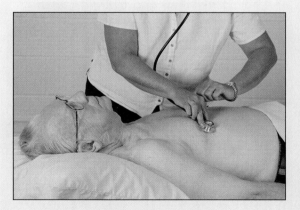

Common sites for palpation of pulses to determine vascular patency are the brachial, popliteal, posterior tibial, and dorsal pedal pulses. These pulses are reported as present or absent.

(continued)

The pulse of the brachial artery is palpated on the medial aspect of the arm midway down the shaft of the humerus.

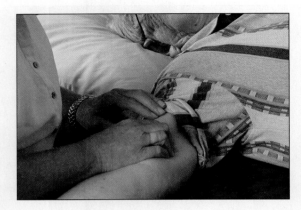

The pulse of the femoral artery is palpated in the femoral triangle. Although a strong pulse, the femoral artery lies close to several large muscles, making palpation difficult. When preparing to palpate the femoral artery, explaining to patients what you are about to do will decrease surprise and reduce risk of embarrassing patients. Palpation of the femoral artery that is too firm can cause pain.

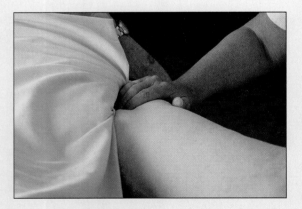

Location of the remaining arteries, and avoiding obliteration of the pulse with excessive pressure, can be difficult, even in healthy patients. These pulses are commonly susceptible to degradation of strength in patients with peripheral vascular insufficiency.

The pulse of the popliteal artery is palpated at, or just above, the posterior aspect of the knee.

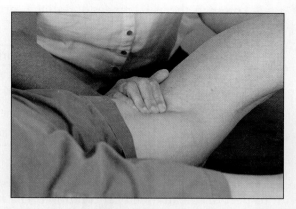

The pulse of the posterior tibial artery is palpated posterior or inferior to the medial malleolus.

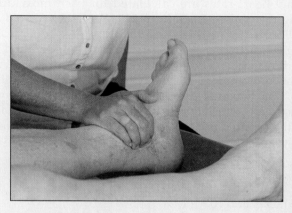

The dorsal pedal pulse is palpated on the dorsum of the foot over the cuboid bones.

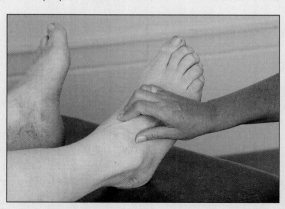

■ **Take Note**
The best sites to monitor patency are the brachial, popliteal, posterior tibial, and dorsal pedal arteries.

The normal resting heart rate for infants and young children is between 80 and 100 bpm. A very slow resting heart rate, or **bradycardia**, is a heart rate of less than 60 bpm. A very fast heart rate, or **tachycardia**, is a heart rate greater than 100 bpm. Bradycardia or tachycardia at a resting state may be indicative of disease or side effects of medication. ■ Table 5–1 presents the usual ranges of resting heart rate.

TABLE 5–1 Usual Ranges of Resting Heart Rate	
Adult normal range	60–100 bpm
Infant/child normal range	80–100 bpm
Bradycardia	Less than 60 bpm
Tachycardia	Greater than 100 bpm

Maximal heart rate is the highest heart rate a person should achieve upon exertion with respect to age and medical condition. The following guidelines for determining maximal heart rate are based on the absence of cardiovascular pathology. Maximal heart rates are calculated for each individual patient based on age, subtracting the patient's age from 220. For a 43-year-old individual, the maximal heart rate is: $220 - 43$, or 177.

Target heart rate is the heart rate that an individual should achieve during exercise for cardiovascular conditioning with respect to age and medical condition. For a patient without contraindications, the target heart rate must fall between 60 percent and 80 percent of the maximal heart rate. Target heart rates for patients with cardiovascular pathology are adjusted by physicians based on clinical findings for individual patients. Thus, the formula used to determine a target heart rate for cardiovascular exercise for the 43-year-old person presented earlier is between 106 and 142 bpm.

$$(0.60) \times (220 - \text{AGE}) \text{ and } (0.80) \times (220 - \text{AGE})$$
$$(0.6)(220 - 43) \text{ and } (0.8)(220 - 43)$$
$$(0.6)(177) \text{ and } (0.8)(177)$$
$$= 106 \text{ and } 142$$

■ **Take Note**

Example maximum heart rate calculation:

- $220 - 60 = 160$

Example target heart rate calculations:

- X% (maximum heart rate)
- $50\% \times 160 = 80$ (deconditioned patient)
- $80\% \times 160 = 128$ (fit patient)

Blood Pressure

Purpose

Blood pressure is a measure of vascular resistance to blood flow. The primary purposes for measuring blood pressure are to determine vascular resistance to blood flow and the effectiveness of cardiac muscle in pumping blood to overcome vascular resistance. There are two values reported as a measurement of blood pressure. The first value represents **systolic pressure**, which is a measurement of pressure exerted by blood against arterial walls when the heart is contracting. The second value represents **diastolic pressure**, which is a measure of the pressure exerted by arterial walls against blood when the heart is not contracting.

■ **Take Note**

Blood pressure numbers:

- Systolic: pressure when heart is contracting
- Diastolic: pressure when heart is at rest

Method

Measure blood pressure by auscultation of an artery using a stethoscope while a sphygmomanometer is applied over the artery being auscultated. A sphygmomanometer consists of an air bladder inside a cuff, a device for inflating the bladder, and a device for measuring the pressure in the bladder (■ Figure 5–3). Blood-pressure measurements are actually measurements of the cuff's air bladder pressure. The pressure corresponds to arterial pressure as arterial blood flows, or attempts to flow, past the restricting cuff.

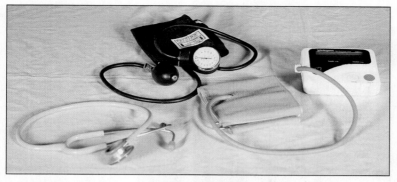

■ **Figure 5–3**   Examples of sphygmomanometers.

Blood-pressure measurements were originally based on the pressure required to raise a column of mercury in a glass tube. Therefore, blood-pressure measurements continue to be reported in mmHg (millimeters of mercury). Sphygmomanometers may provide output using a mechanical gauge or a digital readout. A stethoscope is used to auscultate the sounds of arterial blood flow through the brachial artery as it passes through the antecubital fossa.

Blood-pressure sounds to be monitored are called Korotkoff sounds. Blood-pressure readings are reported as the systolic pressure over the diastolic pressure. A systolic pressure of 120 mmHg and a diastolic pressure of 80 mmHg is documented as 120/80 mmHg and verbally reported as "120 over 80."

■ **Take Note**

$$\text{Blood pressure} = \frac{\text{Systolic}}{\text{Diastolic}}$$

Site

The most common site for measuring blood pressure is the left upper arm. This site corresponds closely to the level of the tricuspid valve of the heart, which is considered the "reference level for pressure measurement." Although body position may change blood pressure, such changes are accurately measured when using the left upper arm as the reference. Initially, physical therapists/assistants should take blood-pressure measurements in both arms, and subsequent blood-pressure measurements should be taken in the arm with the highest reading. Documentation should include the arm in which measurement was taken and the position of the patient.

PROCEDURE 5–2   Measuring Blood Pressure

① Prior to placing a cuff around a patient's left upper arm, consider the size of the cuff. Inaccurate readings will be obtained if the wrong size cuff is used. Cuff sizes range from pediatric to large adult. The bladder of a cuff should cover approximately 80 percent of the circumference of the upper arm, and the width should be approximately 40 percent of the circumference of the upper arm.[1]

② A blood pressure cuff is placed snugly around the upper arm with the bladder centered over the anterior surface and with the lower border approximately 2–3 cm above the antecubital fossa.

③ Support the patient's arm, either on a table or by resting on the physical therapist's/assistant's arm, so the cuff is at the patient's heart level.

(continued)

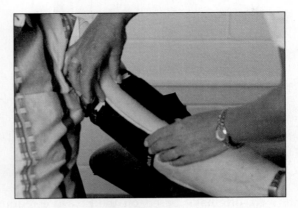

④ Hold the inflation bulb and its attaching tube, and the stethoscope and its tubing, so that the tubes do not touch each other. When the respective tubes touch each other, sounds can be distorted.

⑤ With the patient's arm supported, a physical therapist/assistant locates the brachial artery on the anterior medial surface of the elbow as the artery crosses the antecubital fossa.

⑥ A pulse is palpated as the bladder is inflated. Note the pressure when the pulse can no longer be palpated.

⑦ The cuff is deflated.

⑧ Place the stethoscope drum or bell over the artery and inflate the cuff to about 30 mmHg greater than that noted when the pulse could no longer be palpated. When a cuff is inflated beyond the systolic blood pressure, the artery is totally occluded. Therefore, no sounds of blood flow come from the artery.

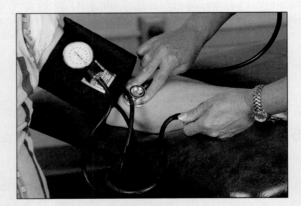

⑨ Air is evacuated from the cuff by slowly opening the pressure-relief valve.

⑩ As pressure in the cuff falls to the level of the systolic pressure, blood flows through the artery during systole (contraction phase) but not during diastole (noncontraction phase). Physical therapists/assistants listen for Korotkoff sounds that are created by systole. The first sounds heard through the stethoscope are usually described as tapping sounds. Initially, the tapping sound may be difficult to hear, as these sounds may be faint or soft and may not occur evenly. As cuff pressure falls, tapping sounds become more distinct and clear. The tapping nature of the sound is a result of the start of blood flow during systole and the stopping of blood flow during diastole. The tapping sounds occur because at this level of cuff pressure, arterial flow can occur only during systole. When the first tapping sounds are heard, a pressure reading is noted and represents the value of systolic blood pressure.

11 As more air is evacuated from a cuff, pressure falls toward the diastolic level. When cuff pressure is at a diastolic pressure level, the distinct and clear tapping becomes muffled, and usually disappears after an additional drop of 5 to 10 mmHg. Muffling of sound occurs at this level of cuff pressure because blood flows through the brachial artery during both systole and diastole. When tapping sounds become muffled, a pressure reading is noted. This reading represents the value of diastolic pressure.

12 At this time, the pressure in the cuff can be released rapidly by opening the pressure-relief valve completely.

13 Then the stethoscope and cuff can be removed from the patient.

14 Document both the systolic and diastolic values as blood pressure.

Throughout this procedure, take care not to maintain pressure on the artery for more than 2 or 3 minutes without relief. If cuff occlusion occurs for more than 2–3 minutes without relief, patients may experience symptoms of tingling or numbness, such as when an arm or leg "falls asleep."

Norms

As a reference point for blood pressure, 120/80 mmHg has been considered ideal. New guidelines emphasize a range rather than set numbers. ■ Table 5–2 presents ranges of normal and abnormal blood pressures for an adult.[2] Blood pressure will change with stress, physical activity, and age. Lower levels are considered to indicate the existence of hypotension. Clinical judgments or clinical decision making based on the values presented in Table 5–2 must also include consideration of age and medical status and should take into account all available data concerning patient status. Clinical decision making with respect to the impact of medical status on patient-care intervention is in the realm of the physical therapist. Physical therapists are to provide the acceptable range of blood pressure changes when directing physical therapist assistants in administering patient care.

Changes from resting blood pressure can result as patients change position or increase activity. Red flags, which are indications to stop activity and examine cardiac status, include (1) failure of systolic pressure to rise in proportion with increased intensity of activity, (2) a decrease in systolic pressure greater than 10 mmHg, (3) a systolic pressure greater than 240 mmHg, or (4) an increase greater than 20 mmHg for diastolic pressure during activity.

■ **Take Note**
Red flags are an indication that physical therapist assistants must notify physical therapists immediately and that physical therapists may need to refer such patients to another practitioner.

TABLE 5–2   Blood Pressure Ranges for Adults

	Systolic (mmHg)	Diastolic (mmHg)
Normal	Less than 120	Less than 80
Pre-hypertension	120–139	80–89
Stage 1 hypertension	140–159	90–99
Stage 2 hypertension	At or greater than 160	At or greater than 100

Respiration

Purpose

Respiratory rate is the rate of breathing. Each respiratory cycle includes one inspiration and the subsequent expiration. Respiratory rate can be measured, and the quality of respiration can be observed.

Methods

Methods of measuring respiratory rate are auscultation and observation. Auscultation is auditory by stethoscope, and observation is visual, auditory, or palpation. Unobtrusive visual and auditory observations can be made just prior to, or just after, taking a pulse. In situations where shallow or quiet breathing patterns make visual or auditory observation difficult, auscultation with a stethoscope may improve auditory observation.

PROCEDURE 5–3   Measuring Respiratory Rate

Palpation of a patient's thorax permits determination of the rise and fall of the chest during respiration.

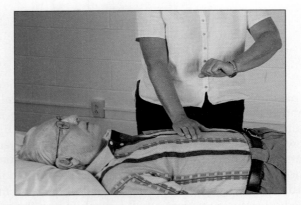

An alternative method of palpation requires placing the dorsum of one's hand close to, but not touching or occluding, a patient's mouth and nose. Changes in the direction of air flow during respiration can be felt as slight changes in pressure or temperature on the dorsum of one's hand.

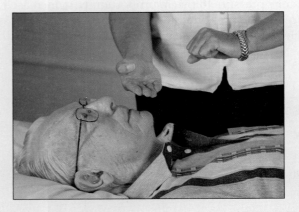

Respiratory rate (RR) is measured as the number of breathing cycles per minute. To measure respiratory rate, use a watch or clock that displays time in seconds. Count respiratory cycles for a set period of time. Only complete respiratory cycles, those consisting of both complete inspiratory and expiratory phases, are counted. Measurements may be over a 60-second time period, or shorter time periods may be used. Problems of accuracy noted previously for determining heart rate when using shortcut methods also apply to measurements of respiratory rate. Respiration is measured as cycles per minute but is reported without the use of units. A respiration rate of 12 respirations per minute is reported as 12 RR.

Duration of inspiratory and expiratory phases can also be measured, and expiratory phases are usually longer than inspiratory phases. Depth of inspiration, regularity of inspiration, and use of accessory muscles of respiration can be observed as indicators of the quality of respiration, measures that are more subjective than respiratory rate. Document information concerning depth, regularity, and use of accessory muscles with specific measurements of respiratory rate.

Norms

Normal breathing patterns are even and relatively quiet, and have a slight pause between the end of expiration and the initiation of inspiration. Only a very low-level hiss of air movement through the nose or mouth should be evident. Small variations may be noted, depending upon an individual's level of physical training and state of anxiety. Normal resting respiratory rate for adults is considered 12 breaths per minute. Normal resting respiratory rate of children is considered 20 breaths per minute. The ratio of inspiratory time to expiratory time within one respiratory cycle (I/E ratio) is normally 1:2. Resting respiratory rates of less than 10 breaths per minute or greater than 20 breaths per minute are considered abnormal.

Following periods of exercise, or during respiratory distress, respiration may increase to 25 to 35 breaths per minute for short periods of time. With increased respiratory rates, breathing will be more shallow, and accessory muscles of respiration are more likely to be involved.

■ **Take Note**
Normal respiratory rates:
Adults 12, children 20.

■ **Take Note**
Inspiratory time is less than expiratory time.

Temperature

Purpose

Body **temperature** provides information concerning basal metabolic state, potential presence of infection, and metabolic response to exercise. Physical therapists/assistants may not routinely measure a patient's body temperature but need to know the methods and norms. Skin temperature provides information concerning circulatory status, potential peripheral nerve injury, and local inflammatory responses. Physical therapists/assistants frequently measure skin temperature for these reasons.

Methods

A variety of devices are available for measuring patient temperatures (■ Figure 5–4). Thermometers originally were constructed of a graduated glass tube with a bulb at one end to hold a small quantity of mercury. Increases in temperature cause mercury to expand, and decreases in temperature cause mercury to contract. The degree of expansion or contraction is indicative of specific temperatures.

Electronic thermometers with disposable probes or probe covers take little time to measure temperature and have supplanted glass thermometers. Electronic thermometers produce a reading of the temperature and often make a sound when the maximum temperature is attained. Digital displays of temperature readings will hold the value of

■ **Take Note**
Methods for temperature measurement: thermometers (electronic, heat-sensitive strips) or palpation.

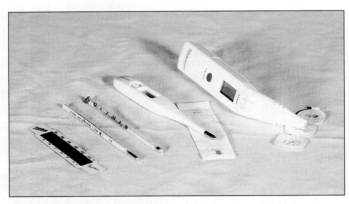

■ **Figure 5–4** Examples of devices for measuring temperature.

the highest temperature until an instrument is reset. Heat-sensitive strips that indicate a temperature range rather than a specific degree are available. When used on extremities, such strips can indicate adequacy of peripheral circulation.

Reusable thermometers must be cleansed and sterilized between uses and inspected to ensure patient safety and measurement accuracy. When probes are used, a new probe cover must be used with each patient.

In all situations, patients should remain quiet during the time temperature is being measured. Close supervision of young children and patients with decreased cognition is necessary for safety and to obtain accurate measurements. Temperature measurements may be recorded in degrees Fahrenheit or degrees Celsius. Documentation must indicate which temperature scale was used.

Sites

Oral temperature measurements were used most commonly for measurement of body temperature. Oral temperature is taken by placing a thermometer probe under the tongue. Place the tip of the thermometer probe as far back as is comfortable for the patient. Tympanic temperature measurements are taken by placing the instrument carefully into the external auditory canal.

Palpation of skin temperature is performed using the dorsal surface of the hand. Place the dorsum of the hand lightly on the site to be examined. Move the hand slowly from distal to proximal, noting temperature changes. Comparison of one extremity to another, such as left arm to right arm, may provide information concerning differences in temperature.

Norms

Normal ranges of body temperature are centered at 98.6°F or 37°C. An individual's temperature will fluctuate throughout a 24-hour period, but these fluctuations should not be more than a few degrees. Depending upon time of day, site of measurement, and level of activity, normal body temperatures vary within general ranges. Therapeutic treatments of heat and cold will cause variations of local site temperatures of several degrees Fahrenheit. ■ Table 5–3 presents temperature ranges for various situations.

Patients with a normal body temperature of 98.6°F are considered to be **afebrile** when oral temperature remains below 100°F (37.8°C). When oral temperature in these patients exceeds 100°F, they are considered to be **febrile**. **Hyperthermia** is defined as a rectal temperature greater than 106°F (41.1°C). **Hypothermia** is defined as a rectal temperature less than 94°F (34.4°C).

TABLE 5–3 Temperature Ranges for Different Activities

Situation	Oral	
	°F	°C
Usual normal range	98.6 to 99.5	36.0 to 37.5
Morning/cold weather	95.0 to 96.8	35.0 to 36.0
Hard work/emotion/a few normal adults/many active children	99.7 to 101.0	37.6 to 38.3

Pain

Pain is a subjective perception described by patients and, thus, is difficult to measure. Perceptions of pain are unique to each individual and may depend upon previous experiences, type of injury or disease (laceration, crush, burn, migraine headaches, arthritis, etc.), body part affected, age, time since onset, and ethnic background. There may also be situations in which pain is expressed when an injury or disease does not truly present pain. Since pain is a subjective symptom, assessment is difficult.

Purpose

The purposes of measuring perceptions of pain are to determine (1) diagnosis, (2) prognosis, (3) appropriate interventions, and (4) responses to interventions. Measurements of perceptions of pain that assist in diagnosis seek to determine type of pain (burning, tingling, sharp, dull, etc.), location (specific joint or limb), extent of painful location, intensity, duration, and frequency.

Method

The most commonly used method of measuring pain is an adaptation of a visual analog scale (VAS). A **visual analog scale** is a straight horizontal line with 0 at the left side and 10 at the right side. The left side, 0, represents a complete absence of pain. The right side, 10, represents the worst pain a patient can imagine. Patients are asked to mark on the horizontal line the point that corresponds with their perception of their current pain. A common adaptation of the visual analog scale is for patients to be asked to provide a number between 0 and 10 that represents where they rank their current perception of pain, rather than being asked to mark an actual scale.

Young children can have difficulty with the concept of ranking pain perceptions. Often a series of faces, from very happy to very unhappy, is used. Children are asked to select the face that represents their perception of pain. This is analogous to selecting a number that represents a perception of pain.

■ **Take Note**

Visual analogy scale (VAS)

0 = no pain;

1, 2, 3 = minimal pain;

4, 5, 6 = moderate pain;

7, 8, 9, 10 = severe pain.

Site

Body diagrams can be used to document the site of pain. Document each site in which pain is perceived, including type, intensity, duration, and frequency. Each site of pain is marked, and types of pain are noted by different markings. Intensity may be noted by different colors.

Norms

A range of pain scoring that is generally used lists 0 as nonexistent, 1–3 as minimal, 4–6 as moderate, and 7–10 as severe.

Anthropometrics

Purpose

An important aspect of health care is monitoring a patient's height and weight, as well as other **anthropometric measures**. Changes of weight, either increases or decreases, in adults can indicate changes in health status. For children, physical development is assessed by height and weight charts.

Methods

To determine levels of physical child development, height and weight are measured carefully using rulers and scales. Measurements may use either U.S. or metric units. Comparison is made to growth charts to determine percentiles for child development.[3]

Body mass index (BMI) is used to classify a person's weight and height relationship with respect to being underweight, normal, overweight, and obese. BMI is calculated in two different manners, depending on whether U.S. units or metric units are used.[4] When U.S. units are used, the formula is $(703.1)(\text{weight in pounds})/(\text{height in inches})^2$. When metric units are used, the formula is $(\text{weight in kilograms})/(\text{height in meters})^2$.

It should be noted that BMI can be misleading. A person with significant muscular development can have a high BMI but may not be overweight or obese. This can occur because the increased weight of muscle mass is not distinguishable from fat.

Norms

For child development, a table of correlations of height and weight may be found at the Centers for Disease Control and Prevention web site, www.cdc.gov/. (In the A-Z index, click on G > Growth Charts > under Educational Materials click on Tools to Calculate BMI > in the left menu click on Introduction.)

Calculations and tables related to Body Mass Index may be found at www.nhlbi.nih .gov/. (In the search box, type BMI > click the link for Calculate Your Body Mass Index [BMI].) NHLBI is the acronym for the National Heart Lung and Blood Institute, a component of the Department of Health and Human Service's (DHHS) National Institutes of Health (NIH).

Current norms used by the CDC for BMI are presented in ■ Table 5–4.

TABLE 5–4 BMI Classifications

Underweight	BMI of less than 18.5
Normal	BMI between 18.5 and 24.9
Overweight	BMI between 25.0 and 29.9
Obese	BMI greater than 30

Chapter Review

Review Questions

1. Define pulse rate, and list the common sites at which pulse rates are measured.

2. What are the purposes for determining pulse rates and quality of pulses?

3. What are the normal and abnormal ranges of heart rate?

4. Describe how to determine a target heart rate.

5. Define respiratory rate, and list the common methods for measuring respiratory rate.

6. What are the normal and abnormal ranges of respiratory rate?

7. Define blood pressure, and list the usual site at which blood pressure is measured.

8. What are the normal and abnormal ranges for blood pressure?

9. Define body temperature, and list the common sites at which body temperature is measured.

10. What are the normal and abnormal ranges of body temperature?

11. What are the units used when documenting heart rate, respiratory rate, blood pressure, and temperature?

12. What are commonly used methods for measuring pain?

13. What are the four categories and their ranges of body mass index?

Suggested Activities

1. Demonstrate the proper methods to measure pulse, patency, respiratory rate, blood pressure, and temperature.

2. Practice measuring vital signs of classmates in the proper position of sitting or lying quietly.

3. Properly document the results from Activity 2.

4. Compare results from Activity 2 to norms to determine if the values obtained are in the normal range.

5. Practice assessing vital signs of classmates before, during, and after activities such as riding a stationary bike, running on a treadmill, or lifting weights.

6. Properly document the results from Activity 5.

7. Compare results from Activity 5 to norms to determine if the values obtained are in the normal range.

Case Study

Mr. Rangarajan is a 47-year-old construction worker. Four days ago he fell from the roof framing of a two-story house under construction. His fall was through the unfinished floor/ceiling framing to the first floor, landing on a pile of used lumber with nails. Upon admission to the hospital, Mr. Rangarajan was diagnosed with two fractured ribs on his right side, a fractured left radius, puncture wounds to his right chest and forearm, a dislocated right shoulder, and a Grade 2 concussion.

A referral for physical therapy services has been forwarded to the Physical Therapy Department.

1. For your first visit, what vital signs would you measure and record?

2. What methods and sites would you use to perform the measurements?

3. What method of measurement of pain perception would you use?

References

1. Bickley LS. *Bates' Guide to Physical Examination and History Taking*, 8th ed. Philadelphia: Lippincott Williams & Wilkins, Philadelphia, 2003.
2. National Heart, Lung, and Blood Pressure Institute. *The Seventh Report of the Joint National Committee on Prevention, Detection, Evaluation, and Treatment of High Blood Pressure* (JNC 7), nhlbi.nih.gov/guidelines/hypertension/index.htm.
3. www.cdc.gov/nccdphp/dnpa/growthcharts/ Accessed 27 April 2008.
4. www.nhlbisupport.com/bmi/ Accessed 27 April 2008.

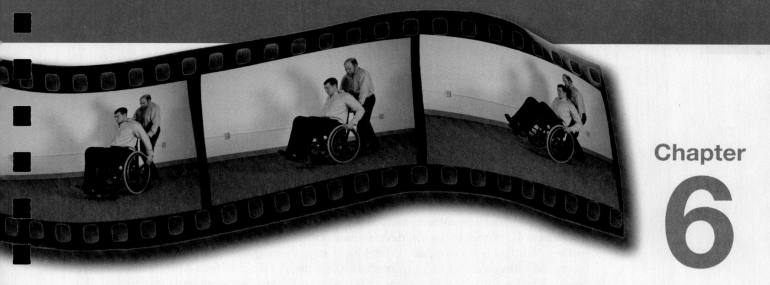

Chapter

6

Wheelchairs

Learning Objectives

Upon completion of this chapter, you will be able to:

1. Identify different components of a wheelchair, including:
- Anti-tipping components
- Armrests
- Front rigging
- Pelvic positioners
- Wheels
- Wheel locks

2. Identify different types of wheelchairs, including:
- Amputee-frame
- Fixed frame
- Folding
- One-arm drive
- Reclining-back
- Standard
- Tilt-in-space

3. Describe the purpose or function of wheelchair components and types.

4. Describe and demonstrate how wheelchair components and types are manipulated.

5. Describe and demonstrate how to measure an individual to determine correct size and components required for a wheelchair.

Key Terms

Anti-tipping devices
Armrests
Caster wheels
Drive wheels
Fixed frame
Folding frame
Footrest
Front rigging

Heel loops
Legrest
One-arm drive
Pelvic positioners
Reclining back
Sacral sitting
Tilt-in-space
Wheel locks

Introduction

In situations when an individual will use a wheelchair as his or her primary means of mobility, a wheelchair is usually specifically fabricated for that individual. Careful measurement of an individual, and the selection of appropriate components with respect to specific needs, provides the user of a wheelchair with a piece of equipment that allows the individual to function with the most independence and safety possible. Guidelines for selection of a wheelchair design indicate that wheelchairs have a short wheelbase and be as light and narrow as possible. These features make propulsion and maneuvering require less user effort.

Wheelchairs incorporate many common features, but there are a variety of mechanisms that can be selected to meet the needs of each individual. This chapter presents selected components, selected types of wheelchairs and other mobility devices, and illustrates how to measure a patient for a wheelchair.

Wheelchair Components

Wheel Locks

One of the most important safety features on a wheelchair is the wheel-lock system (■ Figure 6–1). **Wheel locks** are devices that stabilize the wheels of a wheelchair *after* the wheelchair has been stopped. Wheel locks usually employ a cam and lever system. In some situations, a slot-locking mechanism is used rather than a cam-locking mechanism. Previously, wheel locks were referred to as brakes. Some patients understood that to mean that wheel locks functioned as braking devices, such as on an automobile, which is not correct.

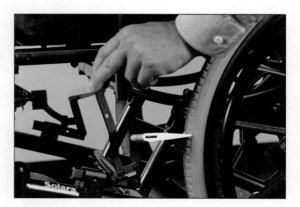

■ **Figure 6–1**   Wheel lock.

A general safety rule is that wheel locks must be engaged whenever an individual is moving into, or out of, a wheelchair. Engaging wheel locks on the rear wheels prevents forward and backward movement of a wheelchair. Wheel locks on front caster wheels minimize side-to-side movement. Although wheel locks are available for front caster wheels, they are not typically placed on wheelchairs. Therefore, slight side-to-side movement of a wheelchair may result as an individual moves into, or out of, a wheelchair when front caster wheels are not secured.

To work properly, wheel locks must make secure contact with tires to prevent movement of the wheels. Effectiveness of wheel locks is reduced if they do not make adequate contact with tires. This may occur when pneumatic tires are not inflated sufficiently or when entire wheel-lock mechanisms become loose or slide forward on the wheelchair frame.

The direction of the force needed to engage or release wheel locks can be selected during wheelchair ordering to match a patient's abilities. Wheel locks are usually engaged by pushing a lever on each side forward (■ Figure 6–2), while pulling the levers backward releases the wheel lock (■ Figure 6–3). The reverse mechanism, engaging wheel locks by pulling levers backward, and releasing them by pushing levers forward, is an

■ **Take Note**

Safety: Engage wheel locks before moving in/out of a wheelchair.

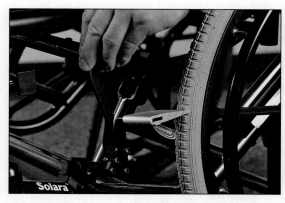

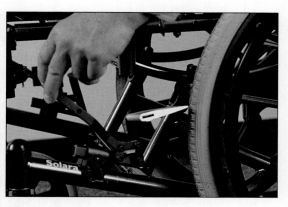

■ **Figure 6–2**   Engaging wheel locks.

■ **Figure 6–3**   Releasing wheel locks.

option. A decision as to which method to use is made by a physical therapist and patient, with respect to the patient's strength and balance. The direction of a patient's greatest strength is the direction of movement that should engage the wheel locks.

Extensions for wheel-lock levers are available (■ **Figure 6–4**). Extensions increase the mechanical advantage of a wheel-locking mechanism by increasing the length of the wheel-lock lever. Increasing the length of the wheel-lock lever increases the length of

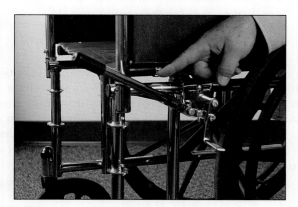

■ **Figure 6–4**   Wheel lock handle extension.

the force arm with respect to the resistance arm of the cam. This increase in mechanical advantage decreases the force required of a patient for engaging or disengaging the wheel lock.

On some reclining-back wheelchairs, the anterior/posterior dimension of the wheelbase increases when the back is reclined. When the wheelbase is enlarged as the back reclines, the relationship of the wheel lock and the tire is altered, resulting in an ineffective wheel lock because wheel-lock contact with the tire is decreased. An additional wheel lock is necessary for these wheelchairs. The additional lock is attached to the back upright of the wheelchair so it is effective when the wheelchair is in the reclined position.

Pelvic Positioners

Pelvic positioners are devices that stabilize a patient's pelvis in the proper position while seated in a wheelchair (■ Figure 6–5). Pelvic positioners are not intended to be used to prevent a patient from falling out of a wheelchair. Rather they are part of a positioning system designed to provide proper positioning of a patient in a wheelchair. Pelvic positioners also are not intended to be used as restraints to keep patients from getting out of a wheelchair unexpectedly.

Three mechanisms are used for fastening pelvic positioners: Velcro straps; latching buckles, such as those used for seat belts in airplanes; and push-button buckles, such as those used for seat belts in automobiles.

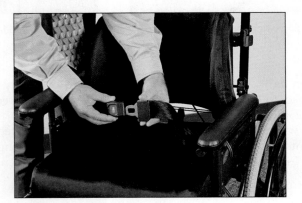

■ **Figure 6–5** Pelvic positioner.

Caster Wheels

Caster wheels are the small front wheels of a wheelchair. Two basic styles of tire are available—standard solid rubber and pneumatic. Pneumatic tires are filled with air, providing some shock absorption, and thus a smoother ride (■ Figure 6–6). Pneumatic tires are wider than standard solid rubber tires, making travel easier on soft, or uneven, surfaces such as sand or gravel. Some wheelchair owners use "rollerblade" wheels for front caster wheels (■ Figure 6–7). Typically these owners are users of ultralight, or sport, wheelchairs. Because of their construction and materials, "rollerblade" wheels are

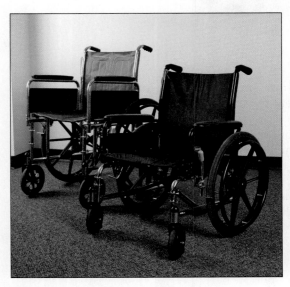

■ **Figure 6–6** Pneumatic caster wheels.

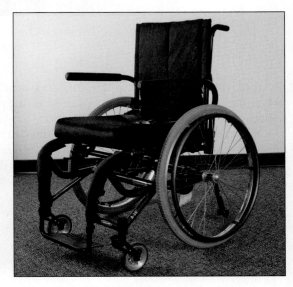

■ **Figure 6–7** "Rollerblade" caster wheels.

small, very durable, and have excellent quality bearings. A trade-off, however, is that smaller wheels may become caught in sidewalk cracks.

Drive (Push) Wheels

Drive wheels are the large rear wheels of a wheelchair, which are used for propulsion. Rear tires may be one of two basic types—standard solid rubber or pneumatic. Pneumatic tires may or may not have tread (■ Figure 6–8). Treads are used on wheelchairs that are often used outdoors and require more traction than smooth tires provide. Pneumatic tires have been modified to reduce the potential for flat tires.

Drive wheels have inner and outer rims. The inner rim is for mounting tires. The outer, or hand, rim is used for propelling the wheelchair. Adaptations of the outer rim, such as projections, are available for use by individuals who do not have sufficient ability to grasp (■ Figure 6–9). Projections add weight and width to the wheelchair and may make maneuvering in small spaces difficult. Nonslip coatings, rather than projections, are more commonly used on hand rims to assist propulsion when an individual does not have sufficient ability to grasp.

■ **Take Note**

Hand rim projections may be horizontal, angled, or vertical.

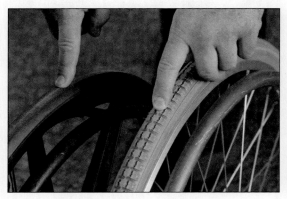

■ **Figure 6–8** Drive wheels—smooth (left), tread (right).

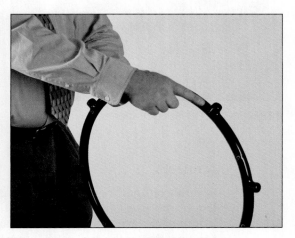

■ **Figure 6–9** Drive wheel rim with projections.

Drive wheels come in two types—standard or "mags" (■ Figure 6–10). Standard wheels are fabricated with multiple steel or aluminum spokes. Spokes are thin and individually adjustable to maintain proper alignment of a wheel. Mag wheels do

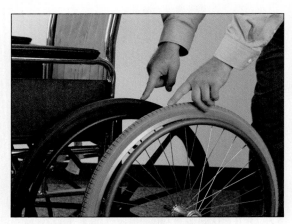

■ **Figure 6–10** Drive wheels—mag (left), spoke (right).

not use spokes but usually have eight thicker struts that connect the outer rim to the hub. Mag wheels were named after their fabrication from magnesium, a very strong, lightweight metal. Mag wheels have the material strength to maintain their original alignment, eliminating the need for multiple adjustable spokes. Because of their design and material, maintenance of mag wheels is easier than standard wheels.

Drive wheels on some chairs are easily removable (■ Figures 6–11 and ■ 6–12), making the chair lighter and smaller, increasing the ease of maneuvering the wheelchair into, and out of, a vehicle.

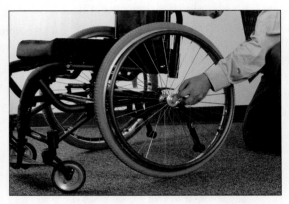 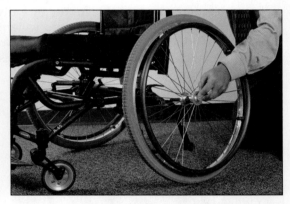

■ **Figure 6–11**   Releasing quick-release drive wheels.   ■ **Figure 6–12**   Removing quick-release drive wheels.

Armrests

Several configurations of **armrests** are available. Armrests are either full length or desk length (■ **Figure 6–13**). The height of full-length armrests is the same along the entire length of the armrest. Desk-length armrests have two heights. In a standard setup, the front portion of the armrest is lower than the rear portion, permitting a wheelchair to be rolled under a table or desk. Most desk-length armrests can be removed and reversed, placing the higher part of the armrest toward the front of the wheelchair. Reversing a desk armrest provides a higher support for patients when pushing to standing or when performing other transfers.

■ **Take Note**

Desk armrests allow a person to get close to tables and desks.

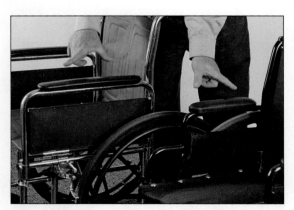

■ **Figure 6–13**   Full-length (left) and desk-length (right) armrests.

Lap trays are available and can be secured to, or rest on, armrests. Full-length armrests offer greater support for lap trays than do desk-length armrests.

Both types of armrests have an option for adjustable height with respect to the top of the seat (■ Figures 6–14 and ■ 6–15). Proper adjustment of armrest height permits the person sitting in the wheelchair to rest his or her forearms on the armrest with the elbow flexed to approximately 90 degrees.

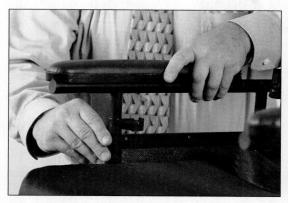

■ **Figure 6–14** Lowered elevating armrest.

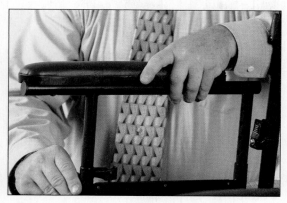

■ **Figure 6–15** Raised elevating armrest.

Armrests, both full length and desk length, can be either removable or fixed. Non-removable armrests usually result in a lighter, and narrower, wheelchair. Removable armrests may be designed so that they wrap around the back uprights of the wheelchair, decreasing wheelchair width (■ Figure 6–16). When a wrap-around design is used, the posterior upright of the armrest is directly behind the upright of the wheelchair back. Removable armrests often allow easier performance of transfers and permit a patient to sit even closer to a table or desk than desk-length armrests allow. Wrap-around desk-length armrests cannot be reversed to place the higher portion toward the front of the wheelchair.

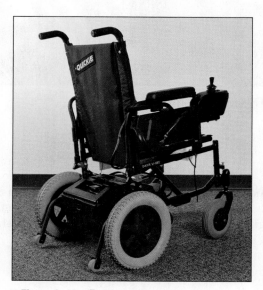

■ **Figure 6–16** Removable wrap-around armrest.

Several types of mechanisms are used to lock armrests in place for patient safety. Both the location and type of armrest-locking mechanisms vary. A common type of lock is operated by a lever that is either pushed down or rotated to release the lock (■ Figures 6–17 and ■ 6–18).

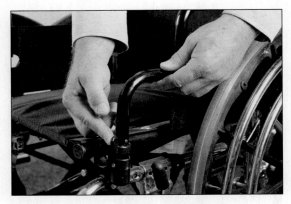

■ **Figure 6–17**   Removable armrest lock.

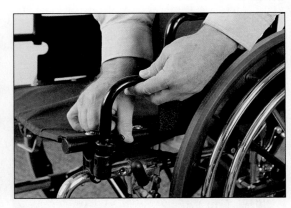

■ **Figure 6–18**   Releasing removable armrest.

Once released, the lever remains in the released position. Thus, only one hand is required to unlock, and then remove, the armrest (■ Figure 6–19).

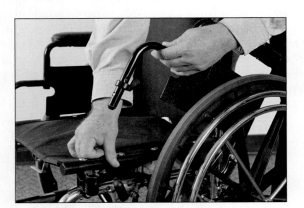

■ **Figure 6–19**   Armrest being removed.

Front Rigging

Front rigging on a wheelchair consists of a footplate attached to either a footrest or an elevating legrest. The purpose of front rigging is to provide support for the lower extremities. Front rigging with a footplate only is called a **footrest**. Front rigging with a footplate and calf pad support is called a **legrest**.

Footplates.   Patients' feet rest on footplates, which are available in several sizes to accommodate feet of different sizes. **Heel loops**, constructed of strapping or webbing, attach to footplates and prevent the feet from sliding off the footplates and under the wheelchair (■ Figure 6–20). Ankle and toe loops, also constructed of strapping or webbing, may also be used to maintain the feet on footplates.

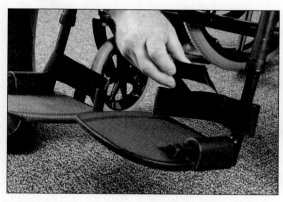

■ **Figure 6–20**   Heel loop on footrest of front rigging.

Footplates are raised to allow patients to transfer safely in and out of a wheelchair (■ Figures 6–21 and ■ 6–22). When raising footplates, push heel loops forward to allow the footplates to be raised completely. Doing this prolongs the life of heel loops by preventing heel loop material from being crushed.

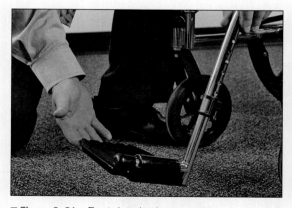

■ **Figure 6–21**   Footplate in down position.

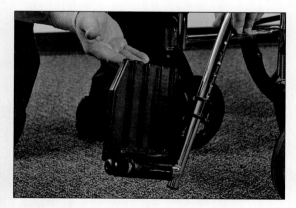

■ **Figure 6–22**   Footplate in up position.

Footrests. The distance from seat to footplate for both footrests and legrests can be adjusted to match a patient's lower leg length and to provide proper support for the entire lower extremity. There are several different types of mechanism for making this adjustment. The method illustrated uses a push-button release and a clamp to ensure that the desired position is maintained (■ Figures 6–23 and ■ 6–24).

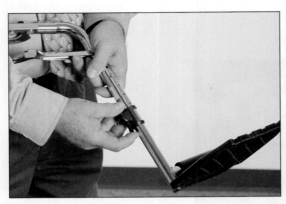

■ **Figure 6–23** Preparing to lengthen front rigging— securing lever and button adjustment.

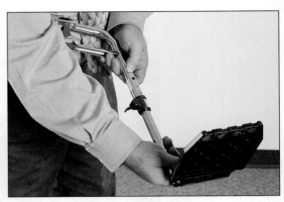

■ **Figure 6–24** Adjusting front rigging length— lengthening while holding button.

Other types of mechanisms use clamps, or tension-adjustment screws, located inside the footrest or legrest tube. The adjustment screws are accessible from the underside of the footrest or legrest.

Footrests can be fixed or removable. Fixed footrests are usually less expensive and result in a lighter wheelchair. Fixed footrests are part of a unitized construction design in standard wheelchairs. In this design, footplates can be raised, but the footrest itself cannot be removed.

Footrests for fixed-frame wheelchairs are part of a unitized construction design and cannot be adjusted (■ Figure 6–25). In this design, footplates are typically bolted to a bar that is positioned so the knees are flexed 90 degrees or more. This results in a shorter overall dimension for the wheelchair. Fixed-frame wheelchairs are usually ultra light-weight sport models.

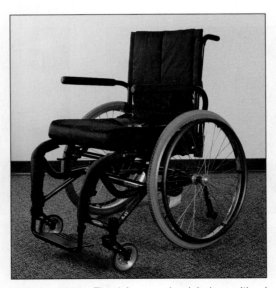

■ **Figure 6–25** Fixed-frame wheelchair—unitized footrest construction.

Removable footrests typically pivot to the sides of wheelchairs, where they can be removed. Several types of locks are used to secure pivoting footrests (■ Figure 6–26).

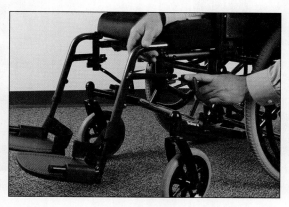

■ **Figure 6–26**   Preparing to release pivoting footrest.

Pivoting footrests use pivot pins as the center of rotation. To remove a pivoting footrest, the footrest is unlocked or released, pivoted to the side, and then lifted from the pivot pins (■ **Figures 6–27** and ■ **6–28**).

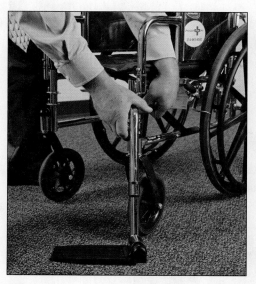

■ **Figure 6–27**   Pushing lever to release pivoting footrest.

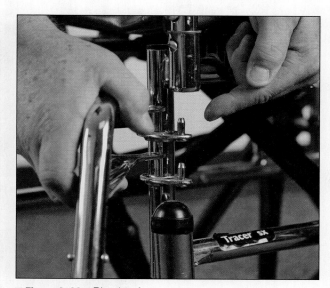

■ **Figure 6–28**   Pivoting footrest.

Elevating Legrests.   Elevating legrests are necessary when a patient is unable to flex his or her knee, when a dependent position of the leg contributes to swelling, or with a reclining-back wheelchair. A calf pad support provides a cushion for the calf and support for the leg.

The height of the legrest position is adjustable. Legrest height position is maintained by a locking mechanism. The lock is released and activated by a lever. The legrest position is adjusted by releasing the lock with one hand while raising or lowering the legrest with the other hand (■ Figures 6–29 and ■ 6–30).

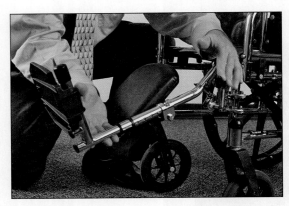

■ **Figure 6–29** Preparing to raise elevating legrest by pushing lever.

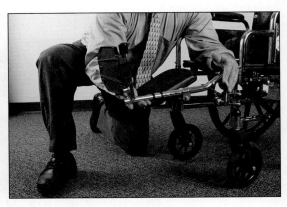

■ **Figure 6–30** Elevating legrest in up position.

To remove an elevating legrest, pivot the calf pad support out of the way. The calf pad support must be pivoted before the footplate is raised (■ Figures 6–31 through 6–33). Failure to use this sequence will keep the calf pad support from moving completely out of the way.

Swing-away removable elevating legrests are removed in a similar manner as swing-away removable footrests are removed.

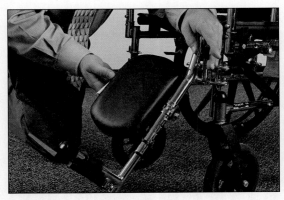

■ **Figure 6–31** Calf pad support in down position.

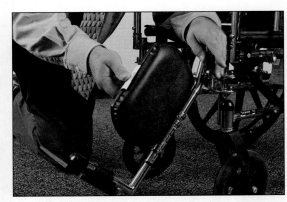

■ **Figure 6–32** Calf pad support pivoted to up position.

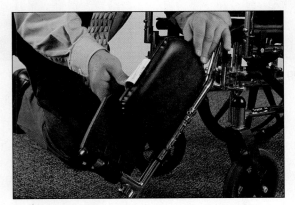

■ **Figure 6–33** Raising footplate with calf pad support in up position.

Anti-Tipping Devices.   **Anti-tipping devices** (■ Figure 6–34) are small extensions, with or without wheels, attached to the lower horizontal support bar. These devices are used to prevent accidental backward tipping of the wheelchair. Anti-tipping devices must permit some tipping of the wheelchair so front casters can roll up and over doorsills, curbs, or other low obstructions.

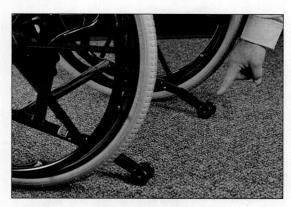

■ **Figure 6–34**   Anti-tipping device.

Wheelchair Types

Different styles of wheelchairs have been developed to meet specific patient needs. Some styles are minimal modifications of standard wheelchairs. Other styles required extensive re-engineering of basic wheelchair design. Several, but not all, types of specialized wheelchairs are discussed in this section. In addition to manual wheelchairs, motorized wheelchairs and scooters are available.

Folding Wheelchair

Folding-frame wheelchairs that can be folded or collapsed for storage or transport use a similar method for folding (■ Figures 6–35 and ■ 6–36). Raising footplates and pulling up on the handles located on either side of the seat will fold most wheelchairs. Do not pull up on the middle of the wheelchair seat upholstery to fold a wheelchair because it will weaken the upholstery, and, eventually, the seat will tear. Push down on the horizontal bars of the seat to unfold the wheelchair.

■ **Take Note**

Wheelchairs should be folded by pulling up on the handles at the edges of the seat.

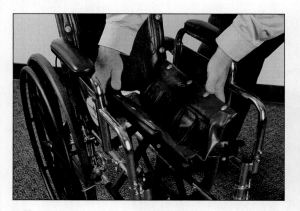

■ **Figure 6–35**   Mid-position of folding a wheelchair.

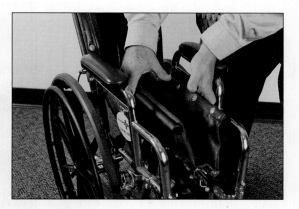

■ **Figure 6–36**   End position of folding a wheelchair.

Standard Wheelchair

A standard wheelchair comes with basic features. This wheelchair is durable and is the standard for facility use. Standard wheelchairs are available in several sizes to fit patients ranging from pediatric to adult to bariatric. Seat-to-floor height can be varied, with a lower seat height facilitating propulsion for individuals who propel the wheelchair with their feet (■ Figure 6–37).

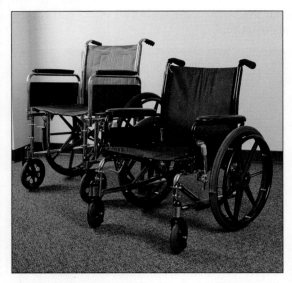

■ **Figure 6–37** Seat height—standard (left), low (right).

Fixed-Frame Wheelchair

A **fixed frame** means the wheelchair frame is solid and cannot be folded (■ Figure 6–38). The front rigging is often part of the frame and not removable. Back height is often lower than on a standard wheelchair, and many individuals who use fixed-frame wheelchairs do not use armrests. Overall frame length in fixed-frame wheelchairs is reduced because the front rigging is an integral part of the frame, and the front rigging is placed further back on the frame. This improves maneuverability, which is important in small spaces. There are fewer components and the materials used to construct them are lighter than standard wheelchairs. Thus fixed-frame wheelchairs are usually ultra lightweight. One disadvantage of the fixed frame is reduced shock absorption because the frame in a unitized design is rigid.

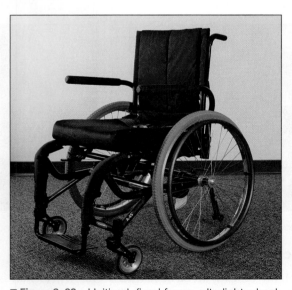

■ **Figure 6–38** Unitized, fixed frame, ultralight wheelchair construction.

Reclining-Back Wheelchair

Reclining-back wheelchairs are indicated when a patient is unable to sit erect for long periods of time or at all. There are two variations of reclining-back wheelchairs—those that recline completely and those that recline only partially. An extended back is used with both types of reclining-back wheelchairs. An extended back provides support for the upper body when the wheelchair back is in a reclined position. Head support is also required when the back is reclined. Reclining-back wheelchairs usually have elevating legrests, permitting patients to be in a mostly supine position when the back is reclined. A reclining-back wheelchair takes much more space to maneuver when reclined because of the increase in overall length (■ Figures 6–39 and ■ 6–40).

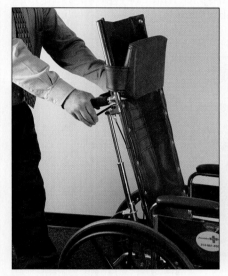

■ **Figure 6–39** Reclining-back wheelchair in upright position.

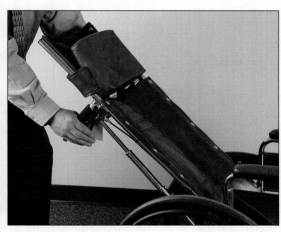

■ **Figure 6–40** Reclining-back wheelchair in reclined position.

There are several types of mechanisms for unlocking and adjusting the angle of inclination of the wheelchair back. To change the wheelchair's back angle, the locking mechanism is released, the angle of the back is adjusted, and the locking mechanism is activated.

A bar across the back of a reclining-back wheelchair provides support and stability. Several different methods of securing the support bar exist. To fold a reclining-back wheelchair, the back support bar must be removed (■ Figures 6–41 and ■ 6–42). Then a

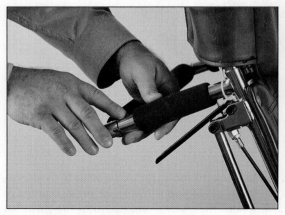

■ **Figure 6–41** Releasing support crossbar to fold reclining-back wheelchair.

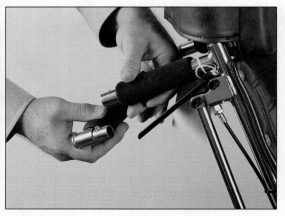

■ **Figure 6–42** Lowering support crossbar on reclining-back wheelchair.

reclining-back wheelchair can be folded following the same steps used when folding a standard wheelchair.

When a reclining-back wheelchair's back is lowered, the seat-to-back angle increases. As the seat-to-back angle increases, the wheelbase increases to maintain stability. Traditionally placed wheel locks will not engage the tires in this situation. Therefore, a reclining-back wheelchair typically has two sets of wheel locks. The second set of wheel locks is usually located on the back of the wheelchair to be able to engage the tires and for easy use by an attendant because the individual using a reclining-back wheelchair will not be able to engage the wheel locks during this maneuver.

Tilt-in-Space Wheelchair

A variation of a reclining-back wheelchair is a **tilt-in-space** frame (■ Figures 6–43 through 6–45). A tilt-in-space wheelchair has a fixed seat-to-back angle, even when reclined.

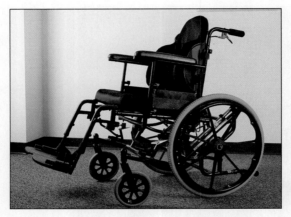

■ **Figure 6–43** Tilt-in-space wheelchair in upright position.

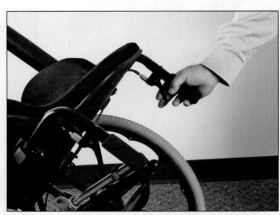

■ **Figure 6–44** Releasing mechanism to reposition tilt-in-space wheelchair.

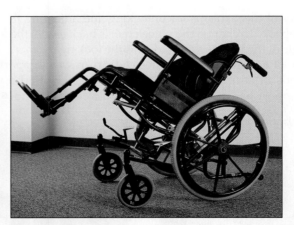

■ **Figure 6–45** Tilt-in-space wheelchair in a reclined position.

Maintaining this relative seat-to-back angle is useful for individuals who require customized seating systems on their wheelchair. The tilt-in-space frame permits changes of orientation for pressure relief, or for different activities, while maintaining the postural control provided by the customized seating system.

One-Arm Drive Wheelchair

A patient with only one functional upper extremity may achieve self-propulsion using a one-arm drive wheelchair. **One-arm drive wheelchairs** have two hand rims on one drive wheel (■ Figure 6–46). A linking mechanism between the drive wheels provides control for both drive wheels using one upper extremity. With both hand rims on one drive wheel, the two hand rims are used simultaneously to achieve forward or backward propulsion. Applying force to one rim at a time turns the wheelchair.

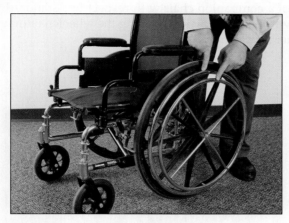

■ **Figure 6–46**   One-arm drive wheelchair.

Amputee Wheelchair

An amputee wheelchair frame has the drive wheels set behind the vertical back supports (■ Figure 6–47). This configuration moves the posterior boundary of the base of support further to the rear. A lower extremity amputation moves the individual's center of mass posteriorly when seated in a wheelchair, necessitating a change in the wheelchair's base of support. If the wheelchair's base of support is not moved posteriorly with respect to the individual, the wheelchair will be less stable and more likely to tip backward.

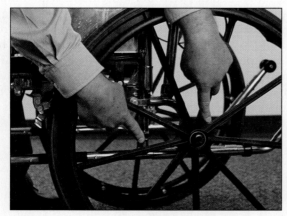

■ **Figure 6–47**   Backset drive wheels on frame of amputee wheelchair.

Propulsion by a patient is more difficult with the drive wheels placed further to the rear. Rather than using a wheelchair with an amputee frame to avoid tipping to the rear, two other methods can be used. Anti-tipping devices can be added to a standard frame, or weights can be added to the front of the wheelchair frame.

Companion Wheelchair

A companion chair, also called a travel chair, is a lightweight wheelchair that does not have drive wheels (■ Figure 6–48). The rear wheels are the size of caster wheels, so all four wheels are the same size. Smaller wheels, and the use of lightweight components, reduce the weight of a companion chair with respect to a standard wheelchair. A companion pushes the wheelchair. The person using the wheelchair may also be able to propel it using his or her feet.

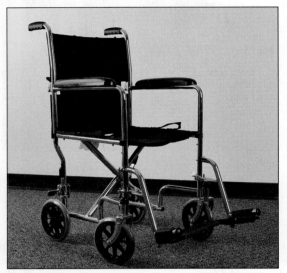

■ **Figure 6–48** Lightweight travel or companion wheelchair.

Motorized Wheelchairs and Scooters

A variety of motorized or power devices are increasingly available (■ Figures 6–49 and ■ 6–50). Although expensive, motorized devices offer individuals with minimal or limited functional abilities an opportunity to have independent mobility. There are a large number of choices and complexities in making decisions concerning motorized devices. In addition to determining available components, such as armrests, headrests, and front rigging, the method of power activation must be determined. Given the number of choices, and the complexity involved in making choices for specific patients, a discussion of the types of, and indications for, various methods of power activation and the various configurations of power devices is beyond the scope of this text.

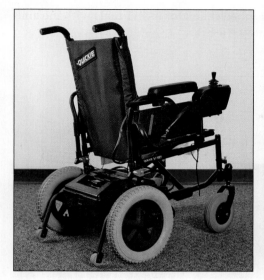

■ **Figure 6–49**   Standard power wheelchair.

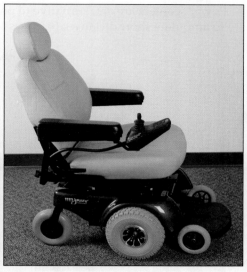

■ **Figure 6–50**   Power wheelchair with reclining back.

Some motorized wheelchairs also have the capability to use a power mechanism to recline the back of the wheelchair (■ **Figure 6–51**). This permits an individual to change position for different activities and provides for pressure relief.

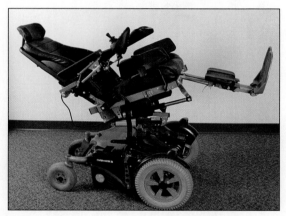

■ **Figure 6–51**   Power wheelchair with reclining back in reclined position.

Power scooters are an alternative to power wheelchairs for individuals with the ability to ambulate short distances (■ Figures 6–52 and ■ 6–53).

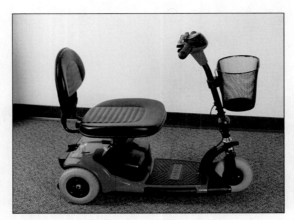

■ **Figure 6–52** Power scooter without armrests.

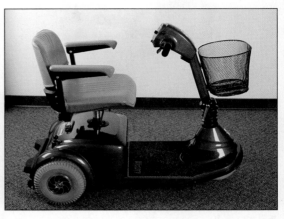

■ **Figure 6–53** Power scooter with armrests.

Power-Assist Chair

A newer type of wheelchair is a hybrid power-manual wheelchair (■ Figure 6–54). The individual propels the wheelchair using the drive wheels. The power-assist mechanism provides additional propulsion, increasing the duration or distance that may be attained.

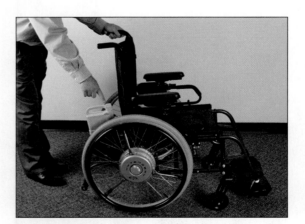

■ **Figure 6–54** Hybrid power-manual wheelchair.

PROCEDURE 6–1   Measuring to Determine Wheelchair Size

Selection of the type, size, and components of a wheelchair for an individual depends on a variety of information. Discussion with the patient and caregivers and determination of the environments in which the device will be used are critical to successful decision making. The decision-making process is the responsibility of a physical therapist, using the patient/client management process. Specific measurements of the individual are necessary for this decision-making process. Taking of measurements may be delegated to physical therapist assistants.

Wheelchair size is determined by selected measurements of the individual. Be careful to use measuring equipment properly and to read a tape measure or ruler accurately. Accurate measurement requires a physical therapist/assistant to assume a position that places the tape measure at eye level. The optimal patient position for obtaining accurate measurements is to have the patient sit on a solid flat surface with solid flat back support. Wood inserts can be used in a wheelchair or straight-back chair to ensure accuracy when measuring. Note that in some of the accompanying photographs, the position of the person performing measurements is altered to allow the tape measure to be seen.

Measuring for Seat Depth

Seat depth is one of the two most important measurements for determining wheelchair size. Proper seat depth provides support for the pelvis and thigh. The front edge of the seat should end 2 to 3 inches from the lower leg or knee when the knee is in a position of 90 degrees of flexion.

When seat depth is too short, the thighs are not supported properly, which adversely affects weight distribution and comfort. Seat depth that is longer than appropriate may affect circulation or lead to "sacral sitting" by a wheelchair user. **Sacral sitting** occurs when an individual slouches, sliding the buttocks forward and tilting the pelvis posteriorly. Sacral sitting places the posterior aspect of the sacrum on the seat of the chair, resulting in improper postural alignment. This position increases pressure on the posterior aspect of the sacrum and may lead to skin breakdown. In addition, a sacral-sitting position is not optimal for efficient propulsion.

One measurement and one calculation are necessary to determine seat depth.

1. During measuring, individuals must sit with proper alignment. Proper alignment requires that the individual's hips and knees be flexed to 90 degrees and his or her back be in contact with the flat back support without posterior pelvic tilt.

2. Measure the horizontal distance from the flat back support to the posterior aspect of the lower leg parallel to, and at the level of, the solid seat surface.

3. Subtract two or three inches from this measurement.

4. The result of this measurement and calculation provides the desired seat depth.

5. When a custom back insert is required, seat depth measurements must be calculated to accommodate the anterior/posterior thickness of the custom back insert.

(continued)

Measuring for Seat Width

The second of the two most important measurements for determining wheelchair size is seat width. Proper seat width results in properly positioned drive wheels and armrests, resulting in easy and efficient wheelchair use. Proper upright posture in a wheelchair is also aided by proper seat width.

When a wheelchair is too wide, an individual may have difficulty reaching the drive wheels for effective propulsion and may lean to one side or the other to rest on the armrests. When a wheelchair is too narrow, excessive pressure on the lateral aspects of the pelvis and thighs may occur, causing discomfort or skin breakdown. In addition to body width, space for clothing, such as winter coats, prosthetic or orthotic devices when necessary, and ease of movement, must be provided.

One measurement and one calculation are necessary to determine seat width.

1. With the individual sitting in proper alignment on the solid flat seat, measure the widest aspect of the patient's hips or thighs, whichever is wider, parallel to the solid flat seat.

2. Add two inches to this measurement.

3. The result of this measurement and calculation provides the desired seat width.

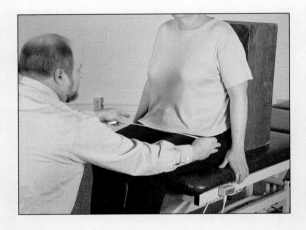

Measuring for Back Height

The amount of back height required depends on how much back support is needed by the individual.

A back height that is too high may restrict an individual's movement. A back height that is not high enough may not provide adequate support. Wheelchair users with adequate sitting balance may choose a low back height. A low back height decreases wheelchair weight and improves mobility within the wheelchair. Some wheelchair users also prefer the low back height for esthetic reasons, as it reduces the visual impact of the wheelchair.

One measurement and one calculation are necessary to determine back height.

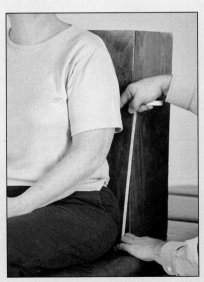

1. Back height is measured with the individual sitting on the solid flat seat in proper alignment.

2. In most cases, the vertical distance, parallel to the back support, is measured from the top of the seat to the inferior angle of the scapula.

3. Add the height of the seat cushion to be used to this measurement.

4. The result of this measurement and calculation provides the desired back height.

Measuring for Armrest Height

Proper armrest height promotes proper positioning and alignment. When armrest height is appropriate, and the individual is sitting with proper alignment, an individual's forearms rest comfortably on the armrests. Some individuals may elect not to use armrests if their sitting balance is adequate. Eliminating armrests decreases the weight of the wheelchair; allows the individual to sit close to surfaces such as sinks, desks, and tables; and reduces the visual impact of the wheelchair.

When armrests are at an improper height, an individual will be unable to rest his or her forearms comfortably on the armrests and maintain proper alignment. Improper alignment may cause an individual to be subjected to unequal pressure on the forearms and ischia and to spinal curvature.

One measurement and one calculation are necessary to determine armrest height.

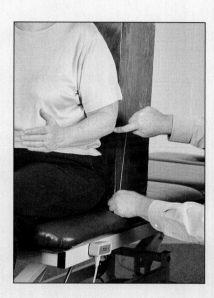

1. Armrest height is measured with the individual sitting on the solid flat seat in proper alignment, the upper arm held against the chest wall, and the elbow flexed to 90 degrees.

2. Measure the vertical distance between the solid seat surface and the individual's forearm, parallel to the back support.

3. Add the height of the seat cushion to be used to this measurement.

4. The result of this measurement and calculation provides the desired armrest height.

Measuring for Seat-to-Footplate Length

Appropriate seat-to-footplate length contributes to proper alignment and support of the lower extremities. When seat-to-footplate length is too great, an individual may sacral sit to rest his or her feet on the footplate. When the length is too short, pressure distribution along the thigh is uneven, forcing excessive weight bearing on the ischia and coccyx. Excessive pressure on the ischia or coccyx may result in skin breakdown.

The seat-to-footplate length is used to determine the type of legrest or footrest selected for the wheelchair in addition to adjusting the seat-to-footplate length. Seat-to-footplate distance and footplate clearance height must be determined in combination with the type of front rigging to be chosen.

Seat-to-footplate length is also a factor when considering the seat-to-floor height of a wheelchair. A minimum of 2 inches between the floor and the under-surface of the footplate are necessary to provide clearance over thresholds and other small obstacles. This distance to be measured is from the lowest point of the footplate to the floor.

One measurement and one calculation are necessary to determine seat-to-footplate length.

(continued)

1. Measure the length of the individual's lower leg, and height of the foot, from the posterior aspect of the thigh at the popliteal fossa to the sole of the foot at the heel.

2. Subtract the height of a seat cushion to be used from this measurement so the total measurement includes the thickness of the seat cushion.

3. The result of this measurement and calculation provides the desired seat-to-footplate length.

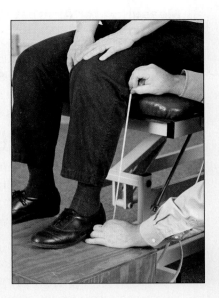

Measuring for Footplate Size

Footplate size is determined by the length of the patient's foot. Supporting the foot provides proper support of the lower extremity and assists in preventing development of deformities of the foot and ankle. While a significant portion of the foot must be supported, footrest length should be kept to a minimum to avoid interference with wheelchair maneuverability.

Footplates for fixed-frame ultra lightweight wheelchairs are often smaller than those used on other frame styles. When footplates on fixed-frame wheelchairs, which may or may not have heel loops, are positioned with the knee in 90 degrees or more of flexion, more of the forefoot than the hindfoot and heel is on the footplate. One measurement is necessary to determine footplate size.

1. The portion of the foot that must be supported by a footplate extends from the calcaneus to the heads of the metatarsals.

2. With the foot supported and the ankle in neutral, measure the horizontal distance from the posterior aspect of the foot (calcaneus) to the head of the first metatarsal.

3. The result of this measurement provides the desired footplate size.

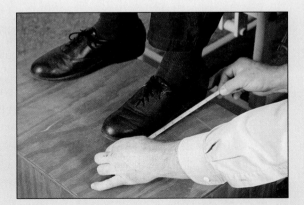

Standard Wheelchair Sizes

■ Table 6–1 provides standard measurements for wheelchairs of different sizes. When a standard-sized wheelchair appropriately fits an individual, the wheelchair is usually less costly and available in a shorter period of time. Custom fabrication, however, has become more commonly used to provide wheelchairs most appropriate for each individual.

TABLE 6–1 Standard Wheelchair Sizes

Size	Seat Depth (inches)	Seat Width (inches)	Seat Height (inches)
Adult	16.0	18.0	20.00
Narrow adult	16.0	16.0	20.00
Slim adult	16.0	14.0	20.00
Tall adult	17.0	18.0	20.00
Hemi or low seat[1]			17.50
Preschool	8.0	10.0	19.50
Tiny tot	11.5	12.0	19.50
Child	11.5	14.0	18.75
	16.0	16.0	18.50

[1]Hemi or low seat can be any adult-size chair with respect to depth and width.

Chapter Review

Review Questions

1. When are wheel locks used?
2. What are the indications for the following variations of wheelchair components?
   a. Desk-length armrests
   b. Full-length armrests
   c. Adjustable-height armrests
   d. Elevating legrests
   e. Footrests
3. How does a tilt-in-space wheelchair differ from a reclining-back wheelchair?
4. How is an amputee wheelchair frame different from a standard frame?
5. Describe how to measure an individual for a wheelchair, including seat width, seat depth, seat-to-footplate length, back height, and armrest height.
6. How do wheelchair cushions affect measurements used to determine wheelchair fit?
7. What are the effects of inappropriate seat depth, seat width, or armrest height on sitting posture?
8. What is the effect of inappropriate footplate-to-seat distance on sitting posture?
9. What are the standard wheelchair sizes?

Suggested Activities

1. Practice as both therapist and patient using a variety of wheelchair components and types.
2. Remove, adjust, and replace all components on the available wheelchairs.
3. Measure available wheelchairs to determine size.
4. Measure several classmates to determine the correct wheelchair size for each person.
5. Review available wheelchairs and discuss which individuals would likely use the wheelchair as it is configured.
6. Practice teaching "patients and families" and other health-care providers how to adjust and handle wheelchairs correctly.
7. Document interventions and wheelchair measurements.

Case Studies

1. An 8-year-old boy with a diagnosis of cerebral palsy presents with spastic quadriplegia. He is nonambulatory and has difficulty adjusting position and maintaining head alignment. Make recommendations for a type of mobility device and components that would be appropriate.

2. A 17-year-old female is 10 weeks post complete T10 spinal cord injury. Prior to her injury, she participated on several elite sport teams. She has indicated that she will use a wheelchair rather than ambulate with crutches and orthosis. Indicate the measurements necessary to determine wheelchair size. Recommend the type of mobility device and components that would be appropriate.

3. A 67-year-old male with right hemiplegia following left CVA presents with slight spasticity and minimal voluntary control over both right extremities. Recommend the type of wheelchair and components that would be appropriate.

4. A 46-year-old female with a 20-year history of rheumatoid arthritis has significant involvement of all four extremities. She is able to walk only a few steps and stand for short periods. Recommend the type of mobility device and components that would be appropriate.

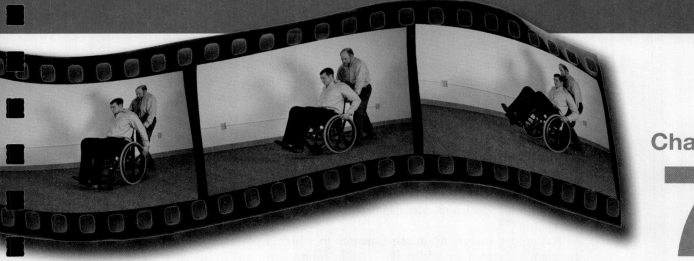

Transfers

Learning Objectives

Upon completion of this chapter, you will be able to:

1. List transfers, indicating those that are dependent, assisted, or independent.
2. Describe and correctly perform dependent, assisted, and independent transfers.
3. Describe types and levels of assistance used when transferring a patient.

Key Terms

Assisted transfers
Close guarding
Contact guarding
Dependent transfers
Gait or transfer belts
Generalizability

Independent transfers
Levels of assistance
Maximum assistance
Minimal assistance
Moderate assistance
Stand-by assistance

Introduction

The purpose of transfers is to permit patients to function in different environments or use different pieces of equipment. A goal of transfer training is generalizability. **Generalizability** means that some skills learned for one transfer can be used for other transfers. For example, the skills for transferring from a wheelchair to a bed are similar to skills for transferring from a wheelchair to a couch. With modifications of basic transfer skills, transfers into and out of bathtubs or cars or on and off toilets can also be achieved.

The transfer of a patient in or out of a wheelchair, bed, car, or cart may require the maximum assistance of several people, minimal assistance of one person, or no assistance at all. Each patient is examined, or a person knowledgeable about the patient's functional capabilities is interviewed, prior to determining an appropriate method of transfer. Physical therapists evaluate the results of the examination, which include strength, ROM, pain, cognitive ability, and movement dysfunction, to select an appropriate method of transfer that can be performed in a consistent, safe, and efficient manner. During rehabilitation, progression through levels, amounts, and types of assistance may occur.

Patient and physical therapist/assistant safety must not be compromised by the selection, or during the performance, of a transfer. Whenever in doubt about the level of assistance necessary to transfer a patient safely, obtain additional assistance. Always stabilize wheelchairs, carts, or beds by securing wheel locks or by other means (i.e., bracing against a wall). Using proper body mechanics reduces the possibility of injury. Before beginning practice of transfers, review material on body mechanics in Chapter 3.

■ **Take Note**
Safety of all involved in transfers is of paramount importance. When in doubt about the safety of a transfer, seek assistance.

Several systems[1] indicating the level, amount, and type of assistance a patient requires are in current use. Regardless of the system used, documentation of levels, amounts, and types of assistance for each patient is required for safe duplication of transfers.

Levels of Transfers

Independent transfers are those transfers in which a patient consistently performs all aspects of the transfer, including setup, in a safe manner and without assistance by additional clinicians. An example of an independent transfer can be a push up transfer.

Assisted transfers are those transfers in which a patient participates actively and requires assistance by additional (one or more) clinicians. Assisted transfers include, but are not limited to, two-person lift, sliding board transfer, squat pivot, and assisted standing pivot transfer.

Dependent transfers are those transfers in which a patient does not participate actively, or participates only minimally, and additional clinicians perform all aspects of the transfer. Dependent transfers include, but are not limited to, sliding transfer from cart to treatment table, three-person carry, dependent standing pivot transfer, and hydraulic lift transfer.

Some transfers may be assisted or independent, depending upon the physical capabilities of a patient. These include, but are not limited to, standing pivot, squat pivot, push-up, sliding board, wheelchair-to-floor, and floor-to-wheelchair transfers.

Levels of Assistance

Indicating the level and amount of assistance required by a patient during a dependent or assisted transfer provides clinicians with information necessary for completing a transfer safely. **Levels of assistance** can be stated as stand-by (supervision), close guarding, contact guarding, minimal, moderate, and maximum assistance. **Stand-by assistance** is indicated for patients who can usually perform the activity without assistance by additional clinicians but do not do so consistently. Examples of stand-by assistance include verbal cues, assistance in problem solving during transfer, or assistance if an emergency arises. In such cases, additional clinicians are not necessarily in close proximity to the patient. **Close guarding** is indicated for patients who can usually perform the activity without assistance by clinicians but have a greater likelihood for needing physical assistance by additional clinicians for support or balance. In such cases additional clinicians are in close proximity to the patient, immediately ready to assist the patient. **Contact guarding** is indicated for patients who can usually perform the activity but have a significant likelihood of requiring physical assistance by additional clinicians for support or balance. In such cases additional clinicians maintain contact with the patient to be able to provide assistance immediately. **Minimal assistance** is indicated for patients who can perform at least 75 percent of the activity. **Moderate assistance** is indicated for patients who can perform at least 50 percent of the activity. **Maximum assistance** is indicated for patients who can perform less than 25 percent of the activity.

Amount of Assistance

When more than one person is required for safe transfers, the number is indicated by adding the number after the level of assistance, such as X2 when two people are required to complete the transfer safely. Therefore, an indication of the level and amount of assistance required when a patient requires moderate assistance of two people during a transfer would be "... moderate assist X2 ..."

■ **Take Note**

Levels of transfers—independent, assisted, dependent.

■ **Take Note**

Levels of assistance—maximum assistance, moderate assistance, minimal assistance, close guarding, contact guarding, stand-by assistance.

Type of Assistance

Type of assistance is indicated as verbal cuing, balance control, and physical assistance for lifting or supporting. For example, one patient may require minimal assistance for balance control. A second patient may require moderate assistance X2 for lifting. Yet a third patient may require stand-by (supervision) assistance for verbal cuing of instructions.

As a patient improves, the type of transfer may progress from dependent to assisted to independent. The amount of assistance may progress from maximum to none as the patient progresses. The type of assistance may progress from the physical therapist/assistant doing

■ Take Note

Types of assistance—physical assist, balance control, verbal cuing.

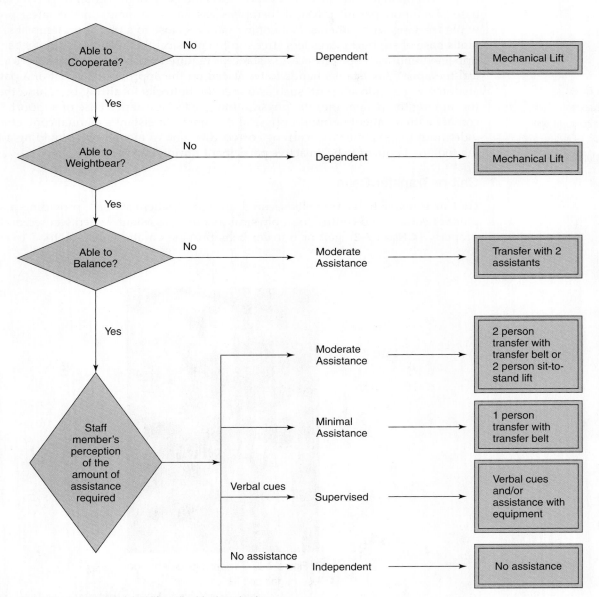

If unsure, use a mechanical lift until told otherwise by a therapist or staff member who can assess the patient and situation.

■ **Figure 7–1** Patient transfer assessment flow chart.

Source: OHSAH, 2002.

all of the lifting to the physical therapist/assistant using only verbal cuing. The goal is for the patient to achieve the maximum level of independent performance of a transfer that is consistent, safe, and efficient.

Algorithms can be used to assist in decision making concerning the selection of the type of transfer depending upon a patient's abilities, which are based on the physical therapist's evaluation. See ■ Figure 7-1.

General Rules

Body Mechanics

Proper attention to body mechanics and the relationship of the center of gravity and the base of support permit physical therapists/assistants to maintain the safest position while working with patients. Positioning patients close to a physical therapist's/assistant's base of support places less stress on the physical therapist's/assistant's back and upper extremities when physical assistance is required. Such positioning allows a physical therapist's/assistant's hands to be placed on the appropriate aspect of a patient's anatomy to provide support, such as under the buttocks for lifting or behind the hips for moving the patient into the physical therapist's/assistant's base of support. Direct contact with a patient permits a physical therapist's/assistant's manual contact to provide input to the patient concerning correct direction of movement, providing a learning tool for a patient to be an active participant during transfers.

■ **Take Note**

Hand placement should provide control of, and feedback to, patients during transfers.

Gait or Transfer Belts

Gait or transfer belts are belts secured around a patient's waist, providing a secure point of contact and control for a physical therapist/assistant. When secured and used properly (■ Figure 7–2), gait or transfer belts provide an alternative method to control

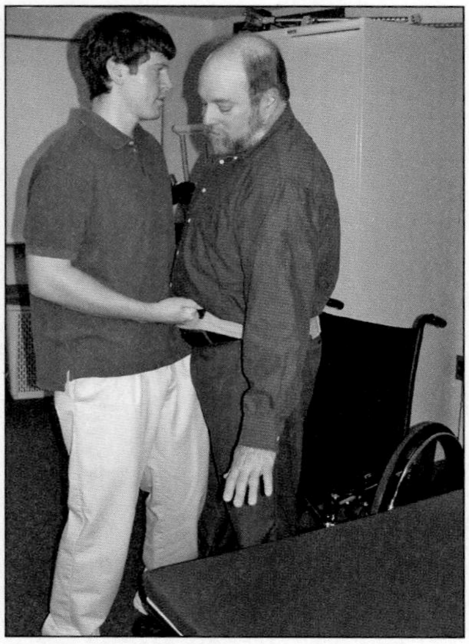

■ **Figure 7–2** Proper placement and use of gait belt for a transfer.

patient motion during transfers. When direct manual contact cannot be safely maintained, such as with an extremely large patient or a patient with wounds or lesions that limit places for contact, a gait or transfer belt provides a safe method of controlling a patient. When a transfer belt is used, patients should be kept in close proximity to the physical therapist/assistant and not at arm's length.

When held at arm's length, a patient is not fully supported and the physical therapist/assistant is at greater risk for injury to the back and upper extremity. This occurs because improper use of gait or transfer belts reduces safety for both patients and physical therapists/assistants by moving a patient's center of mass away from the physical therapist's/assistant's base of support. Gait or transfer belts must not become only a handle for maneuvering patients during transfers. Simply pushing, pulling, or lifting on gait or transfer belts alone does not provide specific support needed by patients during transfers. Gait or transfer belts do not provide the guidance that manual contact can to help patients understand the direction of movement required and to become an active participant in performing a transfer (■ Figure 7–3). Inappropriate use of gait belts during transfers may not allow the gait belt to retain its correct position. Use of a gait or transfer belt should not eliminate a physical therapist/assistant providing appropriate contact to stabilize the supporting lower extremity during transfer (see *Assisting Standing Pivot Transfer*).

■ **Take Note**

When using transfer belts, ensure patients are able to participate appropriately in the transfer.

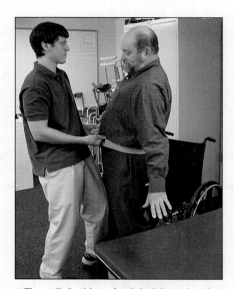

■ **Figure 7–3**   Use of gait belt in a situation where physical therapist/assistant does not retain appropriate manual contacts for the transfer.

In some settings or jurisdictions, gait or transfer belts may be required equipment. Each physical therapist is responsible for determining the administrative and legal requirements of practicing in a specific setting or jurisdiction. Administrative or legal requirements for specific equipment exist in an effort to limit injury or liability. When specific equipment must be used, users must adhere to proper application and use of the equipment.

Preparing the Environment

When preparing the environment for transfers, consider the direction in which the patient will move—to the left or right. Generally, when patients have more involvement on one side than the other, transferring toward the stronger side is easier. This direction can be used during initial transfers to ensure success and bolster a patient's confidence. Patients, however, need to be able to transfer to both sides, and transfers should be practiced to both sides. Specific considerations for preparing the environment for each type of transfer will be covered later in this chapter. Additional considerations for preparing an environment can be found in Chapter 3.

Clinicians performing transfers should avoid wearing jewelry that can become entangled or scratch patients during patient care. Such jewelry must be removed before patient contact is initiated. For example, watches and rings need to be removed before sliding arms under or around a patient.

■ **Take Note**

Patients need to be able to transfer to both sides.

Instructions and Verbal Cues

Patients should always be informed about the transfer to be performed and what they are expected to do. Explanations must be provided in a manner understood by patients, using nontechnical terms and employing a language interpreter if necessary.

Counts and commands are used to synchronize actions of all participants in the transfer. When assistance of more than one person is required for a transfer, the physical therapist/assistant at the head of the patient is in charge and is responsible for successful completion of the transfer. The physical therapist/assistant in charge explains how the transfer will be conducted and indicates the responsibilities of each participant. Counting is used to provide a cue for the ensuing command, allowing all participants to be ready for it. Specific terms, such as "lift," are used to indicate the command. Commands are the specific action word that participants are to perform when the command term is given. An appropriate count and command is "One, two, three, lift." An inappropriate count and command is "One, two, three" because the count "three" is not a specific action command. The physical therapist/assistant in charge describes the counts and commands that will be given and subsequently gives the counts and commands. For example, the sequence of directions and language used by the physical therapist/assistant in charge might be

■ **Take Note**

The person at the patient's head is in charge. Counts are cues for all involved. Commands are action words.

1. "I will count to three and then give the command to lift."
2. "When I say 'lift,' we will lift."
3. The physical therapist/assistant checks visually and verbally to ensure that all assistants and the patient are ready before the transfer is initiated.
4. The physical therapist/assistant says "One, two, three, lift."

Completing the Transfer

A transfer is not complete until the patient is safely and securely in the new position, at which time contact with and control of the patient can be released. Appropriate positioning and draping must be completed, and necessary equipment should be placed within usable reach of the patient. The patient must feel secure in his or her new position. Only then is a transfer considered complete.

■ **Take Note**

Transfers are not complete until patients are safe, appropriately positioned/draped, and the environment is arranged as required.

PROCEDURE 7–1   Sliding Transfer: Cart to Treatment Table

This transfer can be used to transfer a patient between two treatment tables, a treatment table and cart, or a cart and bed. The cart should be positioned parallel to, and against, the treatment table and secured with the patient's head at the head of the treatment table or cart.

When a patient can perform this transfer with stand-by or minimal assistance, one person may assist by stabilizing the cart and, when necessary, providing minimal verbal or physical assistance.

When a dependent transfer is required, three clinicians are needed. A "draw" sheet may be used to move ("draw") the patient from cart to treatment table.

Authors' note: In the following illustrations, two treatment tables are used. The first treatment table represents a cart or gurney and will be referred to as a cart. The second treatment table represents a treatment table or bed and will be referred to as a treatment table.

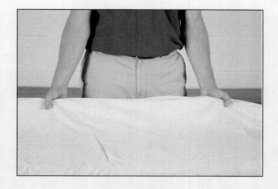

1. A draw sheet is placed under the patient. The strongest and safest way to grasp a "draw" sheet is to supinate the forearms

2. The portion of the sheet to the patient's sides is rolled and grasped close to the patient. A stronger grip is created when grasping with the forearm supinated.

   The physical therapist/assistant at the patient's head should be on the side to which the patient is moving. This physical therapist/assistant is responsible for coordinating the transfer by instructing the patient and assistants, determining when everyone is ready, and issuing the counts and commands.

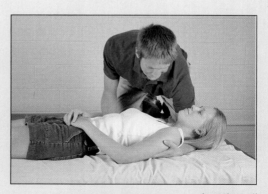

3. When patients are unable to control the head and neck, the physical therapist/assistant at the patient's head supports the patient's head by placing one arm under the patient's shoulders while cradling the patient's head.

(continued)

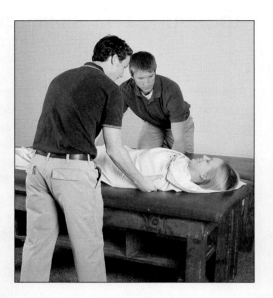

④ When a patient's extraneous movements cannot be controlled during a transfer, or if a patient is agitated, wrap a sheet around the patient to provide control of the patient's extremities.

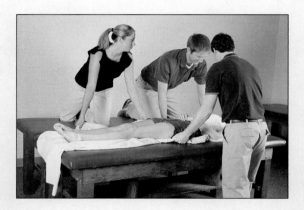

⑤ Two people, the physical therapist/assistant at the patient's head and the assistant at the lower extremities, stand on the side to which the patient is to be moved and grasp the sheet close to the patient. One assistant stands on the other side and grasps the sheet with one hand at the patient's shoulder and the other hand at the patient's hip. When the two people on the side to which the patient is to be moved are not able to reach across the treatment table to lift the patient, they may kneel on the treatment table.

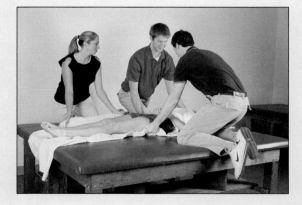

⑥ Upon the physical therapist's/assistant's counts and commands, the patient is lifted and moved part of the way from the cart onto the treatment table.

7 Once the patient has been moved part way onto the treatment table, the people on the side to which the patient is being moved remove themselves from the treatment table. The assistant on the side from which the patient is being moved may kneel on the cart to complete the transfer. The transfer is completed by finishing movement of the patient to the treatment table.

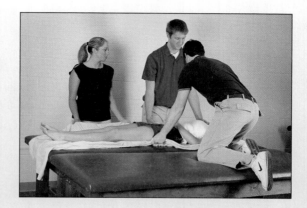

PROCEDURE 7–2 Three-Person Carry

This is a dependent transfer used to transfer a patient between two treatment tables, a treatment table and cart, or a cart and bed. When the two surfaces cannot be arranged parallel to each other, or a sliding transfer is deemed unsafe, a three-person carry is used. As the name of the transfer implies, three people are required to transfer an average-size adult.

A cart is positioned and secured at a right angle to a treatment table, with the head of the cart at the foot of the table or the foot of the cart at the head of the table.

Authors' note: In the following photos, two treatment tables are used. The first treatment table represents a cart or gurney and will be referred to as a cart. The second treatment table represents a treatment table or bed and will be referred to as a treatment table.

■ **Take Note**
Cart-to-treatment-table is a dependent transfer, requiring three people to transfer the patient safely.

■ **Take Note**
A tall or heavy patient may require four people to complete the transfer safely.

1 All three clinicians stand on the same side of the cart and are positioned in such a manner that one can support the head and upper trunk, one can support the midsection, and one can support the lower extremities. The strongest person should be at the patient's head or middle position. The tallest person, if strong enough, should be at the patient's head. The physical therapist/assistant at the head of the patient is responsible for instructing the patient, determining when everyone is ready, and issuing counts and commands. Clinicians stand in stride, with their feet slightly apart and knees flexed.

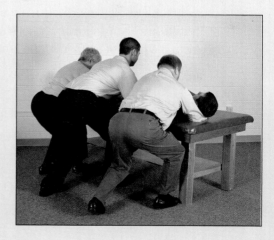

(continued)

2 Clinicians slide their arms under the patient such that their elbows are on the cart and the patient is cradled from head to foot.

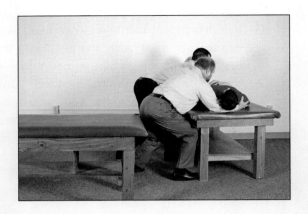

3 Upon command, the patient is moved to the edge of the cart.

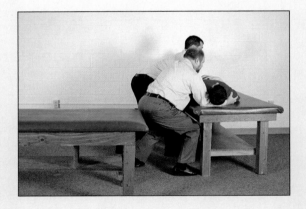

4 By flexing elbows, clinicians log-roll the patient onto his side such that he is facing the clinicians. The patient is now cradled in the bend of the elbows, bringing the patient's weight closer to the base of support of the clinicians.

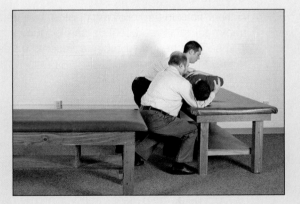

5 Upon command, clinicians stand, lifting the patient from the cart.

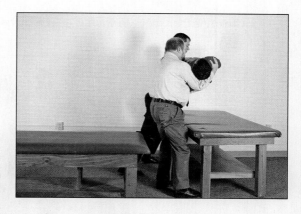

6 Upon command, clinicians walk backward to pivot 90 degrees.

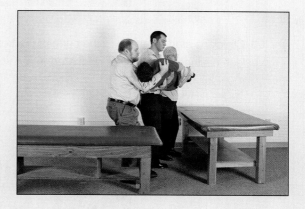

7 Upon completion of the 90-degree pivot, clinicians are aligned parallel to the treatment table.

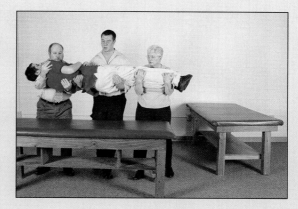

(continued)

8 Clinicians then move forward in unison to the treatment table.

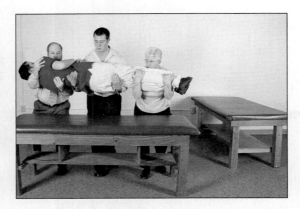

9 Clinicians stand in stride at the edge of the treatment table. Upon command, clinicians flex their legs until their elbows rest on the edge of the treatment table, lowering the patient to the treatment table.

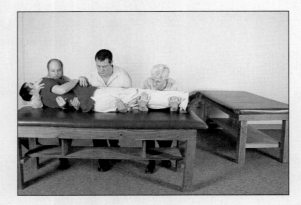

10 The patient is uncradled onto the treatment table, moved to the center of the treatment table, and positioned in proper alignment. Clinicians then remove their arms carefully.

■ **Take Note**

Commands for a three-person transfer—move, curl, lift, pivot, walk, down, done.

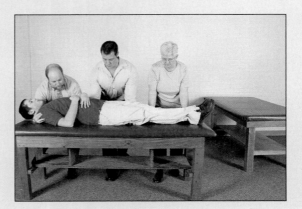

Hydraulic Lift

Hydraulic lifts are mechanical devices that provide a method for one person to transfer a dependent patient. Hydraulic lifts have caster wheels for positioning and maneuvering.

The base of hydraulic lifts can be widened to fit around a wheelchair or other equipment. The base is placed in the narrow position when the patient is being moved to make maneuvering easier. To change the width of the base, the long lever attached to the base is moved from one side to the other (■ Figures 7–4 and ■ 7–5). This lever is locked by either a slotted mechanism at the bottom of the lever or by a cam locking mechanism that is activated and deactivated by twisting the lever.

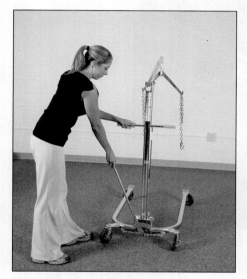

■ **Figure 7–4**   Narrowing the base of a hydraulic lift.

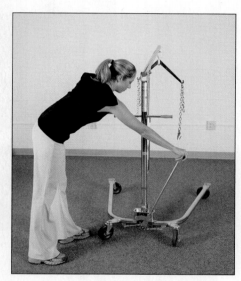

■ **Figure 7–5**   Widening the base of a hydraulic lift.

A hydraulic release valve (■ Figure 7–6) on the front of the lift's upright is closed to allow the arm of the hydraulic lift to be raised and opened slowly to allow lowering of the lift arm. After checking that the hydraulic release valve is closed, a physical therapist/assistant pumps the handle to raise the arm of the hydraulic lift (■ Figure 7–7).

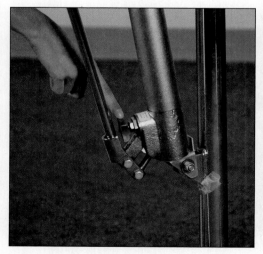

■ **Figure 7–6**   Hydraulic release valve knob for lift arm.

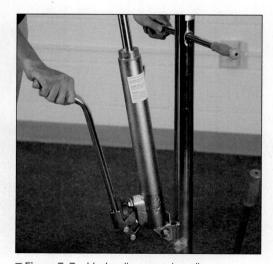

■ **Figure 7–7**   Hydraulic pump handle.

Patients are supported by a sling, which is attached to a spreader bar on the lift arm, by two chains with hooks (■ Figure 7–8). Chain lengths may be adjusted to accommodate the height of each patient. The chains are attached to each side of the spreader bar such that each chain is divided into two unequal segments. The shorter segment will be attached to the upper part of the sling, supporting the patient's back. The longer segment will be attached to the lower part of the sling, supporting the patient's lower extremities. In this way, the patient is lifted in a sitting position.

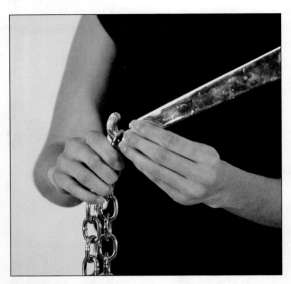

■ **Figure 7–8** Attaching chains to spreader bar.

■ **Take Note**

When a one-piece sling is used, the lower edge of the sling should be just proximal to the knees.

Slings are made of a variety of fabrics. Some are one piece and others are two pieces. Slings are positioned so seams are on the outside, away from the patient, to avoid pressure areas. Chain hooks are attached from the inside of the sling to the outside (■ Figure 7–9). This reduces the likelihood of patients being injured by the hook.

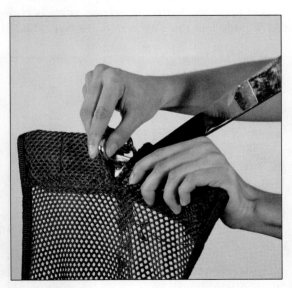

■ **Figure 7–9** Attaching chain hooks to sling.

PROCEDURE 7–3   Using a Hydraulic Lift

The following illustrations present a transfer from a treatment table to a wheelchair.

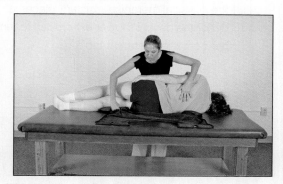

1. When a patient is on a cart, treatment table, or bed, the physical therapist/assistant can position a sling under the patient by rolling the patient onto one side and properly positioning a sling on the treatment table.

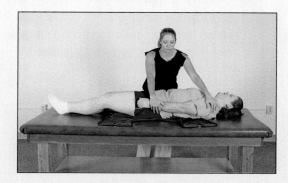

2. The physical therapist/assistant rolls the patient onto the sling. If necessary, the physical therapist/assistant rolls the patient onto her other side to allow proper alignment of the sling under the patient.

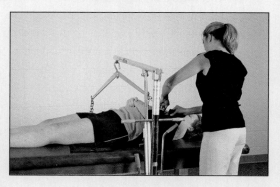

3. Once a patient is positioned on the sling, the physical therapist/assistant moves the hydraulic lift into position with the spreader bar suspended across the patient. Both ends of each chain are attached to their respective sides of the sling.

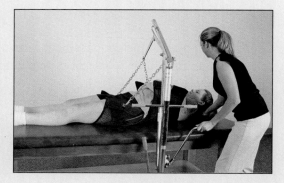

4. With the hydraulic release valve closed, a physical therapist/assistant pumps the handle to lift the patient to a safe sitting position.

(continued)

⑤ As a patient is lifted above the treatment table, the physical therapist/assistant places an arm under the patient's lower extremities to remove her from the treatment table.

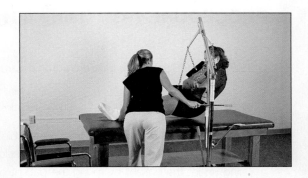

⑥ Cradling a patient's lower extremities, the physical therapist/assistant rotates the lower extremities from over the treatment table and allows the sling to provide full support.

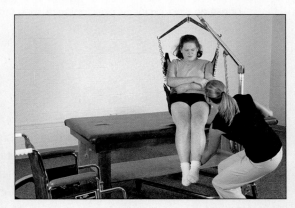

⑦ The physical therapist/assistant may need to steady the patient to prevent excessive sway as the lift, with patient, is maneuvered. The physical therapist/assistant moves the patient to a locked wheelchair. The physical therapist/assistant places the base of the lift in the wide position to fit around the perimeter of the wheelchair.

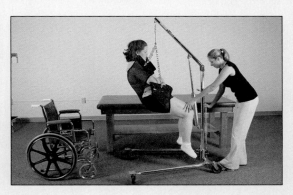

⑧ The physical therapist/assistant maneuvers the lift to position a patient directly over the seat of a locked wheelchair.

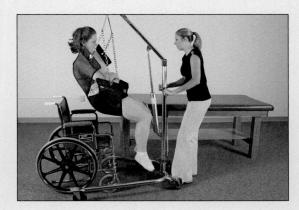

9 The physical therapist/assistant slowly opens the hydraulic release valve to lower the patient into a wheelchair. Seating a patient properly in a wheelchair requires the physical therapist/assistant to apply slight pressure in the horizontal plane at the knees or thighs. This positions a patient into the wheelchair such that her back is resting firmly against the back of the wheelchair.

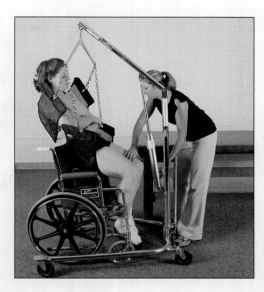

■ **Take Note**
Caution—The wheelchair may tip slightly as the patient is lowered into the wheelchair.

10 Once a patient is seated in the wheelchair, the physical therapist/assistant closes the hydraulic release valve to avoid the potential of the lift arm lowering further and striking the patient.

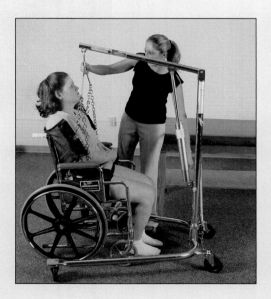

■ **Take Note**
Caution—Control the lift arm to avoid striking the patient.

(continued)

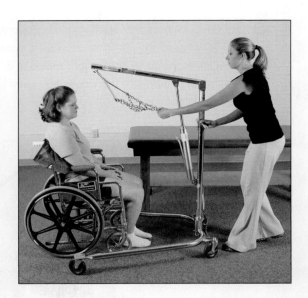

⑪ After determining that a patient can maintain sitting without assistance, a physical therapist/assistant removes the chains from the sling and moves the hydraulic lift away from the patient. The physical therapist/assistant must ensure that the spreader bar and chains do not swing and strike a patient as the lift is removed.

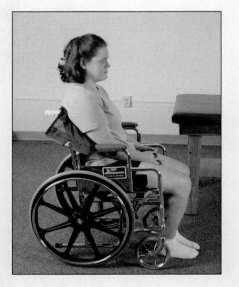

⑫ A one-piece sling is left in place under the patient, hence the initial need to position a sling appropriately to avoid pressure from the seams.

⑬ The physical therapist/assistant secures the wheelchair's pelvic stabilizer and properly places the patient's feet on footrests. When a two-piece sling has been used, the physical therapist/assistant may remove the upper portion of the sling, which is behind the patient's back, while the portion under the patient's thighs remains in place.

PROCEDURE 7–4   Two-Person Lift

Wheelchair to Floor

The two-person lift transfer is an assisted transfer with maximum assistance of two clinicians. This transfer is often used to move a patient between a wheelchair and the floor when the patient has some upper extremity strength and trunk control.

1 A patient participates in this transfer by crossing her upper extremities in front of the trunk. Standing behind the patient, a physical therapist/assistant reaches under the patient's upper extremities and grasps the opposite wrists of the patient (left on right and right on left). This prevents the patient from abducting the upper extremities during the lift. Patients must be able to maintain an upper extremity position of shoulder girdle depression, shoulder extension, adduction, internal rotation, and elbow flexion at approximately 90 degrees to assist in successful completion of the transfer.

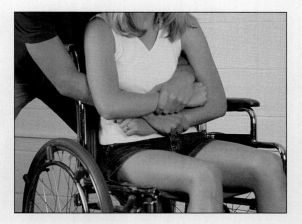

■ **Take Note**
Caution—Be sure to grasp patient's right wrist with your left hand and the patient's left wrist with your right hand.

2 To prepare for a two-person lift transfer, the physical therapist/assistant positions a wheelchair close, and parallel, to the surface to which a patient will be transferred. The physical therapist/assistant engages the wheel locks and removes the patient's feet from the footrests. The physical therapist/assistant raises the footplates and removes the footrests (when possible) or swings the footrests out of the way. The physical therapist/assistant removes the armrest from the side of the wheelchair to which the patient will be transferred.

(continued)

③ The physical therapist/assistant at the head of the patient places one foot on either side of the drive wheel and leans around the push handle on the side to which the transfer will occur. A second physical therapist/assistant faces in the direction of the intended transfer, with feet in stride and hips and knees flexed. This physical therapist/assistant places one arm under the patient's thighs and the other arm under the legs. The position of both physical therapists/assistants may be modified, depending upon the sizes of the patient and physical therapist/assistant and the environment in which the transfer will occur.

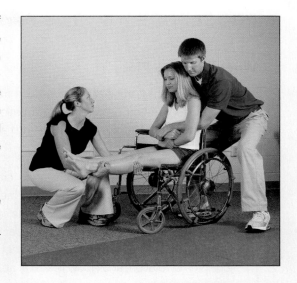

④ On command from the physical therapist/assistant at the head of the patient, both clinicians straighten, lifting the patient to a height that ensures clearance of all parts of the wheelchair.

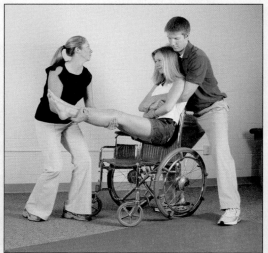

⑤ In unison, the physical therapists/assistants step to the side (physical therapist/assistant at patient's head) or forward (physical therapist/assistant supporting lower extremities), moving away from the wheelchair.

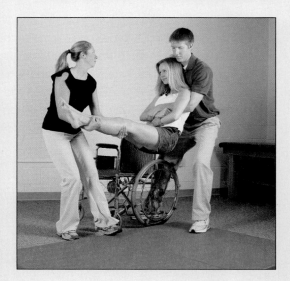

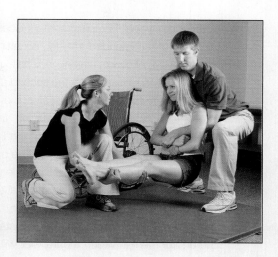

6 Both physical therapists/assistants squat, using good body mechanics to lower the patient to the floor.

7 Physical therapists/assistants continue contact for support until the patient is able to maintain a safe and comfortable position.

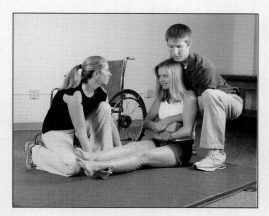

Floor to Wheelchair

To prepare for a two-person lift transfer, the physical therapist/assistant positions a wheelchair close, and parallel, to the surface from which a patient will be transferred. The physical therapist/assistant engages the wheel locks and raises the footplates. The physical therapist/assistant removes the footrests from the wheelchair (when possible) or swings them out of the way. The physical therapist/assistant removes the armrest from the side of the wheelchair closest to the patient.

1 A patient participates in this transfer by crossing her upper extremities in front of the trunk. Squatting behind the patient, a physical therapist/assistant reaches under the patient's upper extremities and grasps the opposite wrists of the patient (left on right and right on left). This prevents the patient from abducting the upper extremities during the lift. Patients must be able to maintain an upper extremity position of shoulder girdle depression, shoulder extension, adduction, internal rotation, and elbow flexion at approximately 90 degrees to assist in successful completion of the transfer.

(continued)

➋ A second physical therapist/assistant faces in the direction of the intended transfer, squatting with feet in stride. Although starting in a half-kneeling position may seem easier for the second physical therapist/assistant, this necessitates movement into a squatting position, increasing the risk of injury to all participants. This physical therapist/assistant places one arm under the patient's thighs and the other arm under the legs. The position of both physical therapists/assistants may be modified, depending upon the sizes of the patient and physical therapist/assistant and the environment in which the transfer will occur.

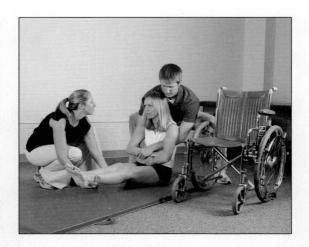

➌ On command from the physical therapist/assistant at the head of the patient, the clinicians lift the patient to a height that ensures clearance of all parts of the wheelchair.

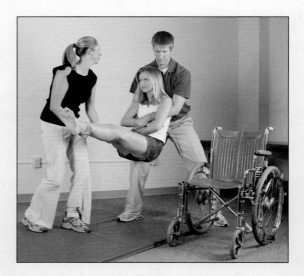

➍ In unison, the physical therapists/assistants step to the side (physical therapist/assistant at patient's head) or forward (physical therapist/assistant supporting lower extremities), moving toward the wheelchair. The physical therapists/assistants move until the patient is centered over the seat of the wheelchair. The physical therapist/assistant supporting the patient's lower extremities gently pulls the patient's lower extremities away from the back of the wheelchair so the patient will clear the upright of the back of the wheelchair. Once the patient clears the back upright of the wheelchair, the patient must be pushed toward the back of the wheelchair for the assumption of proper sitting posture.

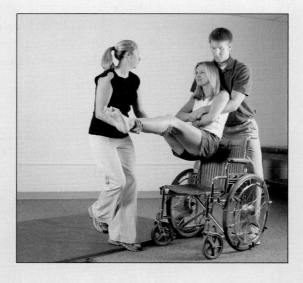

⑤ Physical therapists/assistants continue contact for support until the patient is able to maintain a safe and comfortable position. When the patient is seated in a position she can maintain, the physical therapist/assistant secures the pelvic stabilizer, replaces the armrest and footrests, and places the patient's feet on the footrests.

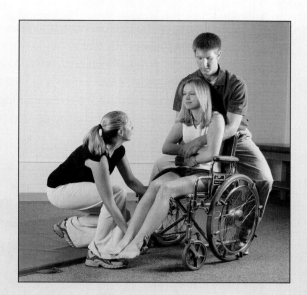

PROCEDURE 7–5   Dependent Standing Pivot

The dependent standing pivot transfer is an assisted transfer with maximum assistance of one person. The dependent standing pivot transfer is used for patients who are unable to stand independently but can bear some weight on their lower extremities. This includes patients with weakness, paresis, or paralysis.

❶ To perform a dependent standing pivot transfer, the physical therapist/assistant places a wheelchair parallel to a treatment table or bed and engages the wheel locks.

❷ The physical therapist/assistant places the patient's feet on the floor, raises the footplates, and removes the footrests from the wheelchair when possible, or swings them out of the way.

❸ The physical therapist/assistant removes the armrest nearest the treatment table.

❹ To facilitate clearing the wheel, the physical therapist/assistant moves the patient to the front edge of the wheelchair seat.

❺ To provide stability for the patient's lower extremities during the transfer, the physical therapist/assistant must "block" the patient's lower extremities. Blocking the lower extremities is performed in different ways for different transfers. In this transfer, the physical therapist/assistant blocks by placing his feet and knees outside the patient's feet and knees, with the physical therapist/assistant holding the patient's knees between his knees. The physical therapist/

(continued)

assistant places the foot closest to the treatment table a little behind the other foot, placing the physical therapist's/assistant's feet in stride. After the physical therapist/assistant blocks patient's lower extremities, the physical therapist/assistant places his hands under the patient's buttocks. The physical therapist/assistant must create and maintain a static spinal posture throughout this transfer. The position of a physical therapist/assistant may be modified, depending upon the sizes of patient and physical therapist/assistant and the environment in which the transfer will occur.

■ **Take Note**
Caution—Protect your back by performing isometric contraction of trunk muscles and lifting using the leg muscles.

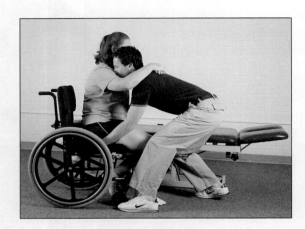

6 The patient rests her head on the shoulder of the physical therapist/assistant. It is best if the shoulder used is the shoulder on the side of the physical therapist/assistant opposite the direction in which the pivot will occur.

An alternative is to have the patient place her upper extremities around the physical therapist's/assistant's upper back and **not** around the physical therapist's/assistant's neck. The purpose of the placement of the patient's arms in this method is to provide control for the patient's upper trunk, and not for the patient to "pull" on the therapist. To avoid injury, the physical therapist/assistant maintains static spinal posture throughout the transfer.

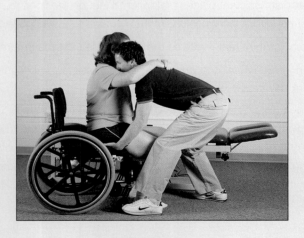

7 To synchronize the efforts of the physical therapist/assistant and patient, the physical therapist/assistant provides counts and commands ("One, two, three, up."). As the physical therapist/assistant counts, he initiates a rocking motion in time with the counts to develop momentum. On the command "up," the physical therapist/assistant lifts the patient from the wheelchair. The lift is only high enough to clear the wheelchair and the height of the treatment table.

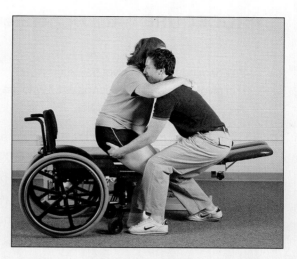

8 The physical therapist/assistant pivots toward the treatment table, rotating the patient to the proper position for sitting on the table. The physical therapist/assistant lowers the patient to a sitting position.

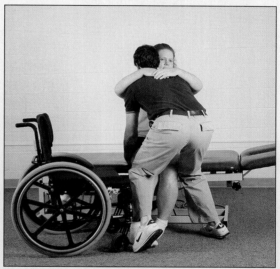

9 A physical therapist/assistant must continue contact for support until a patient is able to maintain a safe and comfortable position.

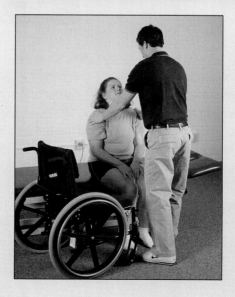

PROCEDURE 7–6   Dependent Sitting Pivot

The dependent sitting pivot transfer is a variation of the standing pivot transfer. The dependent sitting pivot transfer is used for patients who are unable to stand independently but can bear some weight on their lower extremities. This includes patients with weakness, paresis, or paralysis.

❶ To perform a dependent sitting pivot transfer, the physical therapist/assistant places a wheelchair parallel to a treatment table or bed and engages the wheel locks.

❷ The physical therapist/assistant places the patient's feet on the floor, raises the footplates, and removes the footrests from the wheelchair when possible, or swings them out of the way.

❸ The physical therapist/assistant removes the armrest nearest the treatment table.

❹ To facilitate clearing the wheel, the physical therapist/assistant moves the patient to the front edge of the wheelchair seat.

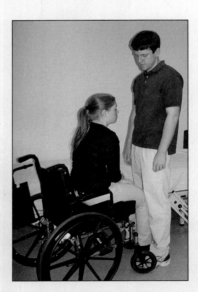

❺ To provide stability for the patient's lower extremities during the transfer, the physical therapist/assistant must "block" the patient's lower extremities. Blocking the lower extremities is performed in different ways for different transfers. In this transfer, the physical therapist/assistant blocks by placing his feet and knees outside the patient's feet and knees, with the physical therapist/assistant holding the patient's knees between his knees. The physical therapist/assistant places the foot closest to the treatment table a little behind the other foot, placing the physical therapist's/assistant's feet in stride. The physical therapist/assistant must create and maintain a static spinal posture throughout this transfer. The position of a physical therapist/assistant may be modified, depending upon the sizes of patient and physical therapist/assistant and the environment in which the transfer will occur.

6 The patient flexes forward and rests her head and upper body on her legs or on the hip/thigh of the physical therapist/assistant. It is best if the hip/thigh used is the hip/thigh on the side of the physical therapist/assistant opposite the direction in which the pivot will occur. After the patient's lower extremities are blocked and the patient has flexed forward, the physical therapist/assistant places his hands under the patient's buttocks.

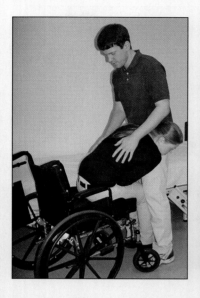 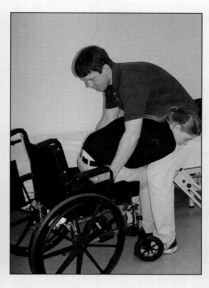

■ **Take Note**
Caution—patient must have flexibility of the spine and hips to achieve the starting position.

7 To synchronize the effort of the physical therapist/assistant and patient, the physical therapist/assistant provides counts and commands ("One, two, three, move."). As the physical therapist/assistant counts, he initiates a rocking motion in time with the counts to develop momentum. On the command "move," the physical therapist/assistant lifts the patient from the wheelchair. The lift is only high enough to clear the wheelchair and the height of the treatment table.

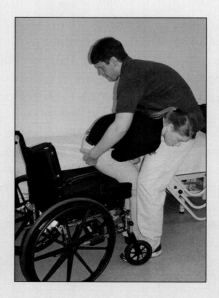

(continued)

8 The physical therapist/assistant pivots toward the treatment table, rotating the patient to the proper position for sitting on the table. The physical therapist/assistant lowers the patient to a sitting position. Physical therapists/assistants must continue contact for support until patients are able to maintain a safe and comfortable position.

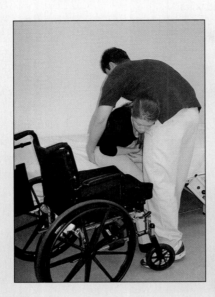 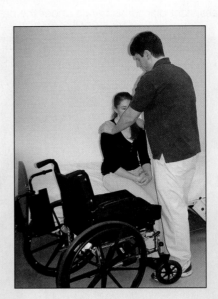

PROCEDURE 7–7 Sliding Board

The sliding board transfer is an assisted or independent transfer that may require moderate assistance of two clinicians to no assistance at all. The sliding board transfer is used when patients have enough strength to lift most of the weight off the buttocks and sufficient sitting balance to move in a sitting position, but are not able to perform push-up transfers.

■ **Take Note**

Hand placement—To assist with lifting, place hands under patient's buttocks. To assist with balance, place hands on patient's shoulders.

When performing a one-person assisted transfer, a physical therapist/assistant guards a patient by standing in front of the patient and may block the patient's knees to prevent the patient from sliding off the sliding board. When assistance in lifting is required, a physical therapist/assistant does so by placing the hands under a patient's buttocks and lifting as the patient performs the push-up. When a patient needs assistance for balance, a physical therapist/assistant can place the hands on the patient's shoulders. Assistance for lifting or balance is decreased as a patient improves.

Authors' note: In the illustrations presenting the sliding board transfer, assistance is being provided for balance.

1 To perform a sliding board transfer, the physical therapist/assistant positions a wheelchair parallel, or at a slight angle, to a treatment table or bed, and engages the wheel locks. The physical therapist/assistant places the patient's feet on the floor, raises the footplates, and removes the footrests from the wheelchair when possible, or swings them out of the way. The patient moves forward to the front of the wheelchair seat. The physical therapist/assistant removes the armrest from the side nearest the treatment table.

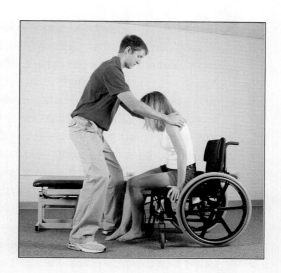

2 The patient leans away from the treatment table and the physical therapist/assistant helps the patient place a sliding board well under the buttocks. Be careful not to pinch the patient between the sliding board and the wheelchair seat.

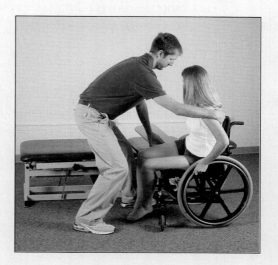

3 The patient returns to an upright sitting position, with the buttock nearest the treatment table resting on the sliding board.

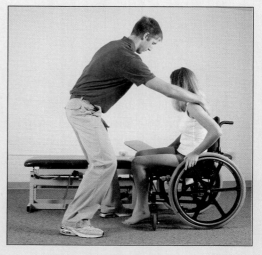

(continued)

④ The patient performs the transfer by doing a series of push-ups and slides sideways. Extending the upper extremities, accompanied by shoulder depression, allows a patient to lift her body and decrease the weight of the buttocks on the sliding board. Reducing body weight on the buttocks, and thus sliding board, allows a patient to slide toward the treatment table. A patient may place palms flat on the sliding board or make a fist and place the outside of the fists on the sliding board to achieve higher lift during push-ups. Wheelchair armrests can be used for the first few push-ups to achieve higher lift. Patients must not grasp the edge of the sliding board, which places the distal ends of fingers under the sliding board, causing fingers to be pinched as push-ups are performed.

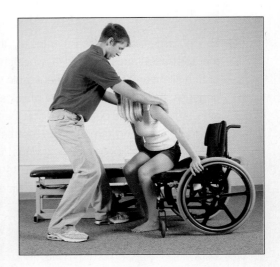

⑤ With the patient repositioning her hands, this sequence is repeated until the patient is on the treatment table and only one buttock remains on the sliding board.

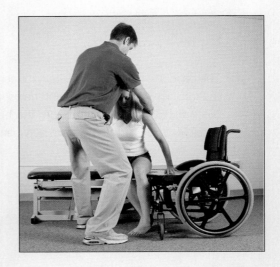

⑥ The patient leans away from the wheelchair to remove the sliding board. A physical therapist/assistant must continue contact for support until the patient is able to maintain a safe and comfortable position.

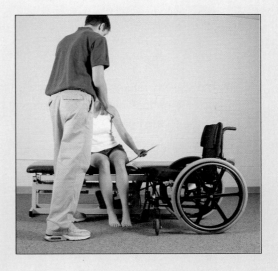

The transfer from treatment table to the wheelchair using a sliding board is essentially the same. Follow the steps below.

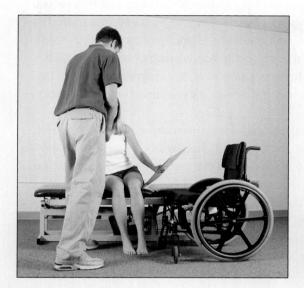

1 Placing sliding board.

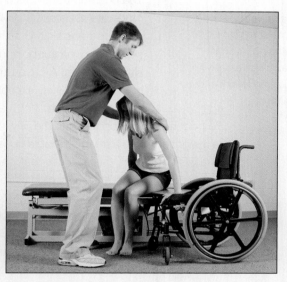

2 Pushing up and sliding.

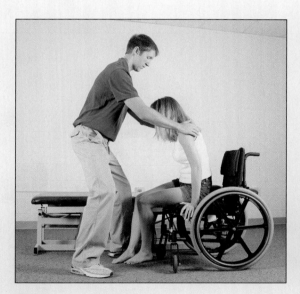

3 Sliding into wheelchair.

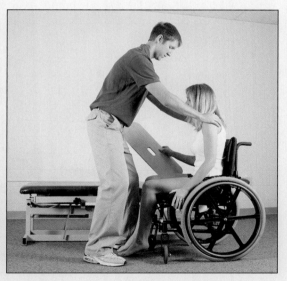

4 Removing sliding board.

PROCEDURE 7–8 Push-Up

■ **Take Note**

Push-up transfers require patients to have more strength and balance than necessary for sliding board transfers.

The push-up transfer is an assisted or independent transfer that may require moderate assistance varying from two clinicians to no assistance at all. The push-up transfer is used when patients have enough strength to lift themselves from the supporting surface and sufficient sitting balance to move in a sitting position. A push-up transfer is performed in a manner similar to a sliding board transfer, except that a push-up transfer does not use a sliding board for support.

To perform a push-up transfer, the physical therapist/assistant places a wheelchair parallel, or at a slight angle, to a treatment table or bed and engages the wheel locks. The physical therapist/assistant places the patient's feet on the floor, raises the footplates, and removes the footrests from the wheelchair when possible, or swings them out of the way. The patient moves forward to the front of the wheelchair seat. The physical therapist/assistant removes the armrest from the side nearest the treatment table.

The patient performs the transfer by doing a series of push-ups and moves sideways. Extending the upper extremities, accompanied by shoulder depression, allow a patient to lift her body and move to the table/bed. The physical therapist/assistant guards at the knees to prevent the patient from sliding too far forward, and at the patient's shoulders for balance. As a patient's capabilities progress, a push-up transfer may be completed using only one push-up.

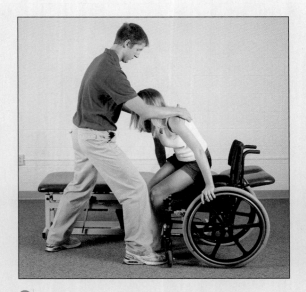

❶ Pushing up to perform push-up transfer.

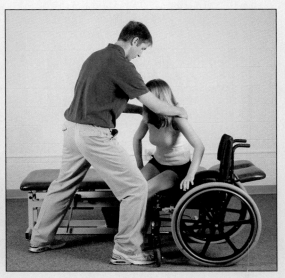

❷ Lowering from a push-up.

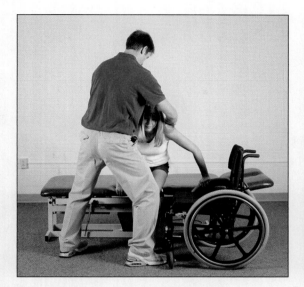

③ Pushing up to treatment table.

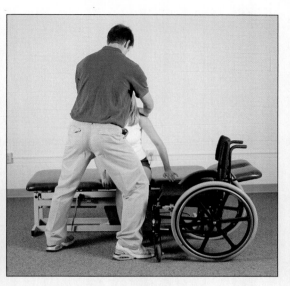

④ Lowering onto treatment table.

A push-up transfer from treatment table to a wheelchair is essentially the same. Follow the steps below.

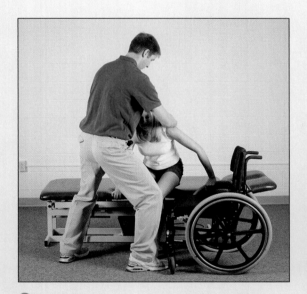

① Starting to return to wheelchair from treatment table.

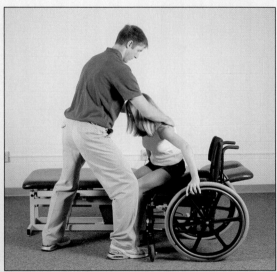

② Midpoint of return to wheelchair from treatment table.

(continued)

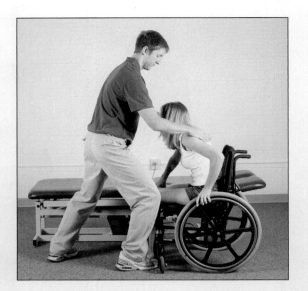

③ Completing return to wheelchair from treatment table.

A physical therapist/assistant must continue contact for support until a patient is able to maintain a safe and comfortable position.

PROCEDURE 7–9 Assist to Front of Wheelchair Seat

A patient must be able to maneuver to the front of a wheelchair seat prior to standing or performing transfers. Sitting on the front of a wheelchair seat allows patients to get their center of gravity over their base of support rapidly and easily as they assume standing. When patients are unable to maneuver forward in a wheelchair independently, several methods can be used to assist. As a patient's ability improves, assistance is reduced until the patient is performing the task independently.

To perform these movements, the physical therapist/assistant positions a wheelchair where desired and engages the wheel locks. The physical therapist/assistant places the patient's feet on the floor, raises the footplates, and removes the footrests from the wheelchair when possible or swings them out of the way.

Side-to-Side Weight Shifting

1 In the side-to-side weight shifting method, a physical therapist/assistant assists a patient to the front of a wheelchair seat by placing one arm around the patient's shoulders from one side and the other arm under the thigh of the opposite lower extremity.

2 The physical therapist/assistant shifts the patient's weight to the side of shoulder support to reduce weight-bearing on the supported thigh and buttock.

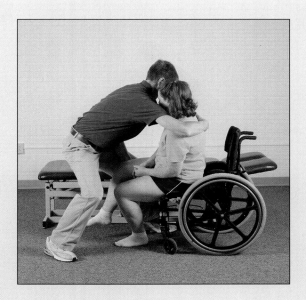

(continued)

❸ While the thigh and buttock are unloaded, the physical therapist/assistant helps the patient move the unloaded thigh and buttock forward.

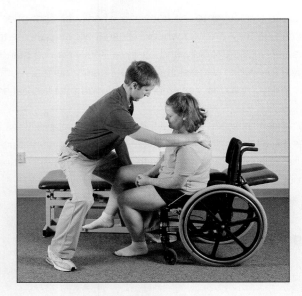

❹ The physical therapist/assistant returns the patient's thigh and buttock that had been supported to the wheelchair seat, and the patient is returned to an erect sitting position.

❺ The physical therapist/assistant reverses arm positions and performs the same maneuver to the opposite side. This sequence is repeated from side to side until a patient is properly positioned at the front of the wheelchair seat. The physical therapist/assistant must continue contact for support until a patient is able to maintain a safe and comfortable position.

■ **Take Note**

Caution—Do not move a patient so close to the front edge of the seat that she is in danger of falling.

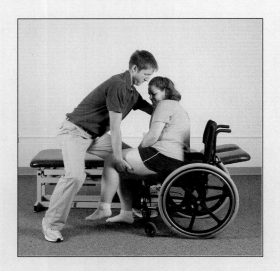

Pelvic Slide

The pelvic slide method of assisting a patient to the front of a wheelchair seat involves moving a patient's pelvis and upper trunk as separate units. The physical therapist/assistant places both hands under a patient's buttocks and assists a patient to lift and slide the buttocks to the front of the wheelchair seat.

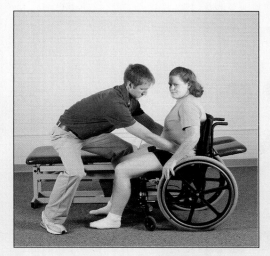

1 Starting position to slide pelvis forward.

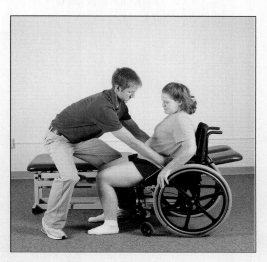

2 Pelvis at front of wheelchair seat.

The physical therapist/assistant then places his hands behind a patient's shoulders and assists the patient in moving her shoulders forward over the pelvis into an erect sitting position. A physical therapist/assistant must continue contact for support until the patient is able to maintain a safe and comfortable position.

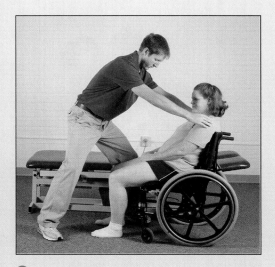

3 Starting position to move shoulders forward.

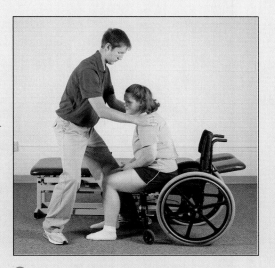

4 Patient sitting erect with shoulders over pelvis.

(continued)

Sitting Push-Up

The sitting push-up method of assisting patients to the front of a wheelchair seat requires a patient to perform sitting push-ups. The physical therapist/assistant may assist by lifting under a patient's buttocks or by guarding at the shoulders. Each time a patient is lowered back to the wheelchair seat, she is lowered closer to the front of the wheelchair seat. The physical therapist/assistant must continue contact for support until a patient is able to maintain a safe and comfortable position.

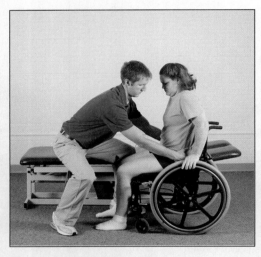

1 Starting position to assist sitting push-up.

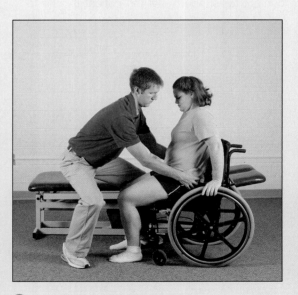

2 Assisting sitting push-up by lifting.

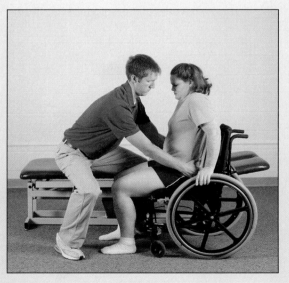

3 Lowered to front of wheelchair seat.

PROCEDURE 7–10   Assist for Moving from Edge of Treatment Table

When patients sit on the edge of a treatment table or bed and are unable to move more completely onto the table, physical therapists/assistants can assist by using a reversal of the side-to-side weight shifting or push-up maneuvers used to move a patient forward on a wheelchair seat. For the side-to-side weight shifting method, physical therapists/assistants assist patients in moving their thighs and buttocks backward onto a treatment table or bed rather than moving the thighs and buttocks forward to the front of a wheelchair seat.

A physical therapist/assistant must guard against a patient sliding off the front of the treatment table as the patient's weight is shifted. The maneuver is repeated side to side as needed. These maneuvers can also be used to assist patients in being seated fully against the back of a wheelchair. As always, the physical therapist/assistant must continue contact for support until a patient is able to maintain a safe and comfortable position.

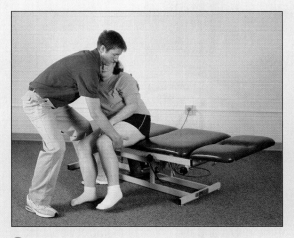
① Shifting patient's weight to one side.

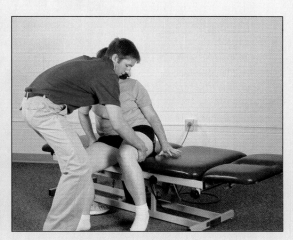
② Moving backward onto treatment table.

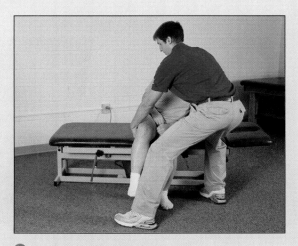
③ Shifting patient's weight to opposite side.

PROCEDURE 7–11   Assisted Standing Pivot

The assisted standing pivot transfer is an assisted transfer that may require moderate to minimal assistance of one person. The assisted standing pivot transfer is used when patients can sit, stand, pivot, and bear some weight on the lower extremities but have some weakness, paresis, paralysis, or loss of balance or sensation, which necessitates assistance to transfer safely. This transfer is also used to teach patients to transfer independently. A physical therapist/assistant reduces the amount of assistance provided to a patient until the highest possible level of independence is achieved.

1 By varying hand position, a physical therapist/assistant can vary the amount and type of assistance provided to a patient performing this transfer. By placing a hand under the buttocks, a physical therapist/assistant can assist by lifting as a patient rises to standing.

■ **Take Note**
Varying hand position will vary the level of assistance provided during the transfer.

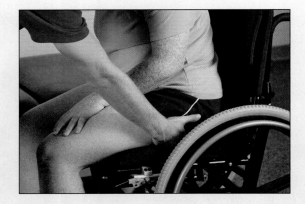

2 By placing a hand on the posterolateral aspect of the pelvis, a physical therapist/assistant can guide as a patient rises to standing. A physical therapist/assistant is in a position to control excessive lateral shift of the pelvis and the physical therapist/assistant can move his hand quickly to the posterior aspect of the pelvis to support a patient when necessary.

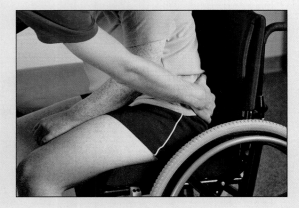

By placing a hand on the anterolateral aspect of the pelvis, a physical therapist/assistant can guide or resist movement as a patient rises to standing. Resistance may provide facilitation, making the activity easier, and teaches patients to bring the pelvis forward as they rise.

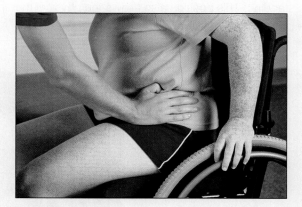

For complete independence, patients must be able to transfer to both sides. When first teaching patients to transfer, moving toward the uninvolved side is easier and safer for many patients because they are moving toward the side in which the lower extremity can provide support. Teaching patients to transfer toward the involved side reinforces a patient's awareness and use of the involved side.

When a physical therapist is unsure of a patient's capability, the physical therapist/assistant guards the patient's uninvolved lower extremity to ensure support on at least one side during the transfer. The physical therapist/assistant always guards the hip and knee on the same side, whether guarding the uninvolved or involved side, by having a knee in contact with the anterolateral aspect of the patient's knee and a hand in contact with the patient's hip.

■ **Take Note**
Caution—When unsure of a patient's capability to transfer, guard the uninvolved lower extremity initially.

Guarding the Right Lower Extremity While Transferring to Right

When transferring from a wheelchair to a treatment table or bed by pivoting to the right, a patient is positioned so the treatment table is to the right during the transfer. The physical therapist/assistant places the wheelchair parallel, or at a slight angle, to the treatment table and engages the wheel locks. The physical therapist/assistant places the patient's feet on the floor, raises the footplates, and removes the footrests from the wheelchair when possible, or swings them out of the way. A patient moves forward to the front of the wheelchair seat (with assistance when necessary) as described previously.

In this example, the physical therapist/assistant is guarding the patient's right knee with his right knee and the patient's right hip with his left hand. This position prevents the patient from collapsing at these joints.

(continued)

1 The physical therapist's/assistant's right hand is on the patient's left shoulder to prevent the patient from falling to the left. The physical therapist/assistant stands in stride with his right foot medial to the patient's right foot. This position provides a base of support in the direction of the transfer and permits both patient and physical therapist/assistant to move without tangling feet once the patient is standing. This position also allows the physical therapist/assistant to move the patient's foot if the patient does not pivot as the transfer proceeds.

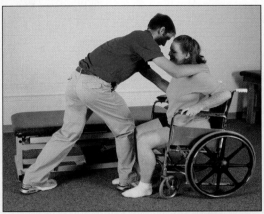

■ **Take Note**
Place your foot medial, and adjacent to, the patient's foot.

2 The patient positions her feet below the front of the wheelchair seat and initiates standing by leaning forward and pushing to standing using the armrest of the wheelchair.

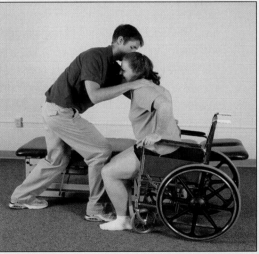

3 The patient attains a full upright position, under control.

■ **Take Note**
Caution—Guard both the hip and knee of the same lower extremity.

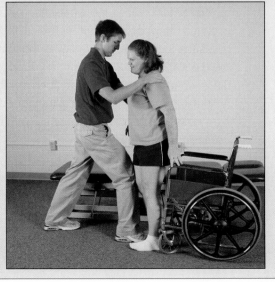

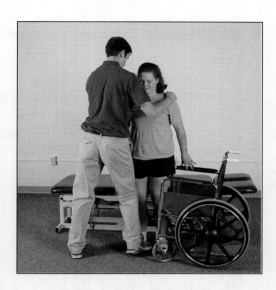

4 The patient pivots to the right, toward the treatment table.

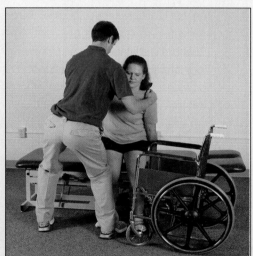

5 The patient lowers to the treatment table. If necessary, the physical therapist/assistant provides assistance.

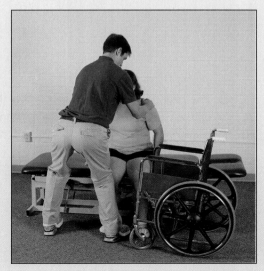

6 A physical therapist/assistant must continue contact for support until the patient is able to maintain a safe and comfortable position.

(continued)

Guarding the Left Lower Extremity While Transferring to Right

When transferring from a wheelchair to a treatment table or bed by pivoting to the right, patients are positioned so the treatment table is to the right during the transfer. The physical therapist/assistant places the wheelchair parallel, or at a slight angle, to the treatment table and engages wheel locks. The physical therapist/assistant places the patient's feet on the floor, raises the footplates, and removes the footrests from the wheelchair when possible or swings them out of the way. Patients move forward to the front of the wheelchair seat (with assistance when necessary) as described previously.

In this example, the physical therapist/assistant is guarding the patient's left knee with his right knee and the patient's left hip with his right hand. This position prevents the patient from collapsing at these joints.

1 The physical therapist's/assistant's left hand is on the patient's right shoulder to prevent the patient from falling to the right. The physical therapist/assistant stands in stride with his right foot lateral to the patient's left foot. This position provides a base of support in the direction of transfer and permits both the patient and physical therapist/assistant to move without tangling feet once the patient is standing. This position also allows the physical therapist/assistant to move the patient's foot if the patient does not pivot as the transfer proceeds.

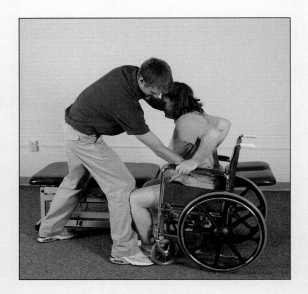

2 The patient positions her feet below the front of the wheelchair seat and initiates standing by leaning forward and pushing to standing using the armrest of the wheelchair.

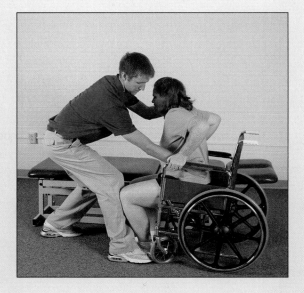

③ The patient pushes to standing using the armrest of the wheelchair.

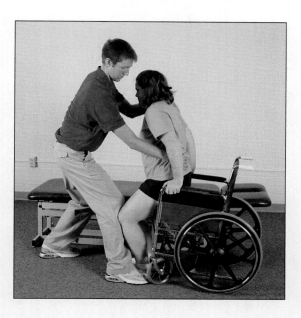

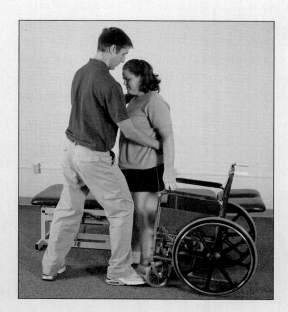

④ The patient attains a full upright position, under control.

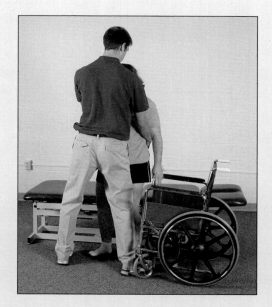

⑤ The patient pivots to the right, toward the treatment table.

(continued)

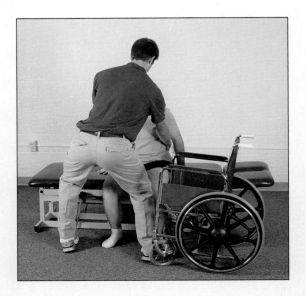

6 The patient lowers to the treatment table. If necessary, the physical therapist/assistant provides assistance. A physical therapist/assistant must continue contact for support until the patient is able to maintain a safe and comfortable position.

Wheelchair to Treatment Table: Using a Step Stool

Transferring patients to a high treatment table requires use of a step stool, especially when a patient is short. The position of the wheelchair, guarding techniques, and activity of coming to standing are performed as in an assisted standing pivot transfer. In the following sequence, the patient is demonstrating a transfer to the right, while the physical therapist/assistant is guarding the left lower extremity. The guarding position and sequence are performed as in an assisted standing pivot transfer to the right while guarding the left lower extremity, as described in the immediately preceding section.

1 The physical therapist/assistant must place a step stool close to himself so he can retrieve and position the step stool while guarding the patient.

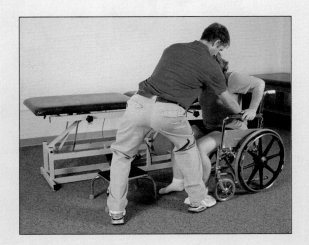

❷ Once the patient has attained a standing position, the physical therapist/assistant places the stool alongside the treatment table and in front of the patient.

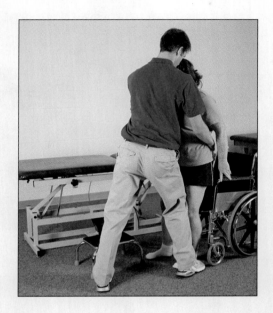

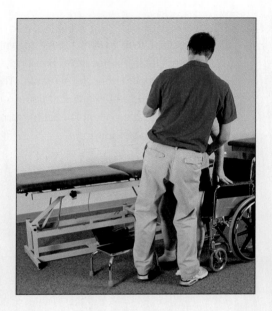

❸ Having attained an erect position, the patient places her hand on the treatment table. With her hand on the table, the patient places the foot of her right lower extremity on the stool. The physical therapist/assistant guards the left lower extremity to ensure adequate support as the patient lifts and places her foot on the stool. The patient steps onto the stool, lifting and pivoting her body over the stool, and raises her pelvis above the level of the treatment table.

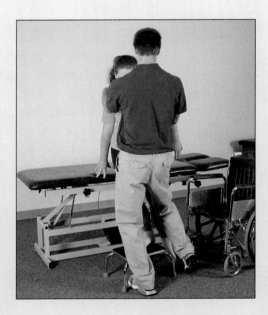

(continued)

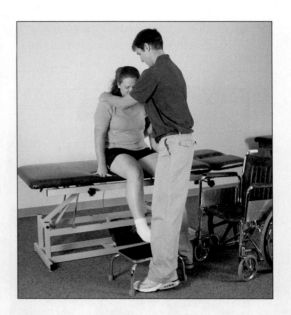

4 The patient then lowers herself to sitting on the treatment table. As described previously, the patient moves completely onto the table. The physical therapist/assistant must continue contact for support until the patient is able to maintain a safe and comfortable position.

5 For the patient to return to a wheelchair from a high treatment table, a stool is not needed. A physical therapist/assistant should be prepared to guard either lower extremity as a patient slides from sitting on the treatment table to standing on the floor in a controlled manner.

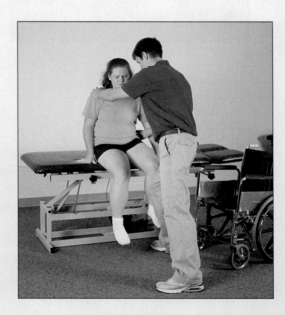

PROCEDURE 7–12   Squat Pivot Transfer

The squat pivot transfer is an assisted transfer that requires minimal assistance of one person. The squat pivot transfer is used when patients can sit, stand, pivot, and bear weight on the lower extremities but have some weakness, paresis, or loss of balance or sensation, which necessitates assistance to transfer safely.

1. When transferring from a treatment table or bed to a wheelchair, the physical therapist/assistant places a wheelchair parallel, or at a slight angle, to the treatment table or bed, and engages the wheel locks. The physical therapist/assistant raises the footplates, and removes the footrests from the wheelchair when possible or swings them out of the way. The patient moves toward the edge of the treatment table (with assistance when necessary) as described previously. A physical therapist/assistant sits on a wheeled stool in front of the patient, blocking both of the patient's knees with her knees. The physical therapist/assistant places her hands on the posterolateral lower thoracic region.

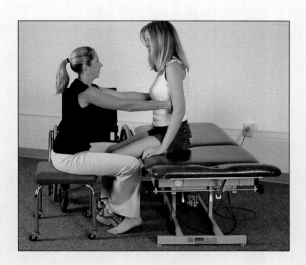

2. The physical therapist/assistant assists the patient to perform an anterior pelvic tilt and extension of the upper back while the patient shifts weight forward onto her feet. This results in the patient being in proper position to rise from the treatment table.

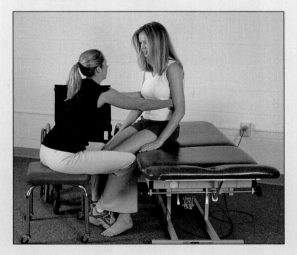

(continued)

3 Without coming to a complete standing position, the patient rises and pivots toward the wheelchair. When not able to move directly to the wheelchair, the patient can use an intermediate move to a new position on the treatment table. The patient repeats the sequence until she is seated in the wheelchair.

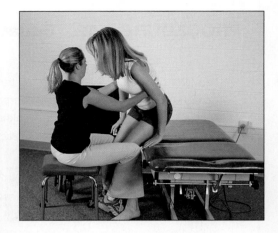

4 As a patient's capabilities progress, the patient may be able to complete the transfer in one pivot movement.

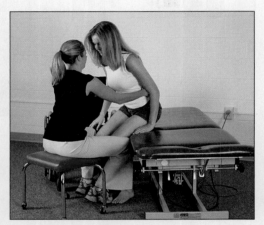

Raising from treatment table.

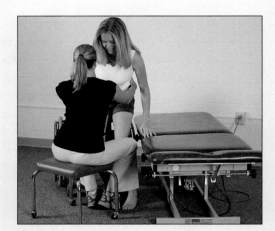

Pivoting to wheelchair.

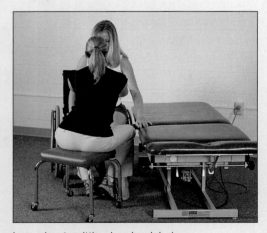

Lowering to sitting in wheelchair.

5 A physical therapist/assistant must continue contact for support until a patient is able to maintain a safe and comfortable position.

PROCEDURE 7–13   Transfers Between Floor and Wheelchair

Transfers between a wheelchair and the floor are necessary when a patient wants to participate in activities on the floor or if the patient should fall out of a wheelchair. Occasionally a patient may fall out of, or tip over, a wheelchair.

Dependent One-Person Transfer: Floor to Wheelchair

When an adult patient is unable to transfer from the floor to a wheelchair independently, either a one-person or two-person transfer may be used to get the patient back into the wheelchair. While a two-person lift is desired, because it is safer for patients and clinicians, a one-person transfer may be necessary. Safe performance of a one-person transfer depends upon the relative sizes of patients and clinicians, the patient's capabilities, and the environment. A physical therapist is responsible for making such a decision and instructing patient and clinicians in proper performance.

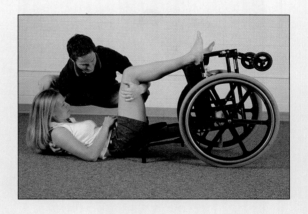

❶ To perform a dependent one-person transfer, the physical therapist/assistant positions a wheelchair on its back at the patient's feet. A physical therapist/assistant places one arm under the patient's lower extremities and the other arm behind the patient's upper back, such that the patient's lower extremities are flexed at the hips and knees.

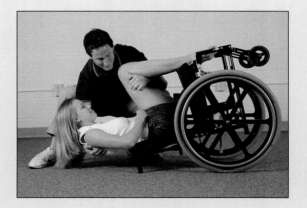

❷ The physical therapist/assistant moves the patient toward the wheelchair seat such that the patient's ankles are placed over the front edge of the wheelchair seat. The physical therapist/assistant performs a series of short lifting and sliding maneuvers to move the patient into the wheelchair.

(continued)

③ When the patient's buttocks are in contact with the wheelchair seat, the physical therapist/assistant moves to the patient's head. He then squats to grasp both handles of the wheelchair while cradling the patient's upper trunk on his forearms.

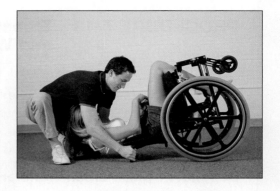

④ The the physical therapist/assistant lifts the patient and wheelchair as a unit as the physical therapist/assistant moves to a standing position. When a patient is tall, or if the back of the wheelchair is low, the physical therapist/assistant may grasp one handle of the wheelchair with one hand and support and lift the patient's trunk with the other hand.

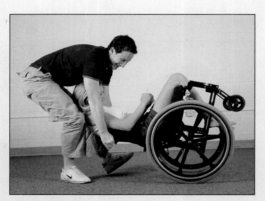

Initiating lift.

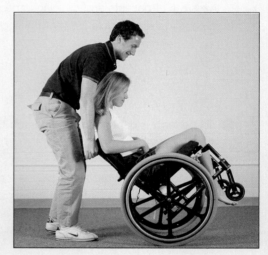

Midposition of lift.

⑤ As the wheelchair approaches an upright position, the physical therapist/assistant shifts one arm to guard the anterior aspect of the patient's upper trunk to prevent her from falling forward.

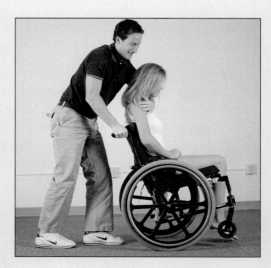

PROCEDURE 7–14   Independent Transfer from Wheelchair to Floor and Return

Many patients can, and must, learn to move safely from a wheelchair to the floor and back into the wheelchair. This type of transfer can be performed using several methods depending upon the capabilities of the patient and the environment. A physical therapist, in conjunction with the patient, selects the appropriate methods of transfer. The physical therapist/assistant must instruct the patient to perform the selected transfers in a safe and efficient manner. The transfers selected may begin as assisted transfers (physical or verbal assistance) and then progress to independent transfers. In the following illustrations, patients are performing the transfers with stand-by assistance.

Preparing the Wheelchair

The initial steps for each of these transfers are similar. The physical therapist/assistant turns the wheelchair casters forward as they would be when a patient is wheeling backward. This increases the base of support of the wheelchair. When casters are not positioned properly, a wheelchair may tip forward as a patient is placed on the front of the wheelchair. After turning the casters forward, the physical therapist/assistant engaes the wheel locks.

Forward Lowering: Wheelchair to Floor

Forward lowering to the floor and a backward lift into a wheelchair requires the most strength and agility of the methods illustrated.

1 The physical therapist/assistant positions a wheelchair and locks the caster wheels forward. The physical therapist/assistant places the patient's feet on the floor, raises the footplates, and removes the footrests from the wheelchair when possible or swings them out of the way. The patient moves to the front of the wheelchair seat and the patient's lower extremities are positioned in front of the patient with knees extended.

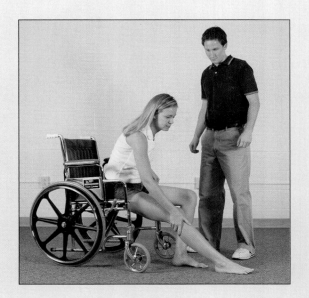

(continued)

2️⃣ The patient positions one hand on the side, and toward the front, of the wheelchair seat or the lower portion of a desk armrest. She places the other hand on the caster or floor. Hand placements depend upon the patient's size, strength, and range of motion (ROM). The patient then lowers to the floor.

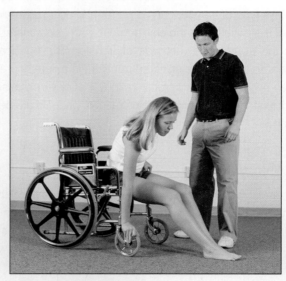

Positioning upper extremities.

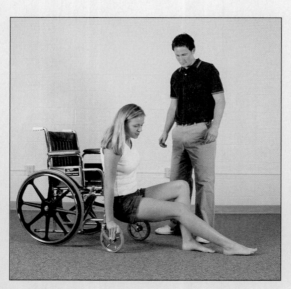

Lowering to floor.

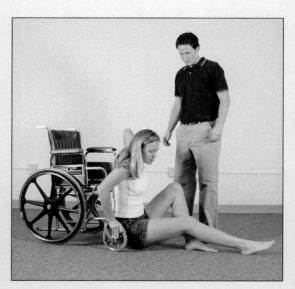

End position on floor.

Backward Lift: Floor to Wheelchair

1 The physical therapist/assistant positions a wheelchair and locks the caster wheels forward. The physical therapist/assistant raises the footplates and removes the footrests from the wheelchair when possible or swings them out of the way. The patient assumes a long-sitting position with her back toward, and close to, the front of the wheelchair. She places one hand on the side, and toward the front, of the wheelchair seat. She places the other hand on the caster or floor. Hand placements depend upon the patient's size, strength, and ROM.

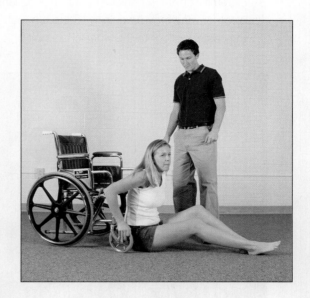

2 The patient pushes up by extending the upper extremities, depressing the shoulder girdles, and flexing the head and neck.

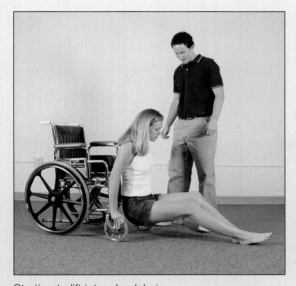

Starting to lift into wheelchair.

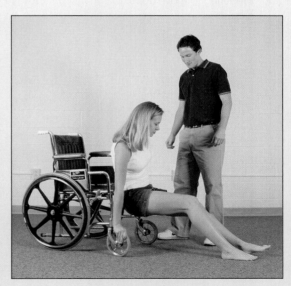

Midposition of lift into wheelchair.

(continued)

3 As the patient's buttocks reach the wheelchair seat, the patient supports herself on the upper extremity on the wheelchair seat. The patient may keep the hand on the wheelchair seat in place or may move it quickly to the armrest. The patient moves the other hand quickly from the caster or floor to the wheelchair seat or lower part of the armrest.

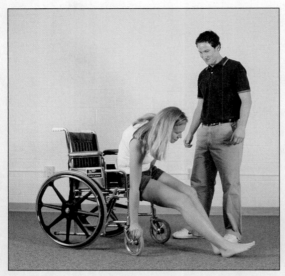

Preparing to move upper extremity from caster to armrest.

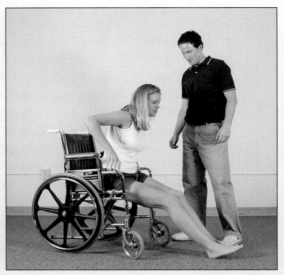

Repositioned arms for movement onto wheelchair seat.

4 Again using both upper extremities, the patient moves well back onto the wheelchair seat.

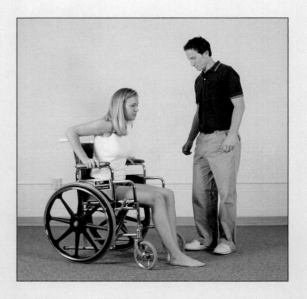

5 The transfer is completed after the physical therapist/assistant attaches the footrests and positions the patient's feet on the footplates, with the patient being in a proper sitting position.

Backward Lift Using a Step Stool: Floor to Wheelchair

When a patient is unable to perform an independent floor-to-wheelchair transfer, a step stool may be used. The reverse of this sequence may be used initially to teach a patient to move from the wheelchair to the floor.

❶ The physical therapist/assistant positions a wheelchair and locks the caster wheels forward. The physical therapist/assistant raises the footplates and removes the footrests from the wheelchair when possible or swings them out of the way. The physical therapist/assistant places a step stool in front of the wheelchair. The patient assumes a long-sitting position with her back toward, and close to, the step stool. She places both hands on the step stool.

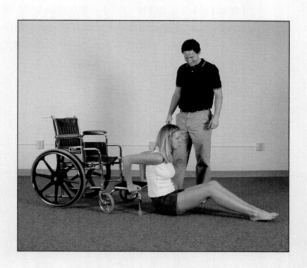

❷ Extending her upper extremities while using scapular depression, the patient pushes upward to lift herself onto the step stool.

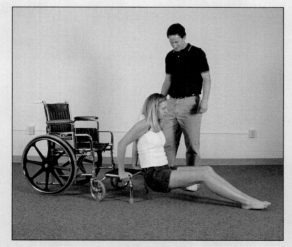

Initiating push-up onto step stool.

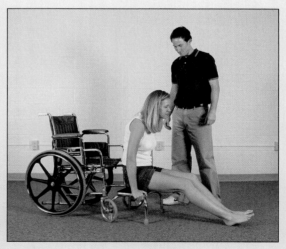

Completing push-up onto step stool.

(continued)

③ Sitting on the step stool, the patient places both hands on the sides and toward the front of the wheelchair seat or the lower part of desk armrests when available. Hand placements depend upon the patient's size, strength, and ROM.

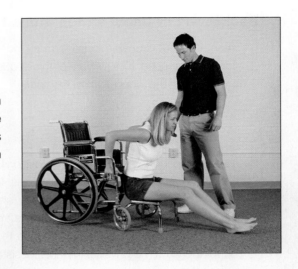

④ Performing another push-up, the patient lifts herself onto the front of the wheelchair seat.

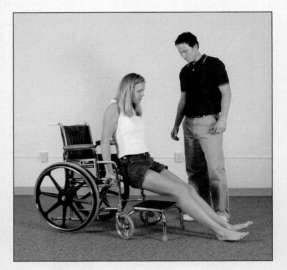

⑤ The patient then moves her hands to the highest part of the armrests. Using the armrests, the patient performs another push-up to lift herself further onto the wheelchair seat.

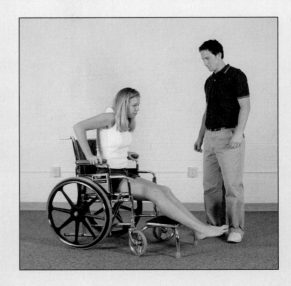

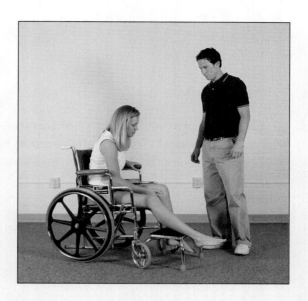

6. Using one hand for support, the patient uses the other hand to position one lower extremity such that her foot rests on the step stool. This maneuver is repeated for the other lower extremity.

7. The patient then adjusts her position in the wheelchair until she is sitting erect, well back on the wheelchair seat. The physical therapist/assistant wheels the wheelchair backward away from the step stool. The physical therapist/assistant positions the footrests and footplates properly and places the patient's feet on the footplates.

Turn Around: Wheelchair to Floor

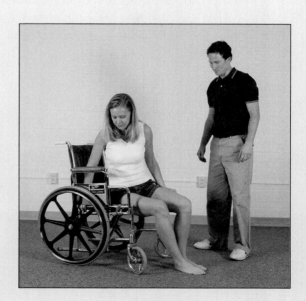

1. The physical therapist/assistant positions a wheelchair and locks the caster wheels forward. The physical therapist/assistant raises the footplates and removes the footrests from the wheelchair when possible or swings them out of the way. The patient moves to the front of the wheelchair seat and turns partially onto one hip.

(continued)

2 The patient moves her right hand behind her to grasp the left side of the seat. She moves her left hand across the front of her body to grasp the right side of the seat.

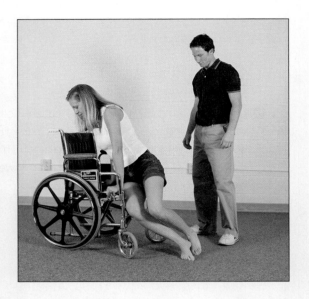

3 Extending her upper extremities while depressing her shoulder girdles, the patient lifts herself and turns to face the back of the wheelchair. She then lowers herself to a kneeling position on the floor in front of the wheelchair.

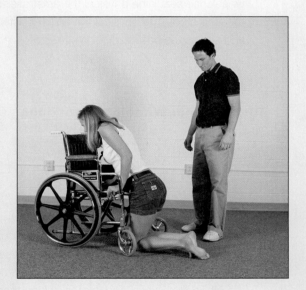

4 From the kneeling position, the patient moves to a hands-knees position and then may assume a side-sitting position.

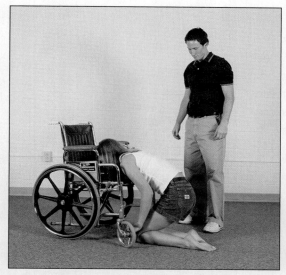

Moving to hands-knees position.

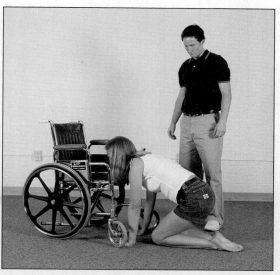

Hands-knees position.

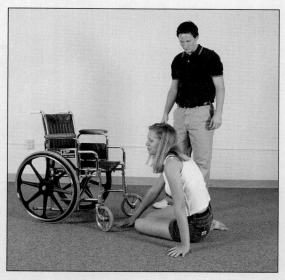

Side-sitting position.

(continued)

Turn Around: Floor to Wheelchair

1 The physical therapist/assistant positions a wheelchair and locks the caster wheels forward. The physical therapist/assistant raises the footplates and removes the footrests from the wheelchair when possible or swings them out of the way. The patient assumes a hands-knees position in front of the wheelchair.

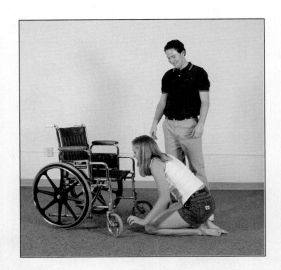

2 The patient places one hand on the side, and toward the front of, the wheelchair seat and the other hand on the caster wheel. She then pushes into a kneeling position.

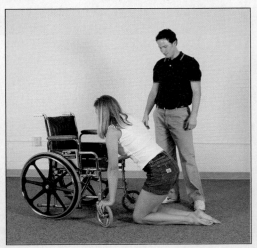

3 The patient moves her hand from the caster wheel to the side, and toward the front of the wheelchair seat, or on the lower part of a desk armrest when available. She is now kneeling in front of the wheelchair.

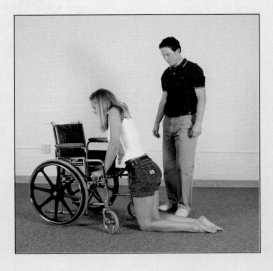

4 Pushing from the wheelchair seat or lower part of the armrest, the patient lifts herself, starts to turn, and then rests on one hip.

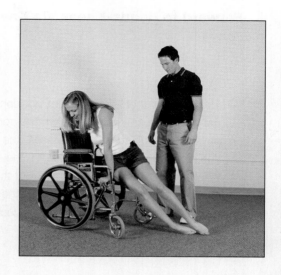

5 The patient repositions her hands onto the appropriate sides of the wheelchair seat, or armrests, and completes the turn.

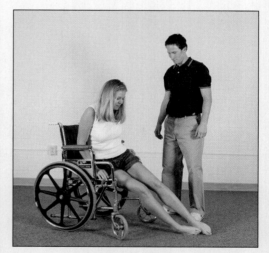

6 The patient can then position herself properly in the wheelchair.

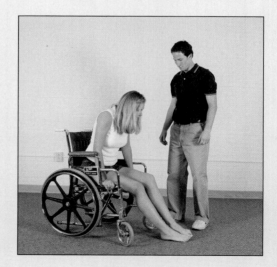

(continued)

Forward to Hands-Knees Via Kneeling: Wheelchair to Floor

1 The physical therapist/assistant positions a wheel-chair and locks the caster wheels forward. The physical therapist/assistant raises the footplates and removes the footrests from the wheelchair when possible or swings them out of the way. The patient moves forward to the front of the wheelchair seat and places her feet on the floor under the front of the wheelchair seat.

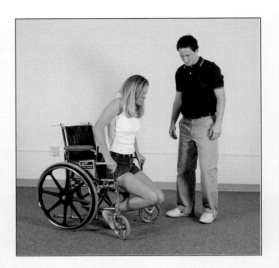

2 Grasping the lower portion of the desk armrests, when available, or the sides of the wheelchair seat, the patient lowers herself to a kneeling position.

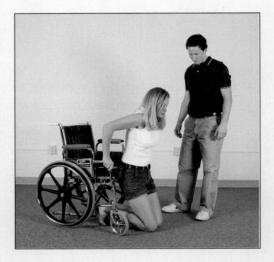

3 Holding the lower portion of a desk armrest with one hand, the patient reaches forward to the floor with the other hand.

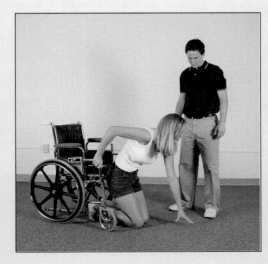

4 When the patient's upper extremity that is reaching to the floor is in a position to support her, she moves her other hand to the floor.

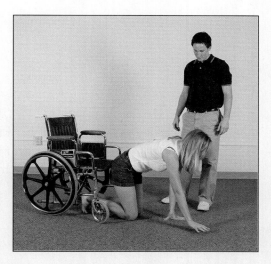

5 The transfer is completed when the patient moves into a hands-knees position. From the hands-knees position, the patient may assume a side-sitting position.

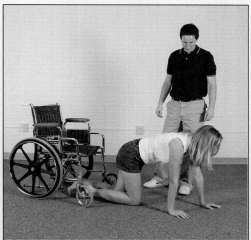

Forward to Hands-Knees: Wheelchair to Floor

1 The physical therapist/assistant positions a wheelchair and locks the caster wheels forward. The physical therapist/assistant raises the footplates and removes the footrests from the wheelchair when possible or swings them out of the way. The patient moves forward to the front of the wheelchair seat and places her feet on the floor under the front of the wheelchair seat.

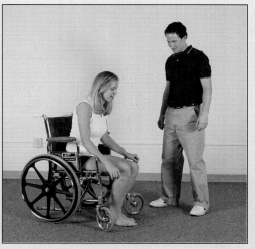

(continued)

2 The patient reaches to the floor with both upper extremities as she moves from the wheelchair seat, creating forward momentum.

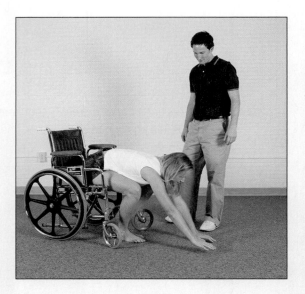

3 With the patient's upper extremities supporting her, momentum shifts weight onto the upper extremities and the patient assumes a hands-knees position on the floor.

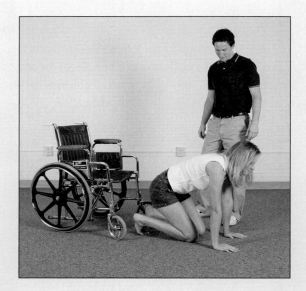

Chapter Review

■■■

Review Questions

1. Differentiate among dependent, assisted, and independent transfers.

2. What are the purposes of verbal commands during transfers?

3. Describe the sequences for performing the following transfers:
   a. Sliding
   b. Three-person carry
   c. Hydraulic lift
   d. Two-person lift
   e. Dependent standing pivot
   f. Dependent sitting pivot
   g. Sliding board
   h. Push-up
   i. Assist to front of wheelchair seat (three methods)
   j. Assist onto treatment table
   k. Assist standing pivot (three methods)
   l. Squat pivot transfer
   m. Independent one-person transfer from floor to wheelchair
   n. Independent transfer from wheelchair to floor and return (seven methods)

■■■

Suggested Activities

1. Demonstrate transfer procedures shown in this chapter.

2. Practice transfers working in groups of two to four people, with each student participating as a patient, lead therapist, and assistant.

3. Practice transfers with partners role-playing the patient. Students should role-play patients with different diagnoses such as CVA (right or left hemiplegia), spinal cord injury (quadriplegia or paraplegia), multiple sclerosis, cerebral palsy, or Parkinson's disease. Students role-playing patients can add "character" to enhance the activity by being cooperative or noncooperative, in pain, hard of hearing, apprehensive, faint, flaccid, or spastic. Students playing the role of a patient must role-play the diagnosis and character consistently.

4. Practice teaching transfers to "patients and families" and other health-care providers.

5. Document treatment.

■■

Case Studies

For the following case studies, develop a sequence of transfers appropriate for progressing a patient from dependent to independent (as much as feasible) transfer status. Note transfer methods and amount and type of assistance.

1. The patient is a 23-year-old female with a diagnosis of multiple sclerosis. She was independent in all ADLs and ambulated with a cane for balance until two weeks ago. At that time, she experienced an exacerbation that has left her totally dependent in all transfers and unable to ambulate. She becomes faint when moved from supine to sitting, or sitting to standing, too quickly. She is expected to recover most of her prior level of independence.

2. The patient is a 63-year-old male with left CVA onset 20 hours ago, presenting with right hemiplegia and global aphasia (both receptive and expressive aphasia). The cause was a blood clot. Because he received immediate medical treatment, recovery is anticipated to be nearly complete. At present, he is dependent in all ADLs, including transfers and ambulation.

3. The patient is a 18-year-old male who sustained a complete T12-L1 spinal cord lesion in a motorcycle accident 2 weeks ago. Following surgery, he is wearing a Thoracic LumboSacral Orthosis (TLSO). He has medical clearance to begin transfer training while wearing his TLSO.

4. The patient is a 23-year-old female with cerebral palsy presenting with spastic quadriplegia. While living with her parents, the patient was lifted by her father for all transfers. Following her recent college graduation, she is living in a group home for the first time. She ambulates by using a power wheelchair. The staff of the group home requests assistance in selecting appropriate transfers. The staff would like a program to assist her in becoming an active participant in her transfers. Would the transfer method selected be different if she was 5 feet tall weighing 250 pounds versus 5 feet tall weighing 96 pounds?

5. The patient is a 49-year-old female with severe rheumatoid arthritis. She is 5 feet 3 inches tall and weighs 175 pounds. Transfers are currently accomplished using a pneumatic lift. She ambulates by using a power wheelchair. Because her arthritis is in remission at this time, she would like to learn to transfer without the pneumatic lift so she can get out in the community more.

■■

References

1. O'Sullivan SB and Schmitz TJ. *Physical Rehabilitation Assessment and Treatment*, 5th ed., chapter 11. Philadelphia: F.A. Davis, 2007.

2. Occupational Health and Safety Agency for Healthcare (OHSAH) in British Columbia. *Safe Patient & Resident Handling—Acute and Long Term Care Sectors Handbook*, 2002, p. 8

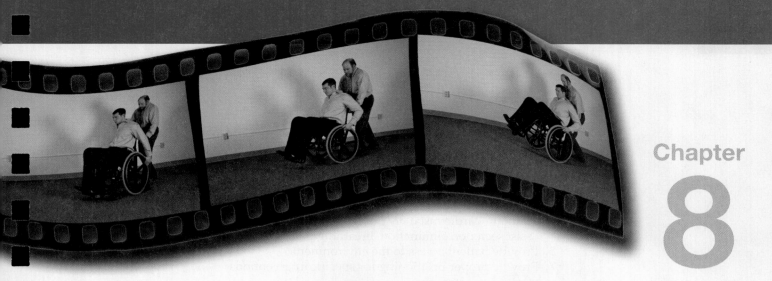

Turning and Positioning

Learning Objectives

Upon completion of this chapter, you will be able to describe:

1. Goals of proper positioning.
2. How to determine the amount of time a patient can spend in a position.
3. General procedures used to properly turn and position a patient.
4. A decision-making algorithm to determine the amount of assistance required for positioning a patient.
5. Specific procedures used to turn a patient to, and to position in, supine, prone, sidelying, and sitting.

Key Terms

Long sitting

Orthostatic hypotension

Prone

Sidelying

Supine

Introduction

Proper positioning is a valuable tool to maintain patient function. Physical therapists/assistants work with other health-care professionals to determine optimal positions for patients. Physical therapists/assistants are responsible for positioning patients properly for physical therapy interventions and for function within a patient's environment. For patients who are unable to change position independently, proper positioning is essential for increasing function and preventing complications.

Goals

The goals of proper positioning are to

1. Ensure patient comfort.
2. Maintain integumentary integrity by preventing development of ulceration as a result of pressure or friction.
3. Maintain musculoskeletal integrity by preventing loss of range of motion.
4. Maintain neuromuscular integrity by preventing peripheral nerve impingement as a result of pressure.
5. Maintain cardiovascular/pulmonary integrity by using changes in position to assist secretion elimination, breathing patterns, and vascular flow.
6. Provide patient access to the environment.
7. Provide proper positioning for specific interventions.

To achieve these goals, patients and environments must be managed properly. Proper positioning includes moving patients into, and out of, desired positions in a safe and effective manner. All health-care providers who have contact with a patient have a responsibility to maintain appropriate patient positioning. Algorithms can be used by physical therapists in the decision-making process.

Time in Positions

The first time a patient is placed in a new position, the patient's skin, particularly over bony prominences that are pressure sites, should be examined after 5 to 10 minutes and frequently thereafter. Observation over time allows determination of tolerance for the position. A general rule is initially to reposition a patient at least every 2 hours to maintain integrity of all four movement systems (integumentary, musculoskeletal, neuromuscular, cardiovascular/pulmonary). Repositioning in less than 2 hours may be required for patients who have additional problems, such as poor circulation, fragile skin, decreased sensation, easily compromised peripheral nerves, difficulty breathing or excreting secretions, or inability to move. Establishment of the positioning schedule is the responsibility of a physical therapist in conjunction with nursing personnel. All health-care providers, including physical therapist assistants, have a responsibility to observe and document changes that may require modification of a positioning schedule.

When a patient is repositioned, skin over the area on which the patient was lying should be inspected and observed for color and integrity. Pay special attention to areas of skin that cover bony prominences, such as the greater trochanter or sacrum. Allow skin redness to resolve before putting pressure on that area of skin again. When recovery from pressure is delayed, reposition patients more frequently. Excessive or prolonged redness indicates tissue damage (Stage 1 ulcer).

When sitting, a patient must relieve pressure on the buttocks and sacrum at least every 10 minutes. Sitting push-ups using the arm rests of a chair, leaning first to one side and then to the other, and leaning forward are methods to relieve pressure on the buttocks in the sitting position. Specialized wheelchairs such as tilt-in-space and reclining-back wheelchairs are used to relieve pressure.

Prolonged periods in one position will affect musculoskeletal structures. Loss of range of motion, compromised joint nutrition, decreased joint stress, and loss of strength will occur if changes in position are not required. Loss of range of motion may occur in two directions, with tissue (muscle, tendon, ligamentous capsule) shortening on one side and lengthening on the other side of a joint. Musculoskeletal structures respond positively to appropriate stresses resulting from movement. Decreased movement eliminates these stresses and contributes to tissue degeneration and compromised function, such as bone demineralization, loss of sarcomeres, and degeneration of cartilage.

■ Take Note
Redness of skin must resolve before positioning on the area again.

Neuromuscular tissue may be affected by prolonged periods in one position. Pressure on peripheral nerves will interfere with function. Pain, decreased sensation, and loss of range of motion may result. Decreased sensation contributes to integumentary problems discussed previously. Loss of range of motion affects neuromuscular tissue as well as musculoskeletal tissue.

Circulation may be reduced by prolonged periods in one position. Decreased blood flow resulting from pressure on vascular structures may exacerbate integumentary problems, cause pain, and decrease nutrition to all tissues distal to compression. **Orthostatic hypotension**, the inability of the cardiovascular system to adapt to upright postures after prolonged horizontal positioning, can be avoided if changes in position include an upright position in the positioning schedule. Breathing is also easier in an upright position. Frequent changes of position aid a patient's capability to excrete lung secretions.

An algorithm for repositioning a patient in bed is presented in ■ **Figure 8–1**, and an algorithm for repositioning a patient in a chair is presented in ■ **Figure 8–2**.

■ **Take Note**
Prolonged periods without repositioning may cause changes in tissues other than just skin.

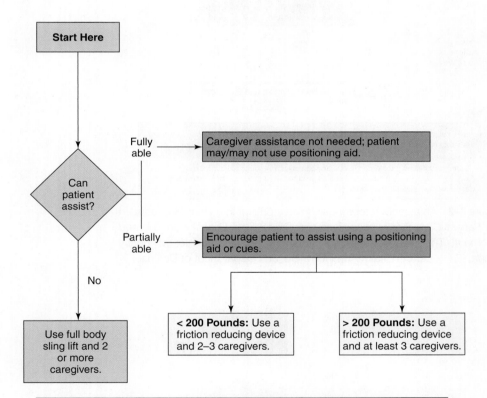

■ **Figure 8–1**   An algorithm for repositioning a patient in bed. Reproduced from *Patient Care Ergonomics Resource Guide: Safe Patient Handling and Movement.* This was developed by the Patient Safety Center of Inquiry (Tampa, FL), Veterans Health Administration, and Department of Defense.

Start Here

Can patient assist?

→ Fully able → Caregiver assistance not needed; Stand by for safety as needed.

→ Partially able →
- If patient has upper extremity strength in both arms, have patient lift up while caregiver pushes knees to reposition.
- If patient lacks sensation, cues may be needed to remind patient to reposition.

No ↓

Can the patient bear weight?

→ Yes → Recline chair and use a friction reducing device and 2 caregivers.

No ↓

Is patient cooperative?

→ Yes → Use full body sling lift or non-powered stand assist aid and 1 to 2 caregivers.

→ No → Use full body sling lift and 2 or more caregivers.

- Take full advantage of chair functions, e.g., chair that reclines, or use arm rest of chair to facilitate repositioning.
- Make sure the chair wheels are locked.
- During any patient transferring task, if any caregiver is required to lift more than 35 lbs. of a patient's weight, then the patient should be considered to be fully dependent and assistive devices should be used.

■ **Figure 8–2** An algorithm for repositioning a patient in a chair. Reproduced from *Patient Care Ergonomics Resource Guide: Safe Patient Handling and Movement.* This was developed by the Patient Safety Center of Inquiry (Tampa, FL), Veterans Health Administration, and Department of Defense.

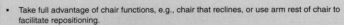

PROCEDURE 8–1   General Procedures

Preparing the environment assists in safe and effective turning and positioning. Preparing the environment means having a clear area for movement and having all necessary supplies, including sheets, pillows, and towels, available within easy reach. A sufficient number of appropriately trained clinicians must be available. Following these general procedures reduces the risk of harm to the patient and clinicians. Before moving a patient, check carefully for tubes, lines, and monitor leads. They must not be disconnected or compromised when turning or positioning.

1 *Smooth all undersheets, towels, and patient clothing.* Avoid wrinkles in the sheets, blankets, and personal clothing because they increase pressure on a small area of skin and cause skin irritation. Such pressure points are uncomfortable for a patient who has sensation but is unable to move independently.

2 *Pillows, rolled blankets, or towels are used to support body parts and to avoid strain or pressure on ligaments, nerves, and muscles.* A sufficient quantity of these items must be available before beginning for safe and efficient positioning. Pillows or towels are used to provide relief to bony prominences or areas most susceptible to ulceration. When patients must be positioned in a specific way for a procedure, be sure to relieve sensitive areas of pressure. Supporting the body segment just proximal and just distal to, but not under, a sensitive area relieves pressure on the sensitive area. This type of positioning is shown in the following photo. Place pillows or towels close to the involved area to prevent contact of the involved area with the supporting surface. In these circumstances, reduce time in the position, as pressure may increase at the site of the pillows or towels, thereby compromising circulation.

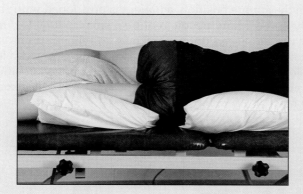

3 *Ensure that enough clear area exists and equipment is ready for moving patients safely.* A clear area allows all personnel involved in moving and positioning a patient sufficient space to move without impediment and without bumping into walls, chairs, and other equipment. Make sure all beds, gurneys, wheelchairs, and other movable equipment are locked or secured prior to initiating moving a patient.

(continued)

④ *Ensure that sufficient personnel trained in moving and positioning patients are present.* When turning and positioning patients, patients must be lifted, rather than dragged, across the sheets. Dragging may result in skin irritation as a result of friction.

⑤ *Draping should allow appropriate positioning while maintaining patient modesty and warmth.* Sheets or blankets are used for draping or covering the patient. Covers tightly tucked at the foot of the bed force the ankle into a position of plantar flexion. This should be avoided to reduce the risk of developing contractures.

⑥ *Whenever possible, patients should participate actively during moving and positioning.* For simple procedures, give explanations and directions before initiation of a procedure. Give commands throughout the procedure. For procedures with many steps, give a general explanation prior to the start of a procedure and then individual commands prior to each step of the procedure. Give additional directions as needed. Providing directions and commands as a complex procedure progresses assists patients who may not be able to remember all steps for an entire procedure while concentrating on the first few steps (see Figures 8–1 and 8–2).

■ **Take Note**

Safety first—Prepare the environment before starting to move a patient.

Descriptions of turning and positioning procedures presented in this chapter are given as if the patient is unable to assist or is able to assist only minimally. Illustrations in this chapter demonstrate a patient on a treatment table or mat. The same procedures are used when turning or positioning a patient in bed. Procedures and positions are modified to accommodate specific needs of each individual patient.

Supine Position

A **supine** position is one in which a person lies on his or her back on a supporting surface. In the supine position, a patient is positioned with shoulders parallel to hips and a straight spine. Many people require a small pillow to support the head for comfort. A pillow can be placed under the knees to relieve strain on the lower back (■ **Figure 8–3**). Positioning with a pillow under the knees, however, can lead to decreased hip and knee extension range of motion as a result of prolonged positioning in hip and knee flexion. A pillow placed lengthwise under the legs will reduce knee flexion and relieve pressure on the heels (■ **Figure 8–4**).

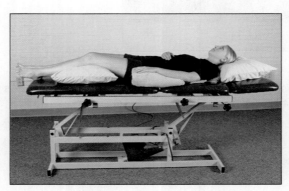

■ **Figure 8–3** Supine position with arm support and a pillow placed crosswise under the knees.

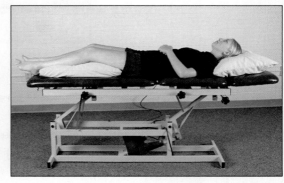

■ **Figure 8–4** Supine position with a pillow placed lengthwise under the legs.

PROCEDURE 8–2 Turning from Supine to Prone

The patient's initial position is supine. The physical therapist/assistant first moves the patient far enough to one side of the treatment table to allow a full turning movement to the prone position without coming too near the opposite edge upon completion of the turning movement. To turn to the left, the physical therapist/assistant first moves a patient to the right side of the treatment table. When segmental movement of the trunk and lower extremities is possible, the physical therapist/assistant moves the patient in stages. When the patient cannot tolerate such movement, more than one person, or specialized beds, will be needed.

To turn a patient from supine to prone, the following steps occur in sequence.

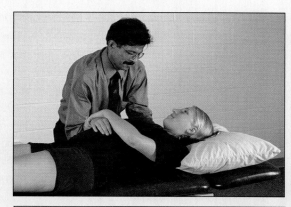

1 Move the patient's upper trunk and head to the right side of the treatment table.

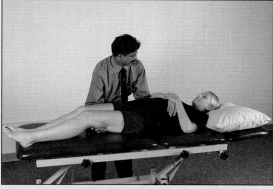

2 Move the patient's lower trunk to the right side of the treatment table.

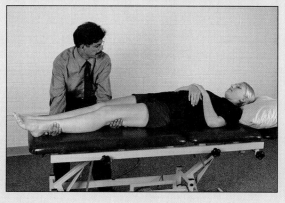

3 Move the patient's lower extremities to the right side of the treatment table.

(continued)

4 Cross the patient's right lower extremity over the left lower extremity, with the right ankle resting on top of the left ankle. The patient's left upper extremity is adducted, placing the hand under the left hip, palm against the hip. This positioning of the extremities applies when a patient is being turned to the left, as presented in these figures. In situations where turning is to the right, the positioning movements must be mirror images of these positions.

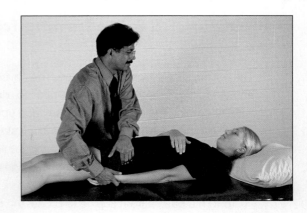

5 The physical therapist/assistant is positioned on the side to which the patient is being turned. When a treatment table is narrow, clinicians assisting in turning the patient should stand next to the patient on the side from which the patient is being turned, to prevent the patient from falling while the physical therapist moves from one side of the treatment table to the other. Clinicians assisting in turning the patient can help with positioning of pillows and turning the patient.

When a pillow will be under the patient while the patient is in the prone position, position the pillow in the proper orientation before the patient is rolled. The right upper extremity is adducted, placing the hand at the right hip, palm against the hip.

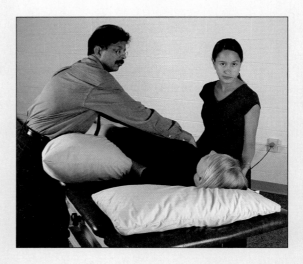

6 When patients have head and neck control, they can assist in turning their head and neck in the direction of the roll as turning is initiated. When patients do not have head and neck control, physical therapists/assistants must be aware that a patient's face may be subject to some rubbing on the mattress or mat during turning. When the physical therapist/assistant is ready to begin the turning movement, he should ask the patient and any assisting clinicians if they are ready. Upon receiving an affirmative reply, a preparatory count is given, followed by a specific verbal command to initiate turning.

As turning is initiated, the physical therapist/assistant has his hands on the patient's back.

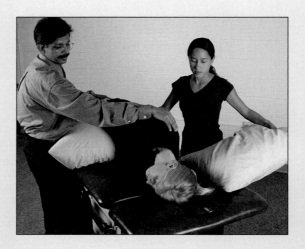

7 When a patient reaches the halfway point, gravity can complete the movement, but will do so in an uncontrolled manner. The physical therapist/assistant must, therefore, rotate and reposition the hands as patients reach the midpoint of the turn. The physical therapist/assistant and other clinicians should reposition their hands to the anterior surface of the patient to control the second half of the turning movement.

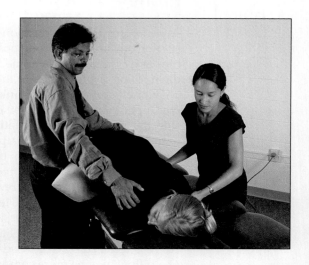

8 When a turn is completed, a patient's head and neck are the first body segments to be repositioned. Place the patient's head in a comfortable position facing the side that will allow best interaction with others and the environment. Positioning the head turned to one side eliminates pressure on the eyes, nose, or mouth but may increase pressure on the external ear. Place a small towel under the temple to relieve pressure on the external ear. In some situations the head may be maintained in the midline, using a small pillow or towel under the forehead to relieve pressure on the eyes, nose, and mouth and to permit unimpeded respiration.

Adjust the position of the pillow under the trunk as needed. Place the arms in a position of slight abduction. Finally, uncross the patient's feet if they remained crossed after the turning movement was completed. Position the patient's lower extremities so the feet are approximately 6 to 8 inches apart.

To turn supine to prone to the right, the previous procedure is used, with the designation of left side becoming right side and the designation of right side becoming left side.

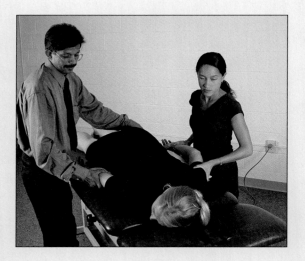

(continued)

Prone Position

A **prone** position is a position in which a person lies on his or her stomach on a supporting surface. In a prone position, patients are positioned with shoulders parallel to hips and with a straight spine. The head may be turned to either side, or maintained in the midline, as described in the previous section. A patient's upper extremities may be positioned alongside the trunk or alongside the head. For some patients, circulation in the upper extremities may be compromised when the patient's arms are placed alongside the patient's head. Position upper extremities alongside the head only when a patient has sensation in the upper extremities and can communicate reliably if a problem arises. When a patient's upper extremities are positioned alongside the head, the physical therapist/assistant should question the patient frequently to determine if the patient is experiencing numbness or tingling.

A pillow may be placed lengthwise or crosswise under the trunk to ensure that spinal curvature is not excessive at any segment. A lengthwise position may be more comfortable when patients have limited neck mobility. The lumbar region's lordotic curve is reduced by crosswise positioning of the pillow. Therefore, a crosswise position of a pillow may be more comfortable for patients with low back pain. Patients with tender or large breasts may also be more comfortable with the pillow in a crosswise position, distal to the breasts. A pillow under the lower legs can also be used to avoid positioning the ankles in plantar flexion (■ Figure 8–5). A pillow under the lower legs places the knees in slight flexion, however, and may promote loss of knee extension range of motion. A patient's feet can be positioned over the end of a treatment table to avoid positioning the ankles in plantar flexion (■ Figure 8–6).

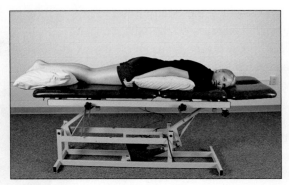

■ **Figure 8–5** Prone position with pillows under the trunk and lower legs.

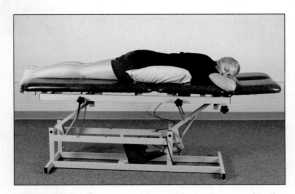

■ **Figure 8–6** Prone position with a pillow under the trunk and feet positioned over the end of the treatment table.

PROCEDURE 8–3   Turning from Prone to Supine

Turning a patient from prone to supine is similar to turning a patient from supine to prone. Since the patient's initial position is prone, the physical therapist/assistant first moves the patient far enough to one side of the treatment table to allow a full turning movement to the supine position without coming too near the opposite edge upon completion of the turning movement. To turn to the right, the physical therapist/assistant first moves a patient to the left side of the treatment table. When segmental movement of the trunk and lower extremities is possible, the physical therapist/assistant moves the patient in stages. When the patient cannot tolerate such movement, more than one person, or specialized beds, will be needed.

To move a patient from prone to supine, the following steps occur in sequence.

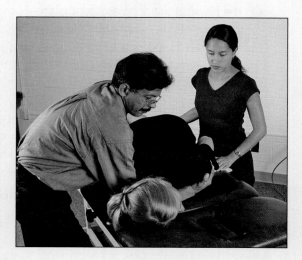

1 Move the patient's upper trunk and head to the left side of the treatment table.

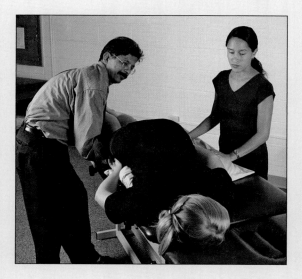

2 Move the patient's lower trunk to the left side of the treatment table.

3 Move the patient's lower extremities to the left side of the treatment table.

(continued)

④ Place the patient's right hand, the hand over which the patient will roll, under the patient's hip with the palm against the body.

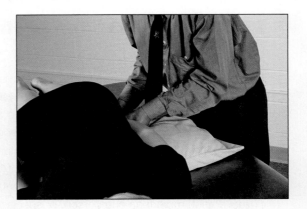

⑤ The physical therapist/assistant is again positioned on the side to which the patient is being turned. When a treatment table is narrow, clinicians assisting in turning the patient should stand next to the patient on the side from which the patient is being turned to prevent the patient from falling as the physical therapist/assistant moves from one side of the treatment table to the other. Clinicians assisting in turning the patient can help with positioning of pillows and turning the patient.

When a patient does not have head and neck control, rubbing of the patient's face on the mattress or mat can be avoided by having the patient start by facing away from the physical therapist/assistant. A patient with head and neck control can assist by looking up and over her shoulder while being turned toward the physical therapist/assistant.

⑥ The patient's left upper extremity is adducted, placing the hand at the hip, palm against the hip. The physical therapist/assistant supports the right upper extremity against the patient's body as the patient is turned.

⑦ As in turning from supine to prone, the physical therapist/assistant must control both phases of the turning motion. Initially, the physical therapist/assistant reaches over the patient, placing his hands on the patient's anterior surface.

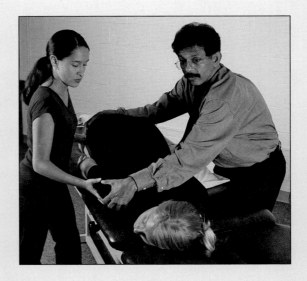

8 When a patient reaches the halfway point, gravity can complete the movement but will do so in an uncontrolled manner. The physical therapist/assistant must, therefore, rotate and reposition his hands as patients reach the midpoint of the turn. The physical therapist/assistant and other clinicians should reposition their hands to the posterior surface of the patient to control the second half of the turning movement.

9 When a turn is completed, a patient's head and neck are the first body segments to be repositioned. The extremities are then positioned as in the supine position.

To turn prone to supine to the left, the previous procedure is used, with the designation of left side becoming right side and the designation of right side becoming left side.

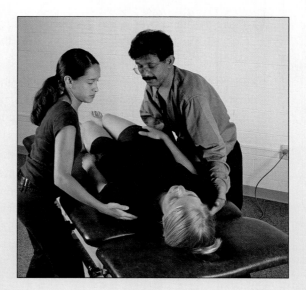

PROCEDURE 8–4   Turning on a Floor Mat

When turning a patient on a floor mat, the same steps and sequence are followed as when turning a patient on a treatment table. Proper body mechanics become more important in preventing injury to physical therapists/assistants when turning a patient on a floor mat.

To turn a patient on a floor mat, the following steps occur in sequence.

1 After a patient is moved to one side of the mat, the physical therapist/assistant should be positioned on the side to which the patient will turn. The physical therapist/assistant should assume a half-kneeling position, with the "down" knee at the level of the patient's hips and the "up" knee at the level of the patient's shoulders.

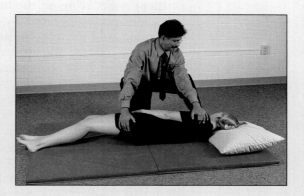

(continued)

2 Place the hand over which the patient will roll against the hip on the same side, with the palm facing the hip.

3 Place the hand that will be on top during the roll against the hip on the same side, with the palm facing the hip. Using the hand closest to the patient's hips, the physical therapist/assistant holds the patient's hand in place against the patient's hip. The physical therapist's/assistant's hand closer to the patient's head is placed on the patient's shoulder. The physical therapist's/assistant's hand position must rotate and reposition at the midpoint of the turn, as described for turning on a treatment table.

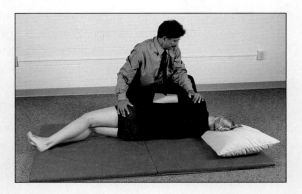

4 The physical therapist/assistant must move out of the patient's way as the turn is completed, allowing the patient to complete the turn without rolling into the physical therapist/assistant.

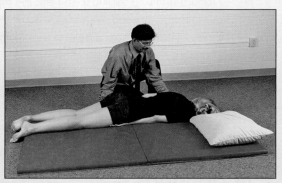

Sidelying

A **sidelying position** is a position in which a patient is lying on one side. The positions of the upper extremities and lower extremities will vary, depending upon whether the patient's upper trunk is rotated forward or backward while in a sidelying position.

In a sidelying position in which the patient's upper trunk is rotated forward (■ Figure 8–7), the lowermost upper extremity is slightly flexed at the shoulder so the patient is not lying on the humerus, the uppermost upper extremity is flexed at the shoulder and supported by a pillow, the lowermost lower extremity is relatively extended, and the uppermost lower extremity is flexed at the hip and knee and supported on pillows. The uppermost lower extremity should be supported by enough pillows so that it is not lowered into adduction. To avoid excessive pressure on the lowermost lower extremity, the uppermost lower extremity should not lie directly on top of the lowermost lower extremity.

In a sidelying position in which the patient's upper trunk is rotated backward (■ Figure 8–8), the lowermost upper extremity shoulder girdle is protracted and the shoulder is slightly flexed so the patient is not lying on the humerus, the uppermost upper extremity is extended and supported by pillows behind the patient, the lowermost lower extremity is flexed at the hip and knee, and the uppermost lower extremity is relatively extended and supported on pillows. The uppermost lower extremity should be supported by enough pillows so that it is not lowered into adduction. To avoid excessive pressure on the lowermost lower extremity, the uppermost lower extremity should not lie directly on top of the lowermost lower extremity.

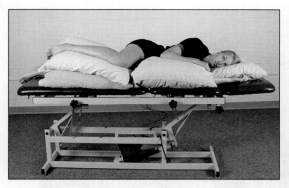

■ **Figure 8–7** Sidelying position with upper trunk rotated forward.

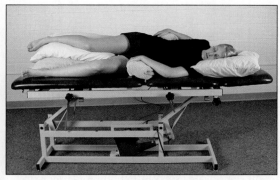

■ **Figure 8–8** Sidelying position with upper trunk rotated backward.

PROCEDURE 8–5   Turning from Supine or Prone to Sidelying

A patient can be turned to a sidelying position from either the supine or prone position. The steps in turning a patient from supine to sidelying are similar to those for turning a patient from supine to prone, with the movement stopping when the patient reaches the midpoint of the turn. The patient is then positioned in the chosen one of the two sidelying positions.

The steps in turning a patient from prone to sidelying are similar to those for turning a patient from prone to supine, with the movement stopping when the patient reaches the midpoint of the turn. The patient is then positioned in the chosen one of the two sidelying positions.

PROCEDURE 8–6   Moving from Supine to Sitting

There are various methods for assisting a patient to assume a sitting position. The method chosen will depend upon a patient's functional abilities, medical problems, and starting position. Whichever method is chosen, patients should not be left unguarded in a sitting position if they cannot maintain the position independently in a safe manner.

Supine to Long Sitting

Long sitting is a position in which a person sits with hips flexed to 90 degrees and knees fully extended on a supporting surface. When patients have sufficient strength, they can assume a long-sitting position by doing a sit-up from supine to sitting. To assist a patient in moving from supine to long sitting, the following steps occur in sequence.

(continued)

1 When minimal assistance is needed, as for patients with generalized weakness, a trapeze bar can be used. In some situations patients can perform a sit-up or use a trapeze bar while a physical therapist/assistant provides assistance. A physical therapist/assistant can place an arm behind a patient's back to assist the patient in changing position. When a trapeze bar is not available, a physical therapist/assistant can stabilize an arm in front of the patient in lieu of a trapeze bar.

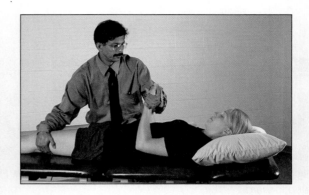

2 A patient can pull up by pulling on a physical therapist's/assistant's arm. The physical therapist/assistant may assist the sit-up movement by placing an arm across a patient's thighs to stabilize the patient's lower extremities.

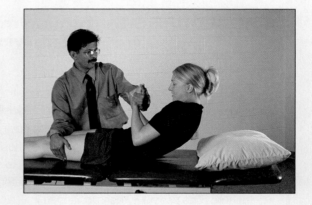

3 The physical therapist/assistant should not move the arm and do the patient's work of pulling up into a sitting position. As necessary, the physical therapist/assistant should move toward the patient's feet to permit the patient to assume a long-sitting position.

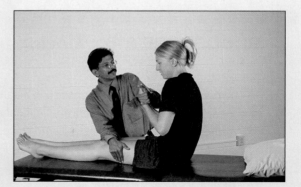

Sidelying to Sitting on Side of Table

To assist a patient in moving from sidelying to sitting, the following steps occur in sequence.

1 The patient assumes a sidelying position to the side of the treatment table on which the patient wishes to sit.

 The patient's hips and knees are flexed 60 degrees to 90 degrees and the patient's lower legs are moved over the edge of the treatment table to act as counterweight to the patient's trunk and upper extremities.

 The physical therapist/assistant assists the patient in assuming a sitting position by placing one arm under the patient's thighs to control the rate of lowering the patient's lower extremities and one arm under the patient's shoulder to assist in coming to sitting.

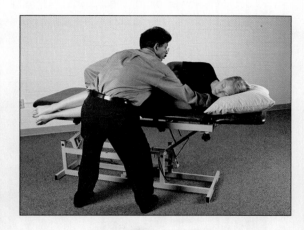

2 With the lower extremities acting as counterweights, the patient uses the upper extremities to push to sitting.

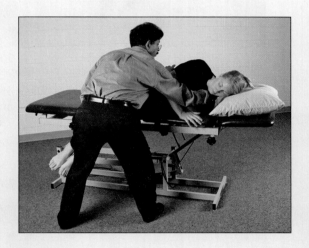

3 The physical therapist/assistant assists by controlling lowering of the patient's lower extremities and lifting the upper trunk as necessary.

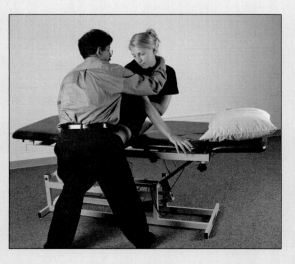

(continued)

Supine to Sitting on Side of Table

When patients are dependent upon higher levels of assistance, the physical therapist/assistant uses the lower extremities as counterweights to provide additional assistance. To move a patient from supine to sitting, the following steps occur in sequence.

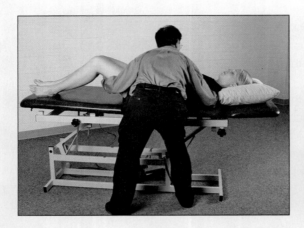

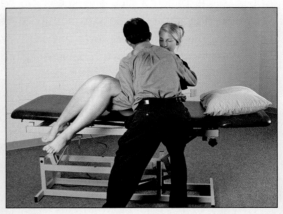

1 Starting in supine position, the physical therapist/assistant places one arm around the upper trunk at the level of the patient's shoulders and the other arm under the patient's thighs.

2 The physical therapist/assistant simultaneously lifts the patient's trunk and lowers the patient's lower extremities over the side of the table.

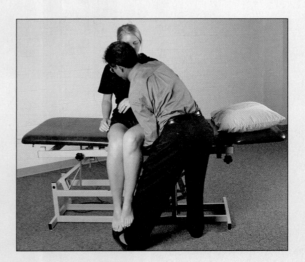

3 The physical therapist/assistant lifts the patient into a sitting position and pivots her to sitting over the side of the table.

Chapter Review

Review Questions

1. List the goals for proper positioning.

2. State the purposes of proper positioning for the four practice patterns: integumentary, musculoskeletal, neuromuscular, and cardiovascular/pulmonary.

3. Describe how physical therapists determine the proper amount of time a patient can be in a position.

4. Describe how to position a patient properly in the supine, prone, and sidelying positions.

5. Describe how to turn a patient properly from supine to prone, supine to sidelying, sidelying to prone, sidelying to supine, and prone to supine.

6. Describe how to assist a patient to sitting from supine.

Suggested Activities

1. Demonstrate the specific procedures presented.

2. Practice specific procedures working in groups of three, role-playing patient, therapist, and assistant.

3. Practice performing turning and positioning while other partners role-play diagnoses (see following case studies). The student role-playing the patient can add "character" to the role by employing behaviors such as being cooperative, noncooperative, in pain, hard of hearing, or faint. The "patient" must role-play the diagnosis and character consistently, so the students must have researched the diagnosis, signs, and symptoms. The student role-playing the physical therapist/assistant should document the "intervention."

4. Monitor vital signs and check for signs of skin irritation as appropriate.

5. Practice teaching "family and patients" and other health-care providers how to perform turning and positioning. Document the intervention.

Case Studies

For the following case study situations, describe and/or demonstrate appropriate turning and positioning procedures. For each procedure or position chosen, provide an appropriate rationale.

1. The patient is a 59-year-old male with right hemiplegia who presents with mild spasticity in both right extremities and expressive aphasia.
2. The patient is a 21-year-old with T12 complete spinal cord injury.
3. The patient is a 12-year-old with moderate spastic cerebral palsy.
4. The patient is a 75-year-old with a fractured right hip status post hip replacement.

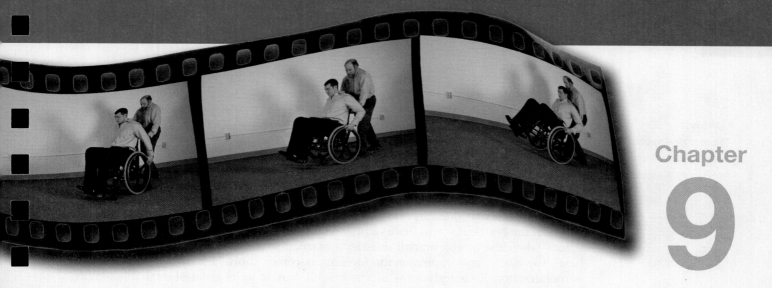

Range of Motion Exercise

Learning Objectives

Upon completion of this chapter, you will be able to:

1. Describe anatomical position.
2. Define the terms used to describe movements in the anatomical planes.
3. Distinguish between joint range of motion (ROM) and muscle ROM.
4. Indicate when passive ROM (PROM), active assisted ROM (AAROM), or active ROM (AROM) intervention is appropriate.
5. Describe different joint end feels.
6. Describe differences in movement when a patient has normal muscle tone, spasticity, rigidity, and pain.
7. Describe general methods used to perform ROM exercises properly.
8. Describe the benefits of using diagonal patterns of motion.
9. Describe the combining components of motion used in proprioceptive neuromuscular facilitation (PNF) patterns.
10. Describe the specific procedures used to perform ROM exercises in the anatomical planes and diagonal patterns of motion.

Key Terms

Abduction
Active assisted range of motion (AAROM)
Active range of motion (AROM)
Adduction
Anatomical planes of movement
Anatomical position
Biarticular
Combining components
Diagonal patterns of movement
End feel
Eversion
Extension
External (lateral) rotation
Flexion
Horizontal abduction
Horizontal adduction

Internal (medial) rotation
Inversion
Joint range of motion
Muscle range of motion
Opposition
Passive range of motion (PROM)
Pronation
Proprioceptive neuromuscular facilitation (PNF)
Protraction
Radial deviation
Range of motion (ROM)
Retraction
Rigidity
Spasticity
Supination
Ulnar deviation
Uniarticular

Introduction

Range of motion (ROM) is movement of each joint and muscle through its available arc of motion. ROM movements are included in plans of care as interventions to prevent development of contractures, muscle shortening, and tightness in capsules, ligaments, and tendons, all of which can limit mobility. ROM interventions also provide sensory stimulation beneficial to patients.

Joint ROM is moving a joint in all planes of motion appropriate for the specific joint. Limitations of joint ROM may result from bony structure of joint surfaces, internal derangement of joint structures, lack of length of soft tissue (capsule,

■ **Take Note**

Joint range of motion: Movement to maintain mobility of joints.

cartilage, ligament, muscle, skin, tendon) surrounding the joint, or pain. Examples include decreased joint ROM resulting from deterioration of joint surfaces, meniscal tears, ligament adhesions, or shortness of single joint (**uniarticular**) muscles.

Muscle ROM is lengthening a muscle through its available length for all appropriate joint motions. To lengthen a muscle, joints must be moved in the direction opposite the shortening action of the specific muscle. This will affect both single joint (uniarticular) and multijoint (**biarticular**) muscles. When a joint is moved through all available ROM, muscle ROM for muscles that cross only that joint (uniarticular muscles) is also achieved. To lengthen muscles that cross more than one joint (biarticular muscles), all joints the biarticular muscles cross must be moved in a manner that achieves full elongation of the biarticular muscles as a final result. An example of decreased muscle ROM occurs when the biceps brachii muscle, a biarticular muscle that flexes the shoulder, flexes the elbow, and supinates the forearm, becomes shortened following prolonged immobilization. To lengthen the biceps brachii muscle to its greatest available length, the shoulder and elbow must be extended and the forearm pronated. These movements may occur simultaneously or in sequence, provided that the end result is having all joint movements at their greatest limit at the same time.

In certain circumstances, a goal of treatment is to allow biarticular muscles to become shortened (not able to be lengthened over all joints at once) to provide a more functional length. Biarticular muscles that cannot be lengthened completely over all joints at the same time will cause these muscles to shorten across one joint when lengthened completely across another joint. This functional use of shortening is called tenodesis action. An example of tenodesis producing function is when shortened long finger flexors cause grasp and release as the wrist is extended and flexed. Patients with quadriplegia use this tenodesis to hold and release utensils, such as a fork, toothbrush, or writing implement.

Physical therapists must differentiate between ROM exercises, which use only the available range of motion, and stretching exercises. Stretching exercises are designed to increase the available range of motion by having an effect on joint structure and soft tissue. Physical therapists determine the appropriate intervention, ROM or stretching. Physical therapist assistants may provide both interventions upon direction by physical therapists.

Joint and muscle range-of-motion exercises may be performed as passive range of motion (PROM), active assisted range of motion (AAROM), and active range of motion (AROM) exercises. **Passive range of motion** exercise is performed with the patient relaxed and a physical therapist/assistant moving the body segment without patient assistance.

Active assisted range of motion is performed by a physical therapist/assistant assisting a patient in performing movement. **Active range of motion** exercises are performed independently by a patient, although they may be supervised by a physical therapist/assistant to ensure correct performance. ■ Table 9–1 indicates the different types of ROM exercises and the impairments patients may have for which specific types of range of motion exercises are indicated.

The limit of ROM is achieved when a body segment cannot be moved farther because of restriction by joint structure or soft tissues or because of patient reports of pain. When a limit of motion is reached, the quality of restriction felt by a physical therapist/assistant is described as "**end feel**." End feel may occur based on a number of variables, including joint structure and soft tissue. Normal end feel may vary depending on the reason for nonpathological limitation of further motion. When further motion is limited by bone abutting bone, the end feel is hard and is called *bony end feel.* An example of a nonpathological bony end feel occurs when complete elbow extension is attained. At this point, movement is halted by contact between the olecranon process of the ulna and the olecranon fossa of the humerus. When further motion is limited by a soft tissue approximation, the end feel is soft. An example of nonpathological soft end feel occurs when elbow flexion is limited by forearm soft tissue approximating the muscle bulk of elbow flexors on the anterior surface of the upper arm. A firm end feel

■ **Take Note**

Muscle range of motion: movement to maintain mobility of multijoint muscles.

■ **Take Note**

Types of range of motion: passive range of motion, active assistive range of motion, active range of motion.

■ **Take Note**

End feel: the "feel" when a joint reaches the end of motion—bony, firm, soft.

TABLE 9–1 Types of Range of Motion and Indications for Use

Type	Use
Passive	Paralysis, paresis, weakness, pain, increased muscle tone.
	When active assisted or active, would cause excessive cardiopulmonary stress.
	When a patient lacks safe control of movement.
	Maintain joint and soft tissue mobility.
	Maintain joint and tissue nutrition.
	Increase kinesthetic awareness.
Active assisted	Paresis, weakness, pain, cardiopulmonary problems, abnormal tone.
	Maintain joint and soft tissue mobility.
	Maintain joint and tissue nutrition.
	Increase kinesthetic awareness.
Active	Patient can move correctly without causing undue stress on any body system.
	Maintain joint and soft tissue mobility.
	Maintain joint and tissue nutrition.
	Increase kinesthetic awareness.

with minimal give is a result of a taut capsule or ligament. This is known as a *capsular end feel*. An example of nonpathological capsular end feel occurs when a nonpathological knee is stress-tested for varus (adduction) and valgus (abduction) strain. When further motion is limited by pain, there is no tissue limitation to motion and the end feel is described as an empty end feel.

Involuntary muscle contractions or pain can interfere with movement. Patients who have upper motor (central nervous system) lesions, or patients trying to avoid pain, may have involuntary muscle contractions. Muscle tone is altered in upper motor neuron lesions, presenting as spasticity or rigidity. Spasticity presents as increased resistance to movement, especially as the velocity of movement is increased. When spasticity is present, a point in the range of motion may be reached where further muscle lengthening is temporarily prevented. If force is maintained, a sudden reduction in tone may occur, and movement through the remaining range of motion is possible. This is referred to as the *clasp-knife phenomenon*. Spasticity usually occurs in antigravity muscles. Rigidity presents as resistance to passive movement that is not affected by movement velocity. Both antigravity and progravity muscles may present with rigidity. In the presence of spasticity or rigidity, slow, maintained movement usually permits movement through the complete range of motion without eliciting interference.

Methods

To assist physical therapists/assistants in maintaining proper posture and body mechanics during ROM exercises, a table or bed of appropriate height for the individual therapist should be used. Preparing a treatment area and the use of proper body mechanics is covered in Chapter 3.

Passive ROM (PROM) exercises during rehabilitation preferably are performed by physical therapists/assistants twice each day. Additional exercise times during each day assisted by other clinicians or family members can be quite useful. A frequently chosen number of repetitions for each movement is ten; however, fewer repetitions still provide benefits. The exact frequency and number of repetitions of PROM exercises needed to maintain tissue extensibility is not known and likely varies for each patient and the need for such exercises. Typically, PROM is performed once or twice a day by a physical therapist/assistant. When a patient can perform active-assisted or active ROM exercises, physical therapists again determine the frequency of treatment periods and the number of repetitions for each movement. Physical therapists/assistants, other clinicians, or family members may participate or oversee sessions when directed by a physical therapist.

ROM exercises are performed by moving the body segments through each **anatomical plane of motion** separately or by combining components of motion. When using anatomical plane movements, multiple joints may be exercised simultaneously. Examples include combinations of hip and knee flexion with ankle dorsiflexion and hip and knee extension with ankle plantar flexion. **Combining components** of motion occurs when more than one plane of joint motion is performed simultaneously. **Diagonal patterns of movement** described by **proprioceptive neuromuscular facilitation (PNF)** are combining components of motion at one joint as well as all the joints of an extremity.

Physical therapists determine whether anatomical planes of movement or diagonal patterns of movement are used. Physical therapist assistants may provide both interventions upon direction by physical therapists. Anatomical planes of movement allow more specific isolation of joint motions and involved musculature. Full joint motion may be more easily accomplished using anatomical planes of movement, which does not usually occur when using diagonal patterns of movement. Diagonal patterns of movement simulate functional joint movement more closely than do anatomical planes of motion.

Gentle but secure manual contact is used to provide support when performing range-of-motion exercises. Hand placement should allow movement of body segments through complete ROM and provide support of all joints with minimal hand repositioning. Velocity of movement should be slow to moderate. Joint ROM exercises should encompass all planes of motion available in a joint. Muscle ROM exercises must result in lengthening biarticular muscles across all joints crossed simultaneously.

Anatomical Planes of Movement

All motions of the body are described in terms of starting from the anatomical position. The **anatomical position** is described as that position in which a person is standing upright, eyes looking straight ahead, arms at the sides with palms facing forward, and the feet approximately 4 inches apart at the heels, with the toes pointing forward (■ Figures 9–1 and ■ 9–2).

■ **Take Note**

Anatomical planes of motion: flexion/extension, abduction/adduction, internal/external rotation.

■ **Take Note**

Combining components of motion: PNF diagonal patterns.

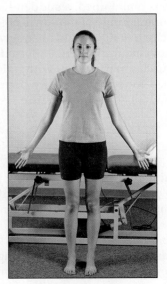

■ **Figure 9–1** Anterior view of anatomical position.

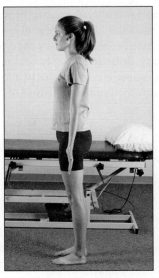

■ **Figure 9–2** Lateral view of anatomical position.

Three anatomical, or cardinal, planes are defined with respect to the anatomical position. The *sagittal* plane divides the body into two sides—left and right. The *midsagittal* plane divides the body exactly into left and right halves. Motions of flexion and extension occur in the sagittal plane. The *frontal,* or coronal, plane divides the body into front and back portions. Motions of abduction and adduction occur in the frontal plane. The only motions of flexion/extension and abduction/adduction that do not occur in their respective planes of motion are motions of the thumb. Thumb flexion and extension occur in the frontal plane, and thumb abduction and adduction occur in the sagittal plane. The *transverse* plane divides the body into upper and lower portions. All movements of rotation, and horizontal abduction and adduction of the shoulders, occur in the transverse plane.

The following definitions assume the starting position is the anatomical position:

Flexion: Except for the thumb, flexion is movement in a sagittal plane. For the neck, trunk, upper extremities, and lower extremities except knee and toes, flexion results in approximation of anterior limb segment surfaces. For the knee and toes, flexion results in approximation of the posterior and plantar limb segment surfaces respectively. Dorsiflexion, moving the foot and toes upward, is the movement of the ankle considered flexion. Thumb flexion is approximation of the palmar limb segment surfaces and occurs in the frontal plane.

Extension: Except for the thumb, extension is movement in the sagittal plane. For the neck, trunk, upper extremities, and lower extremities other than knee and toes, extension results in anterior limb segment surfaces moving away from each other. For the knee and toes, extension results in posterior and plantar limb segment surfaces moving away from each other, respectively. Plantar flexion, moving the foot and toes downward, is the movement of the ankle considered extension. Thumb extension is moving the palmar limb segment surfaces away from each other and occurs in the frontal plane.

Abduction: Except for the thumb, abduction is movement in the frontal plane and is the result of the limb segment surfaces moving away from the midline of the body. Thumb abduction is movement of the thumb away from the palm of the hand and occurs in the sagittal plane. When the wrist is moved such that the hand moves away from the midline of the body, the movement is labeled **radial deviation**.

Adduction: Except for the thumb, adduction is movement in the frontal plane and is the result of the limb segment surfaces moving toward the midline of the body. Thumb adduction is movement of the thumb into the palm of the hand and occurs in the sagittal plane. When the wrist is moved such that the hand moves toward the midline of the body, the movement is labeled **ulnar deviation**.

Horizontal abduction: Horizontal abduction is movement of the upper extremity posteriorly when the shoulder has already been abducted to 90 degrees in the frontal plane.

Horizontal adduction: Horizontal adduction is movement of the upper extremity anteriorly when the shoulder has already been abducted to 90 degrees in the frontal plane.

Protraction: Protraction is multiplanar movement of the scapula around the lateral aspect of the ribs toward the anterior aspect of the thorax. This motion is often termed scapular abduction.

Retraction: Retraction is multiplanar movement of the scapula around the lateral aspect of the ribs as the scapula moves toward the spine. This motion is often termed scapular adduction.

Opposition: Opposition is multiplanar movement of the carpometacarpal joint of the thumb that results in approximation of the tip of the thumb and the tip of a finger of the same hand. There is no term that describes the opposite motion.

Internal (medial) rotation: Internal rotation is movement in the transverse plane that results in anterior limb segment surfaces turning inward, toward the midline of the body.

■ **Take Note**
Exceptions for flexion and extension—thumbs, knees, toes.

External (lateral) rotation: External rotation is movement in the transverse plane that results in anterior limb segment surfaces turning outward, away from the midline of the body.

Supination: Supination is defined differently for the upper and lower extremities. For the upper extremity, supination of the forearm occurs when the arm is stabilized and the forearm is rotated so that the palm of the hand faces anteriorly. This is a uniplanar movement occurring in the transverse plane. Supination of the forearm is the position of the forearm in the anatomical position. For the lower extremity, supination of the foot occurs when the leg is stabilized and the foot is rotated about the oblique axis of the subtalar and other midfoot joints. This is a triplanar motion that incorporates plantar flexion, forefoot adduction, and inversion of the foot.

Pronation: Pronation is defined differently for the upper and lower extremities. For the upper extremity, pronation of the forearm occurs when the arm is stabilized and the forearm is rotated so that the palm of the hand faces posteriorly. This is a uniplanar movement occurring in the transverse plane. For the lower extremity, pronation of the foot occurs when the leg is stabilized and the foot is rotated about the oblique axis of the subtalar and other midfoot joints. This is a triplanar motion that incorporates dorsiflexion, forefoot abduction, and eversion of the foot.

Inversion: Inversion is movement of the foot that occurs in the frontal plane about the long axis of the foot. Inversion occurs when the foot is rotated about the long axis of the foot such that the plantar surface of the foot faces toward the midline of the body.

Eversion: Eversion is movement of the foot that occurs in the frontal plane about the long axis of the foot. Eversion occurs when the foot is rotated about the long axis of the foot such that the plantar surface of the foot faces away from the midline of the body.

Confusion exists concerning the use of the terms supination/pronation and inversion/eversion when describing motion at the ankle and foot. The definitions provided earlier are those used by a majority of clinicians in practice. The clinical definitions are based upon the writing of Root, Orien, and Weed.[2] Using clinical definitions, supination and pronation are terms describing triplanar movements, of which inversion and eversion are uniplanar components. Anatomists Warwick and Williams,[3] however, describe these terms of ankle and foot motion in the opposite manner. Under the anatomical definitions, inversion and eversion are terms describing triplanar movement, of which supination and pronation are uniplanar components. In the text, these terms are used in accordance with the clinical definitions presented by Root et al.[2]

Diagonal Patterns of Movement

Two diagonal patterns of movement have been described for the upper and lower extremities.[1,4] Diagonal patterns of movement are achieved by simultaneously combining components of all three cardinal planes of motion and of multiple joints of an extremity. ■ Figure 9–3 illustrates the difference between two successive cardinal planes of motions on the left and the simultaneous combining of three cardinal planes of motion into a diagonal pattern on the right.

Specific diagonal patterns of motion are described by the combination of motions performed by either the shoulder or the hip joints (■ Figures 9–4 through 9–12). These patterns are modified by varying the position or movement of the elbow or knee, providing the ability to perform both joint ROM and muscle ROM exercises. The two diagonal patterns are commonly referred to as D1 and D2, where "D" stands for diagonal and "1" and "2" refer to specific diagonal patterns.

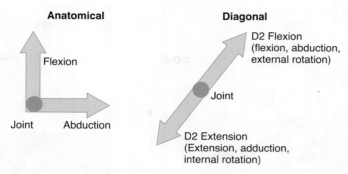

Anatomical

Flexion

Joint   Abduction

Diagonal

D2 Flexion
(flexion, abduction,
external rotation)

Joint

D2 Extension
(Extension, adduction,
internal rotation)

■ **Figure 9–3**   Anatomical vs. diagonal patterns of movement.

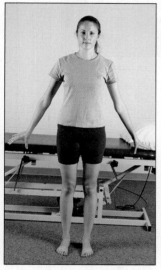

■ **Figure 9–4**   Bilateral upper
extremity D1 extension.

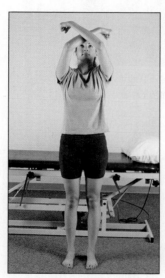

■ **Figure 9–5**   Bilateral upper
extremity D1 flexion.

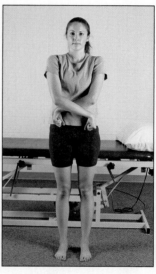

■ **Figure 9–6**   Bilateral upper
extremity D2 extension.

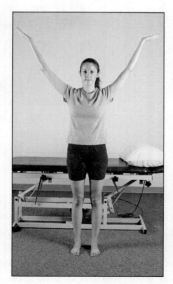

■ **Figure 9–7**   Bilateral upper
extremity D2 flexion.

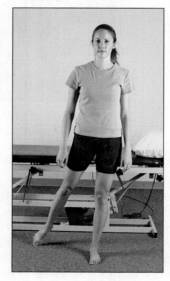

■ **Figure 9–8**   Right lower
extremity D1 extension with
knee extension.

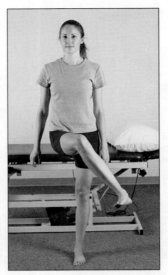

■ **Figure 9–9** Right lower extremity D1 flexion with knee flexion.

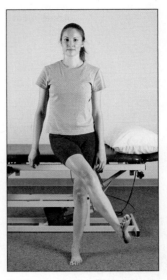

■ **Figure 9–10** Right lower extremity D1 flexion with knee extension.

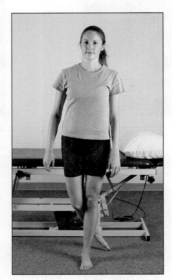

■ **Figure 9–11** Right lower extremity D2 extension with knee flexion.

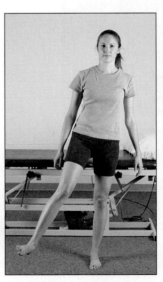

■ **Figure 9–12** Right lower extremity D2 flexion with knee extension.

When combining components of motion are performed, joint movements and muscle lengthening may not occur through as much ROM as when anatomical planes of motion are performed. However, the mobility that is necessary for function is maintained by use of diagonal patterns. Sensory feedback from movement in diagonal patterns is thought to be closer to the sensory feedback provided by normal active movement than movement in individual anatomical planes.

■ Table 9–2 lists the combining components of motion found in the proprioceptive neuromuscular facilitation patterns.

TABLE 9–2 Combining Components of Motion in PNF Diagonals

Diagonal 1 Upper Extremity

Segment	Flexion	Extension
Scapula	Elevation	Depression
	Abduction	Adduction
	Upward rotation	Downward rotation
Shoulder	Flexion	Extension
	Adduction	Abduction
	External rotation	Internal rotation
Elbow	Straight or flexion or extension	Straight or extension or flexion
Forearm	Supination	Pronation
Wrist	Flexion	Extension
	Radial deviation	Ulnar deviation
Fingers	Flexion	Extension
	Adduction	Abduction
Thumb	Flexion	Extension

Diagonal 1 Lower Extremity

Segment	Flexion	Extension
Hip	Flexion	Extension
	Adduction	Abduction
	External rotation	Internal rotation
Knee	Straight or flexion or extension	Straight or extension or flexion
Ankle	Dorsiflexion	Plantar flexion
	Inversion	Eversion
Toes	Extension	Flexion

Diagonal 2 Upper Extremity

Segment	Flexion	Extension
Scapula	Elevation	Depression
	Adduction	Abduction
	Upward rotation	Downward rotation
Shoulder	Flexion	Extension
	Abduction	Adduction
	External rotation	Internal rotation
Elbow	Straight or flexion or extension	Straight or extension or flexion
Forearm	Supination	Pronation
Wrist	Extension	Flexion
	Radial deviation	Ulnar deviation
Fingers	Extension	Flexion
	Abduction	Adduction
Thumb	Extension	Opposition

Diagonal 2 Lower Extremity

Segment	Flexion	Extension
Hip	Flexion	Extension
	Abduction	Adduction
	Internal rotation	External rotation
Knee	Straight or flexion or extension	Straight or extension or flexion
Ankle	Dorsiflexion	Plantar flexion
	Eversion	Inversion
Toes	Extension	Flexion

Directions

Illustrations in this chapter present ROM performed as passive ROM exercises. Presented are the joint(s) for which the exercise is being performed, the movement, and hand placement of the physical therapist/assistant. Where appropriate, precautions have been noted. For procedures specifically involving multijoint muscles, we have listed the muscles involved. Listed are the movements required to *lengthen* muscles, *not* movements produced by the muscles.

The order of presentation will be lower extremity movement in anatomical planes, lower extremity movement in diagonal patterns, upper extremity movement in anatomical planes, upper extremity movement in diagonal patterns, and head/neck/trunk movements.

PROCEDURE 9–1   Lower Extremity ROM Exercises: Anatomical Planes

Joints:	Hip and knee
Motion:	Extension and flexion
Position:	Supine
Hand placement:	Heel and posterior knee
Precaution:	Hip motion is complete when pelvic rotation occurs. Anterior pelvic rotation with hip extension, posterior pelvic rotation with hip flexion. Do not allow pelvic rotation to occur as hip motion is performed.

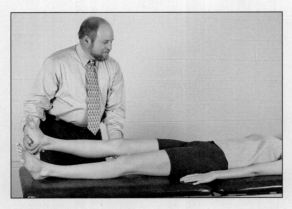

Hip and knee extension.

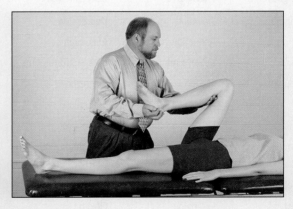

Hip and knee flexion.

Joints:	Hip and knee
Muscles:	Semitendinosus, semimembranosus, biceps femoris
Motions:	Hip flexion with knee extension—straight leg raise (SLR)
Position:	Supine
Hand placement:	Heel and posterior knee
Note:	This maneuver lengthens the multijoint muscles of the posterior thigh across both joints at which they act.
Precautions:	Keep the knee extended. Do not allow the hip to rotate, adduct, or abduct. Do not allow the pelvis to rotate posteriorly.

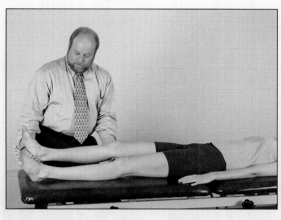

Starting position for straight leg raise (SLR).

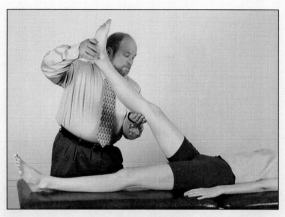

Hip flexion with knee extended (SLR).

Joint:	Hip
Motion:	Extension
Position:	Sidelying
Alternative Position:	Prone
Hand placement:	Place one hand on the pelvis for stabilization. The other hand and forearm support the patient's lower extremity in the anatomical position.
Note:	Maintain the knee in extension.
Precautions:	The end of hip extension is achieved when the pelvis starts to rotate anteriorly.

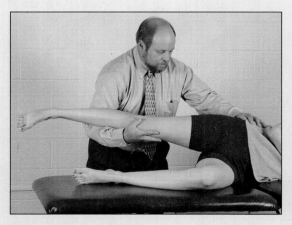

Hip extension in sidelying position.

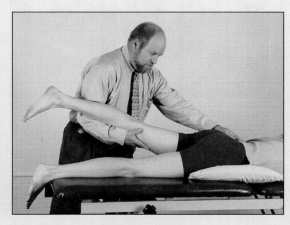

Hip extension in prone position.

(continued)

Joint: Hip
Motions: Abduction and adduction
Position: Supine
Hand placement: Heel and posterior knee
Note: To perform adduction beyond neutral, abduct the opposite lower extremity.
Precaution: Avoid hip flexion, hip rotation, and pelvic motion.

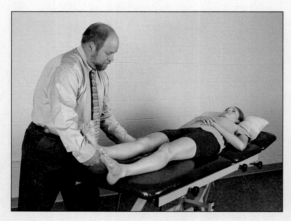

Starting position for hip abduction.

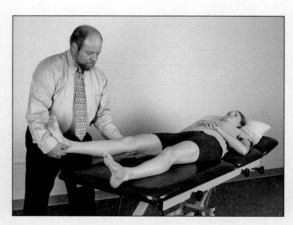

End position for hip abduction.

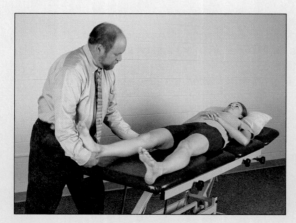

Starting position for hip adduction.

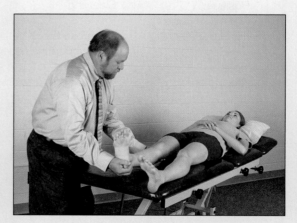

End position for hip adduction.

Joint:	Hip
Muscle:	Tensor facia latae
Motions:	Extension and adduction
Position:	Sidelying
Hand placement:	One hand stabilizes the pelvis. The other hand and forearm support the leg.
Note:	The tensor fascia latae flexes and abducts the hip and may assist in knee extension. Hip extension, adduction, and knee flexion lengthen this muscle.
Precaution:	Do not substitute lateral pelvic motion for hip adduction motion.

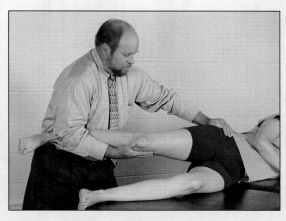

Starting position for tensor fascia latae lengthening.

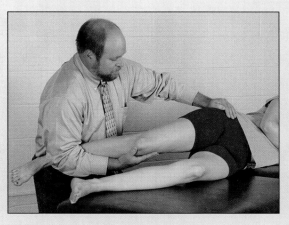

End position for tensor fascia latae lengthening.

(continued)

Joint: Hip
Motions: Internal and external rotation
Position: Sitting
Hand placement: One hand stabilizes the femur. The other hand grasps the distal leg.

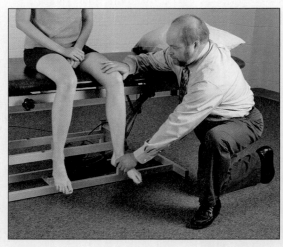

Starting position for hip internal rotation in sitting.

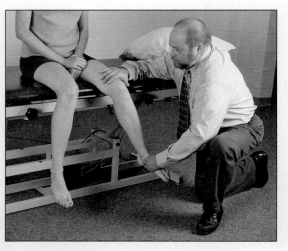

End position for hip internal rotation in sitting.

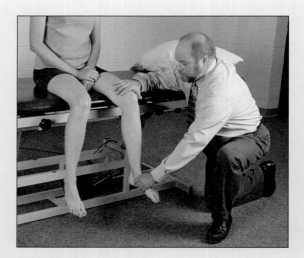

Starting position for hip external rotation in sitting.

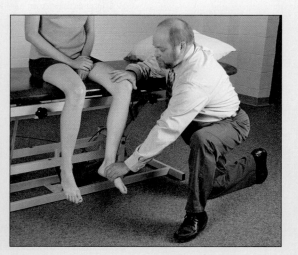

End position for hip external rotation in sitting.

Joint: Hip
Motions: Internal and external rotation
Position: Supine, with hip and knee flexed to 90 degrees
Hand placement: Heel and anterior knee
Alternative placement: Heel and posterior thigh
Precautions: Avoid excessive stress on the medial and lateral structures of the
                                knee. Maintain the pelvis flat on the supporting surface.

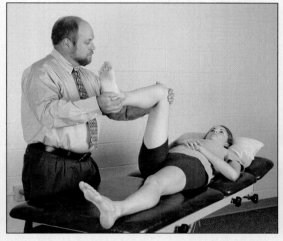

Starting position for hip internal rotation in supine with hip flexion.

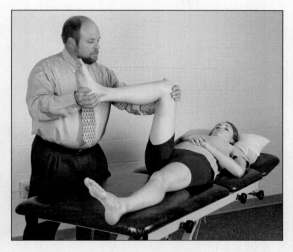

End position for hip internal rotation in supine with hip flexion.

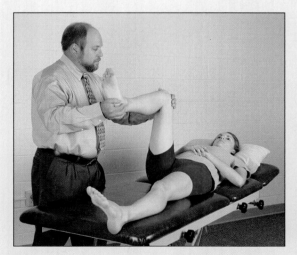

Starting position for hip external rotation in supine with hip flexion.

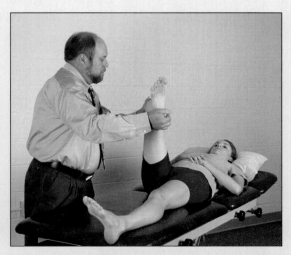

End position for hip external rotation in supine with hip flexion.

(continued)

Joint: Hip
Motions: Internal and external rotation
Position: Supine, with hip and knee extended
Hand placement: Heel and posterior knee
Precautions: Avoid excessive stress on the medial and lateral structures of the knee. Maintain the pelvis flat on the supporting surface.

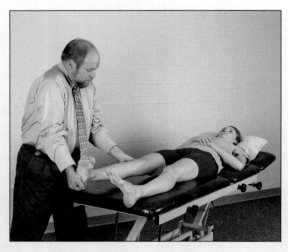

Hip rotation in supine with hip extended.

Joint: Knee
Motion: Flexion
Position: Supine with hip flexed to 90 degrees
Hand placement: Heel and distal femur

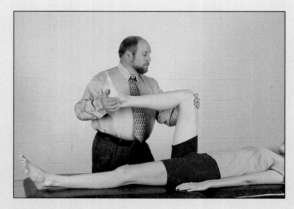

Midposition for knee flexion.

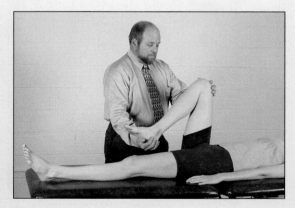

End position for knee flexion.

Joints:	Hip and knee
Muscle:	Rectus femoris
Motion:	Knee flexion with hip extended
Position:	Prone with hip extended
Alternative position:	Supine with knee at the end of the table
Hand placement:	One hand is on the posterior thigh or used to stabilize the pelvis. The other hand is on the distal tibia.
Precaution:	The rectus femoris is a hip flexor and knee extensor. Do not allow anterior pelvic rotation or hip flexion to occur.

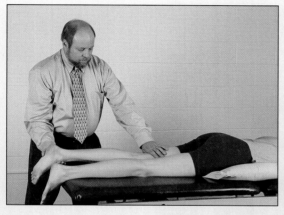

Starting position for rectus femoris range of motion.

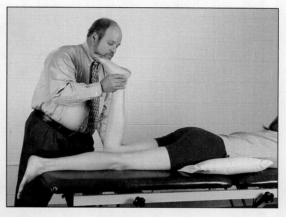

End position for rectus femoris range of motion.

Joint:	Ankle (talocrural)
Motion:	Plantar flexion
Position:	Supine
Hand placement:	Heel and dorsum of foot
Note:	Motion should emphasize movement of the talocrural joint, not midfoot joints.
Precaution:	Apply force to the heel in the superior direction, not to the dorsum of the foot.

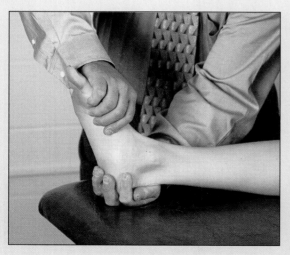

Starting position for ankle plantar flexion.

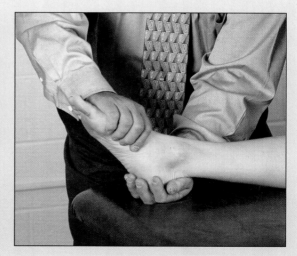

End position for ankle plantar flexion.

(continued)

Joint: Ankle (talocrural)
Motion: Dorsiflexion
Position: Supine with slight knee flexion
Hand placement: Heel and posterior calf
Note: To move structures of the ankle joint and the one joint soleus muscle, flex the knee such that the gastrocnemius muscle does not limit motion.
Precaution: Apply force to the heel in the inferior direction, not to the ball of the foot.

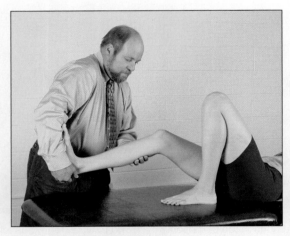

Ankle dorsiflexion.

Joint: Ankle (talocrural)
Muscle: Gastrocnemius
Position: Supine with knee extended
Hand placement: Heel and leg
Note: To move the gastrocnemius muscle simultaneously across all joints over which it acts, keep the knee extended as the ankle is dorsiflexed.
Precaution: Apply force to the heel in an inferior direction, not to the ball of the foot.

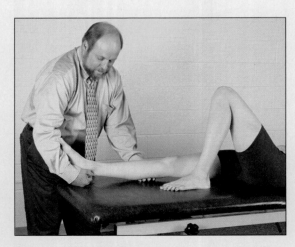 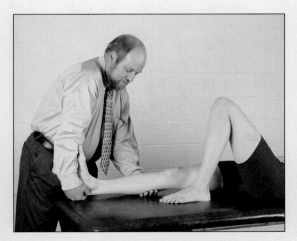

Starting position for gastrocnemius range of motion.   End position for gastrocnemius range of motion.

Joint:	Foot (intertarsal)
Motions:	Inversion and eversion
Position:	Supine
Hand placement:	One hand grasps the heel to stabilize the leg. The other hand grasps the forefoot.

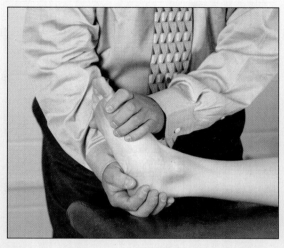

Starting position for foot inversion.

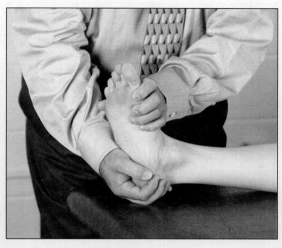

End position for foot inversion.

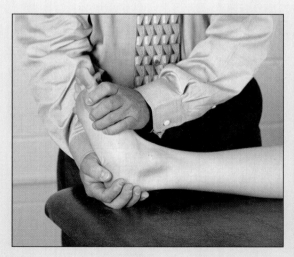

Starting position for foot eversion.

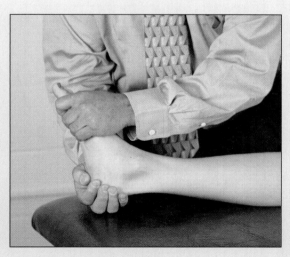

End position for foot eversion.

(continued)

Joints: Toes (metatarsophalangeal and interphalangeal)
Motions: Extension and flexion
Position: Supine
Hand placement: One hand stabilizes the foot and leg. The other hand grasps the toes.

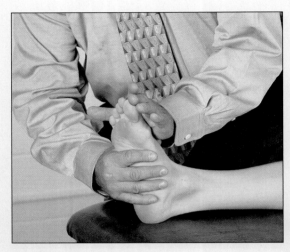

Starting position for toe flexion.

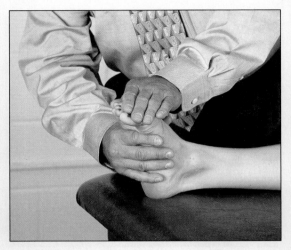

End position for toe flexion.

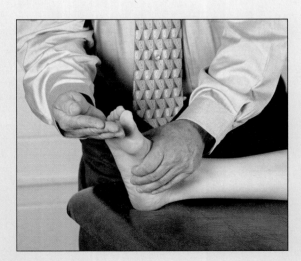

Starting position for toe extension.

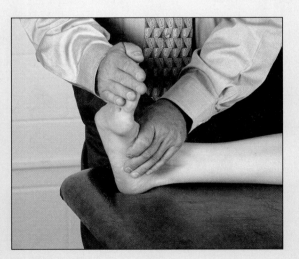

End position for toe extension.

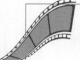

PROCEDURE 9–2 Lower Extremity ROM Exercises: Diagonal Patterns

MEDIALINK Watch the video on the CD for PROM: Lower extremity diagonal patterns under the heading of range of motion.

Pattern:	PNF diagonal 1 (D1) extension with knee extended
	PNF diagonal 1 (D1) flexion with knee extended
Combining components of motion:	D1 extension with knee extended
	Hip: extension, abduction, internal rotation
	Knee: extended
	Ankle and foot: planar flexion, eversion
	D1 flexion with knee extended
	Hip: flexion, adduction, external rotation
	Knee: extended
	Ankle and foot: dorsiflexion, inversion
Position:	Supine
Hand placement:	Heel and posterior thigh
Note:	*Knee extended* (straight) indicates that the knee remains in complete extension throughout the movement of both patterns. In these patterns, motion begins distally and progresses proximally, with the motions occuring more or less simultaneously.

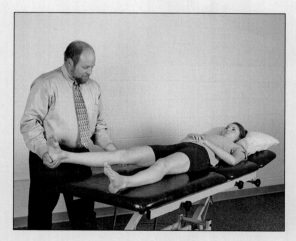

D1 extension with knee extended.

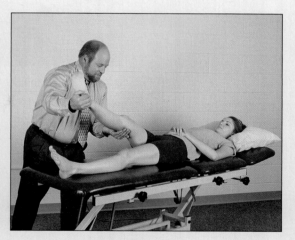

D1 flexion with knee extended.

(continued)

Pattern: PNF diagonal 1 (D1) extension with knee extension
                                   PNF diagonal 1 (D1) flexion with knee flexion
Combining components
of motion: D1 extension with knee extension
                                       Hip: extension, abduction, internal rotation
                                       Knee: extension
                                       Ankle and foot: plantar flexion, eversion
                                   D1 flexion with knee flexion
                                       Hip: flexion, adduction, external rotation
                                       Knee: flexion
                                       Ankle and foot: dorsiflexion, inversion
Position: Supine
Hand placement: Heel and posterior thigh
Note: In these patterns, motion begins distally and progresses proximally,
                                   with the motions occurring more or less simultaneously.

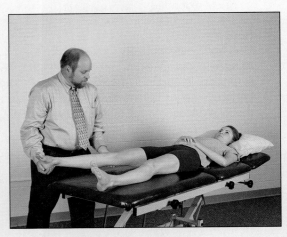

D1 extension with knee extension.

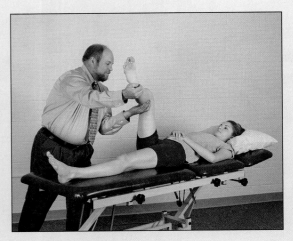

D1 flexion with knee flexion.

Pattern: PNF diagonal 1 (D1) extension with knee flexion
                                 PNF diagonal 1 (D1) flexion with knee extension
Combining components
of motion: D1 extension with knee flexion
                                     Hip: extension, abduction, internal rotation
                                     Knee: flexion
                                     Ankle and foot: plantar flexion, eversion
                                 D1 flexion with knee extension
                                     Hip: flexion, adduction, external rotation
                                     Knee: extension
                                     Ankle and foot: dorsiflexion, inversion
Position: Supine
Hand placement: Heel and posterior thigh
Note: In these patterns, motion begins distally and progresses proximally,
                                 with the motions occurring more or less simultaneously.

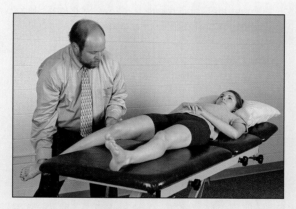

D1 extension with knee flexion.

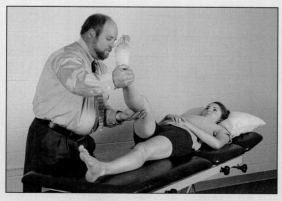

D1 flexion with knee extension.

(continued)

Pattern:	PNF diagonal 2 (D2) extension with knee extended
	PNF diagonal 2 (D2) flexion with knee extended
Combining components of motion:	D2 extension with knee extended
	Hip: extension, adduction, external rotation
	Knee: extended
	Ankle and foot: plantar flexion, inversion
	D2 flexion with knee extended
	Hip: flexion, abduction, internal rotation
	Knee: extended
	Ankle and foot: dorsiflexion, eversion
Position:	Supine
Hand placement:	Heel and posterior thigh
Note:	*Knee extended* indicates that the knee remains in complete extension throughout the movement of both patterns. In these patterns, motion begins distally and progresses proximally, with the motions occurring more or less simultaneously.
Precautions:	When performing PNF D2 patterns, the physical therapist/assistant must step and move to allow a patient's leg to move through the pattern completely and correctly.

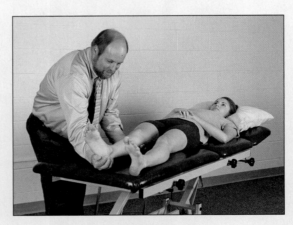

D2 extension with knee extended.

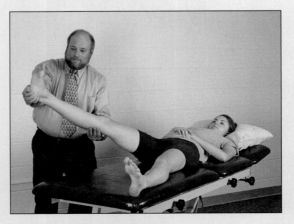

D2 flexion with knee extended.

Pattern: PNF diagonal 2 (D2) extension with knee extension
         PNF diagonal 2 (D2) flexion with knee flexion

Combining components
of motion: D2 extension with knee extension
          Hip: extension, adduction, external rotation
          Knee: extension
          Ankle and foot: plantar flexion, inversion
         D2 flexion with knee flexion
          Hip: flexion, abduction, internal rotation
          Knee: flexion
          Ankle and foot: dorsiflexion, eversion

Position: Supine
Hand placement: Heel and posterior thigh
Note: In these patterns, motion begins distally and progresses proximally,
        with the motions occurring more or less simultaneously.

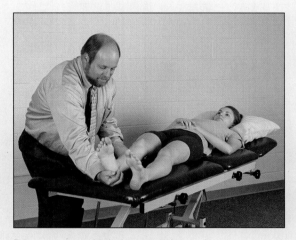

D2 extension with knee extension.

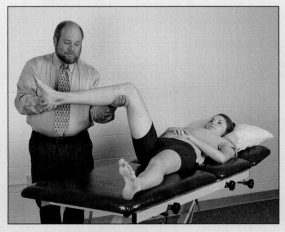

D2 flexion with knee flexion.

(continued)

Pattern:	PNF diagonal 2 (D2) extension with knee flexion
	PNF diagonal 2 (D2) flexion with knee extension
Combining components of motion:	
	D2 extension with knee flexion
	Hip: extension, adduction, external rotation
	Knee: flexion
	Ankle and foot: plantar flexion, inversion
	D2 flexion with knee extension
	Hip: flexion, abduction, internal rotation
	Knee: extension
	Ankle and foot: dorsiflexion, eversion
Position:	Supine, knee flexed over end of the table
Hand placement:	Heel and posterior thigh
Note:	In these patterns, motion begins distally and progresses proximally, with the motions occurring more or less simultaneously.

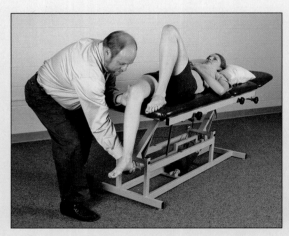

D2 extension with knee flexion.

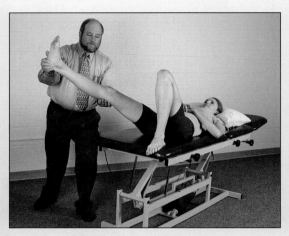

D2 flexion with knee extension.

PROCEDURE 9–3 Upper Extremity ROM Exercises: Anatomical Planes

Joint:	Shoulder girdle (scapulothoracic)
Motions:	Protraction (abduction) and retraction (adduction)
	Elevation and depression
	Upward and downward rotation
Position:	Sidelying
Hand placement:	Place one hand over the acromion process and the other hand at the inferior angle of the scapula.
Note:	The hand placement for each of the three pairs of motion is the same. The only difference is the direction of force applied to the scapula.

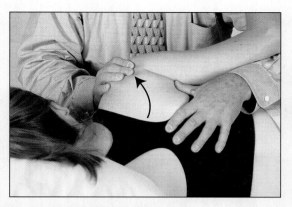

Scapular protraction (abduction).

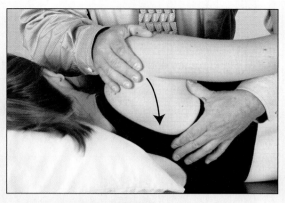

Scapular retraction (adduction).

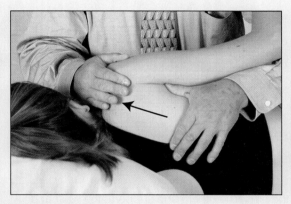

Scapular elevation.

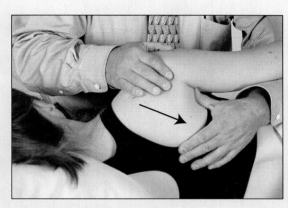

Scapular depression.

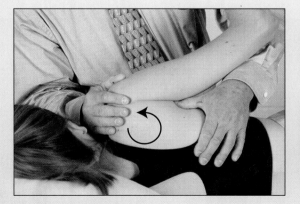

Scapular upward rotation.

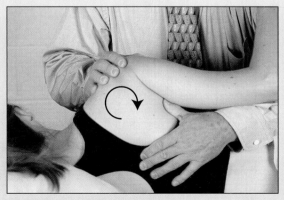

Scapular downward rotation.

(continued)

Joint: Shoulder (glenohumeral)

Motion: Flexion

Position: Supine

Hand placement: One hand supports the arm. The other hand grasps the wrist and hand. Hand placement may need to shift as movement occurs through full flexion.

Precautions: Permit external rotation to avoid impingement.

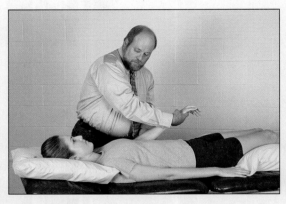

Beginning shoulder flexion.

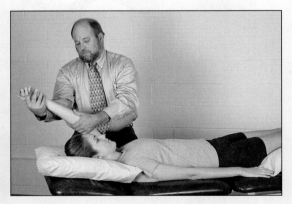

Ending shoulder flexion.

Joint: Shoulder (glenohumeral)

Motion: Extension

Position: Sidelying

Alternative position: Prone

Hand placement: One hand supports the arm. The other hand supports the wrist and forearm.

Precaution: When the end of the range of shoulder extension is reached, shoulder girdle motion will occur.

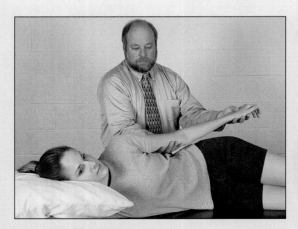

Beginning shoulder extension.

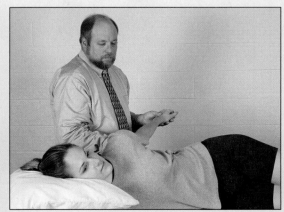

Ending shoulder extension.

Joint: Shoulder (glenohumeral)
Motion: Abduction
Position: Supine
Hand placement: One hand supports the arm and stabilizes shoulder girdle. The other
                  hand grasps the wrist and forearm.
Precautions: Avoid shoulder flexion and internal rotation during shoulder abduction.
                  Permit external rotation to avoid impingement. The physical therapist/
                  assistant must move to allow movement through complete range of
                  motion.

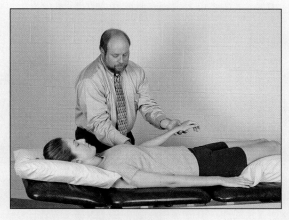

Beginning shoulder abduction.

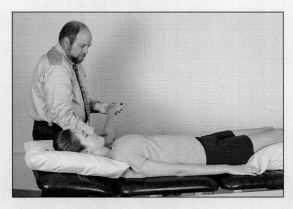

Midpoint of shoulder abduction.

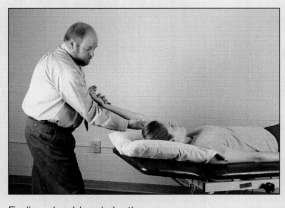

Ending shoulder abduction.

(continued)

Joint:	Shoulder (glenohumeral)
Motion:	Horizontal adduction
Position:	Supine, shoulder abducted to 90 degrees and elbow flexed to 90 degrees
Hand placement:	One hand supports the arm. The other hand grasps the wrist and hand.

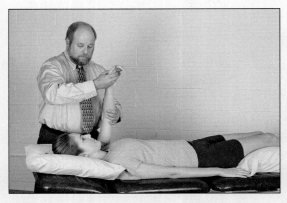

Midpoint of shoulder horizontal adduction.

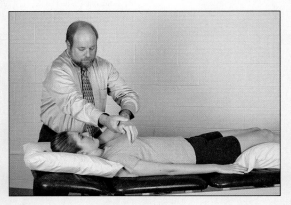

Ending shoulder horizontal adduction.

Joint:	Shoulder (glenohumeral)
Motion:	Internal (medial) rotation
Position:	Supine, shoulder abducted to 90 degrees, elbow flexed to 90 degrees, and the forearm in pronation
Hand placement:	One hand supports the arm. The other hand grasps the patient's wrist and forearm.
Precaution:	When the end of internal rotation ROM is reached, the shoulder girdle will start to move into protraction. Do not allow this to occur.

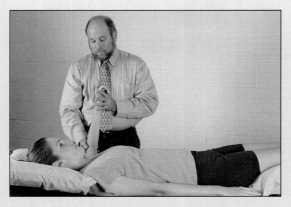

Starting position for shoulder internal rotation.

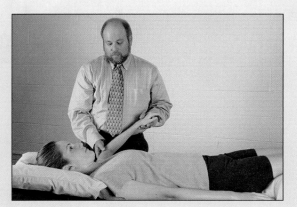

Shoulder internal rotation.

Joint:	Shoulder (glenohumeral)
Motion:	External (lateral) rotation
Position:	Supine, shoulder abducted to 90 degrees, elbow flexed to 90 degrees, and forearm pronated
Hand placement:	One hand supports the arm. The other hand grasps the patient's wrist and hand.
Precaution:	When the end of the range of external rotation is reached, the shoulder girdle will start to move into retraction. The patient may also extend the trunk when motion is limited. Do not allow this to occur.

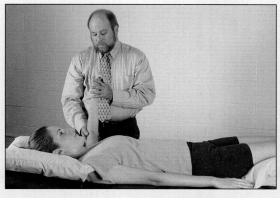

Starting position for shoulder external rotation.

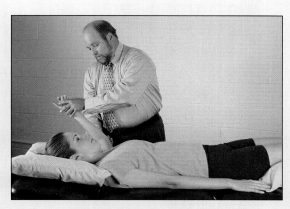

Shoulder external rotation.

Joints:	Shoulder (glenohumeral) and elbow
Muscle:	Triceps brachii
Motion:	Shoulder and elbow flexion
Position:	Supine
Hand placement:	One hand supports the arm. The other hand grasps the patient's wrist and hand.
Note:	To move the triceps muscle across both joints over which it acts requires elbow flexion with the shoulder in flexion. This movement is achieved by first flexing the shoulder through its available ROM and then flexing the elbow through its available ROM while maintaining shoulder flexion.

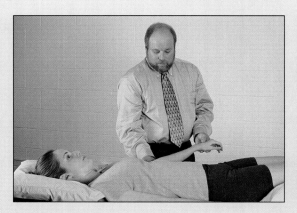

Starting position for shoulder flexion.

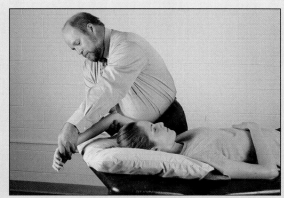

Shoulder flexion with elbow flexion.

(continued)

Joint:	Elbow
Motions:	Flexion and extension
Position:	Supine, upper extremity in anatomical position
Hand placement:	One hand supports the arm. The other hand grasps the patient's wrist and hand.
Note:	In this illustration, the shoulder is slightly flexed to allow visualization of the elbow.

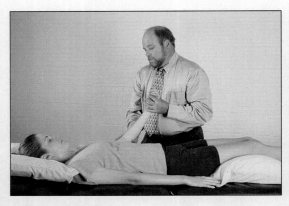

Elbow extension.

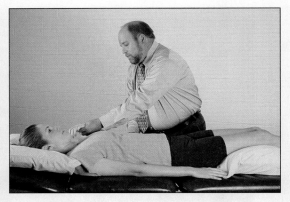

Elbow flexion.

Joints:	Forearm (radioulnar)
Motions:	Pronation and supination
Position:	Supine, elbow flexed to 90 degrees
Alternative position:	Sitting
Hand placement:	One hand stabilizes the arm. The other hand grasps the distal forearm and supports the hand.
Precaution:	This motion occurs in the forearm. Do not apply the force through the wrist by grasping the hand instead of the forearm.

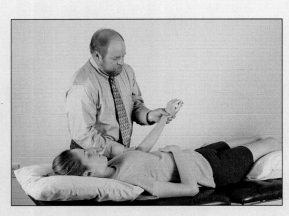

Forearm pronation.

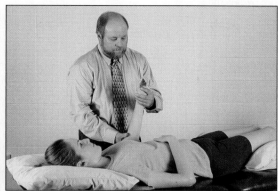

Midposition (neutral) of forearm.

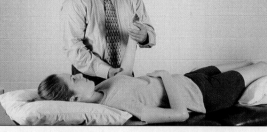

Forearm supination.

Joints: Wrist (radiocarpal and intercarpal)
Motions: Flexion and extension—finger motion is permitted
Position: Supine, elbow flexed, and fingers free to move
Alternative position: Sitting
Hand placement: One hand stabilizes the arm and forearm. The other hand grasps
                         the patient's hand.

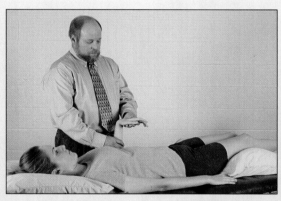

Wrist flexion.

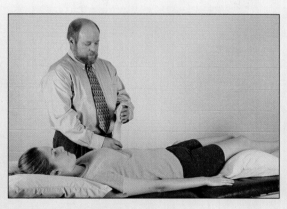

Midposition (neutral) of wrist.

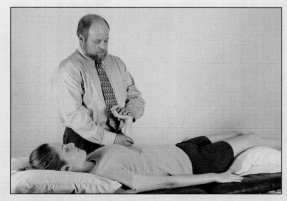

Wrist extension.

(continued)

Joints:	Wrist (radiocarpal and intercarpal)
Motions:	Ulnar and radial deviation
Position:	Supine, elbow flexed, and forearm in mid-position
Alternative position:	Sitting
Hand placement:	One hand stabilizes the forearm. The other hand grasps the patient's hand.
Note:	The ROM for radial deviation is less than for ulnar deviation.
Precaution:	Avoid wrist flexion and extension, and forearm pronation and supination, while performing ulnar and radial deviation motions.

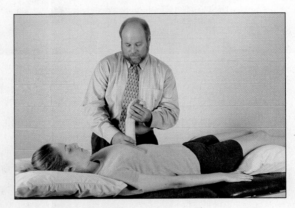

Ulnar deviation.

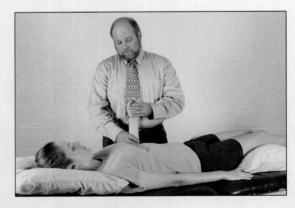

Midposition (neutral) of wrist.

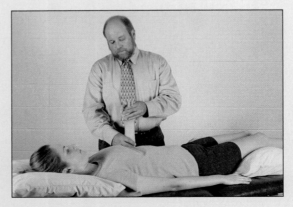

Radial deviation.

Joints:	Fingers (metacarpophalangeal and interphalangeal)
Motions:	Flexion and extension
Position:	Supine, elbow flexed to 90 degrees and wrist in neutral position
Alternative position:	Sitting
Hand placement:	One hand stabilizes the forearm and wrist. The other hand grasps the fingers or an individual digit.
Note:	Digits may be moved through the ROM at all joints and in all directions as a group or individually.

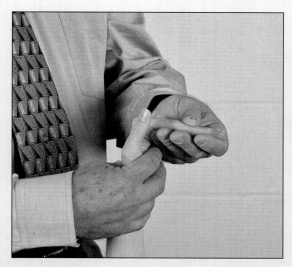

Finger flexion.

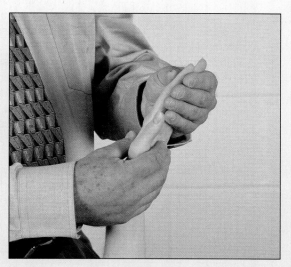

Neutral position of metacarpophalangeal joints with interphalangeal joint extension.

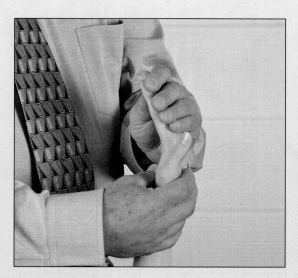

Finger extension.

(continued)

Joints:	Elbow, wrist (radiocarpal and intercarpal), and fingers (metacarpophalangeal and interphalangeal)
Muscles:	Flexor digitorum superficialis
	Flexor digitorum profundus
	Palmaris longus
	Extensor digitorum
	Extensor digiti minimi
	Extensor indicis
Motions:	Wrist flexion with finger extension
	Wrist extension with finger extension
	Wrist flexion with finger flexion
	Wrist extension with finger flexion
Position:	Supine, elbow extended, forearm supinated
Alternative position:	Sitting
Hand placement:	One hand stabilizes the forearm and wrist. The other hand grasps the hand and fingers.
Note:	These motions move (lengthen) multijoint muscles that cross the joints of the elbow, wrist, and fingers, to the fullest extent possible. Although these muscles cross the elbow joint, the full effect of muscle lengthening can usually be achieved without regard for elbow joint position.
Precaution:	Some patients should not have long finger flexors and extensors moved (lengthened) across all joints simultaneously to permit development of tenodesis action.

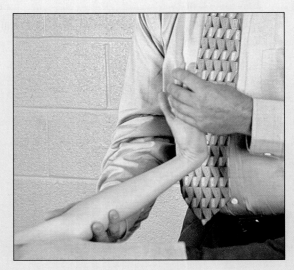

Wrist flexion with finger extension.

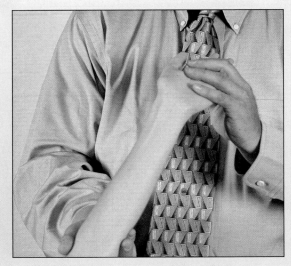

Wrist extension with finger extension.

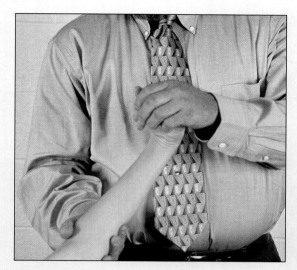

Wrist flexion with finger flexion.

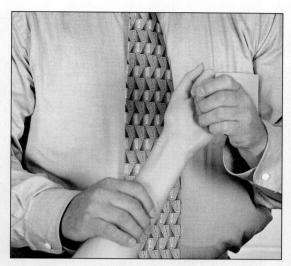

Wrist extension with finger flexion.

Joints:	Fingers (metacarpophalangeal)
Motions:	Abduction and adduction
Position:	Supine, elbow flexed to 90 degrees and wrist in neutral position
Alternative position:	Sitting
Hand placement:	One hand supports the hand and fingers, and the other hand grasps the finger to be moved through the ROM.
Note:	The middle finger is the reference point for abduction and adduction. Movement of the middle finger in both directions is labeled abduction.

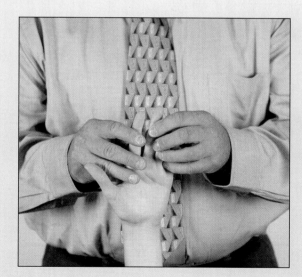

Starting position for finger abduction and adduction.

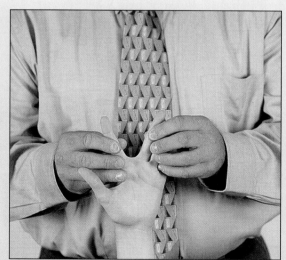

Finger abduction.

(continued)

Joints:	Thumb (carpometacarpal) and fifth finger
Motion:	Opposition
Position:	Supine, elbow flexed to 90 degrees and wrist in anatomical position
Alternative position:	Sitting
Hand placement:	One hand grasps the thumb. The other hand grasps the fifth finger.
Note:	To preserve function of the hand, maintain the arches of the hand. Opposition of the thumb and fifth finger can contribute to maintaining the arches of the hand.

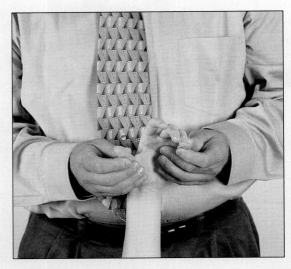

Beginning opposition.

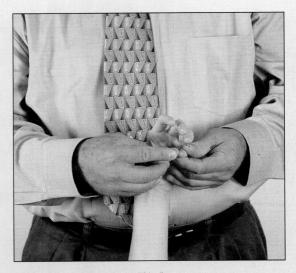

Opposition of thumb to fifth finger.

Joint:	Thumb (carpometacarpal)
Motions:	Abduction and adduction
Position:	Supine, elbow flexed to 90 degrees, wrist in neutral position, and the thumb extended
Alternative position:	Sitting
Hand placement:	One hand grasps the thumb. The other hand grasps the patient's hand.
Note:	Maintaining the "web space" is vital for a functional hand.

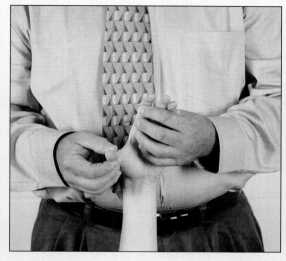

Thumb abduction.

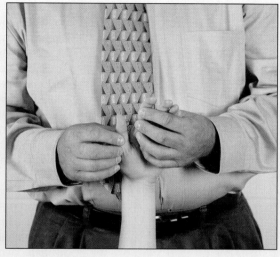

Thumb adduction.

Joint:	Thumb (carpometacarpal and metacarpophalangeal)
Motions:	Flexion and extension
Position:	Supine, wrist in neutral position
Alternative position:	Sitting
Hand placement:	One hand grasps the thumb. The other hand grasps the patient's hand.

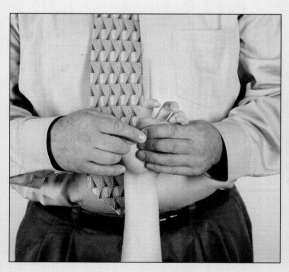

Thumb flexion.

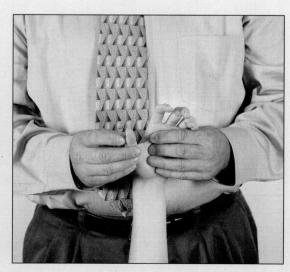

Thumb extension.

PROCEDURE 9–4 Upper Extremity ROM Exercises: Diagonal Patterns

Pattern:
PNF diagonal 1 (D1) extension with elbow extended
PNF diagonal 1 (D1) flexion with elbow extended

Combining Components
of Motion:
D1 extension with elbow extended
  Shoulder: extension, abduction, internal rotation
  Elbow: extended
  Forearm: pronation
  Wrist: extension, ulnar deviation
  Digits: extension, abduction
D1 flexion with elbow extended
  Shoulder: flexion, adduction, external rotation
  Elbow: extended
  Forearm: supination
  Wrist: flexed, radial deviation
  Digits: flexion, adduction

Position:
Supine

Hand placement:
One hand supports the arm. The other hand grasps the patient's hand. When performing ROM of a patient's left upper extremity, the physical therapist's/assistant's right hand controls the patient's left wrist and hand.

Note:
Elbow extended indicates that the elbow maintains extension throughout the movement of both patterns. In these patterns, motion begins distally and progresses proximally, with the motions occurring more or less simultaneously.

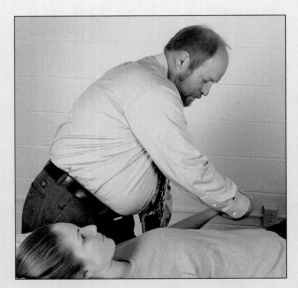

D1 extension with elbow extended.

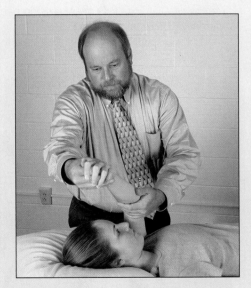

D1 flexion with elbow extended.

Pattern:	PNF diagonal 1 (D1) extension with elbow extension
	PNF diagonal 1 (D1) flexion with elbow flexion
Combining components of motion:	D1 extension with elbow extension

D1 extension with elbow extension
  Shoulder: extension, abduction, internal rotation
  Elbow: extension
  Forearm: pronation
  Wrist: extension, ulnar deviation
  Digits: extension, abduction
D1 flexion with elbow flexion
  Shoulder: flexion, adduction, external rotation
  Elbow: flexion
  Forearm: supination
  Wrist: flexion, radial deviation
  Digits: flexion, adduction

Position:	Supine
Hand placement:	One hand supports the arm. The other hand grasps the patient's hand. When performing range of motion of the patient's left upper extremity, the physical therapist's/assistant's right hand controls the patient's left wrist and hand.
Note:	In these patterns, motion begins distally and progresses proximally, with the motions occurring more or less simultaneously.

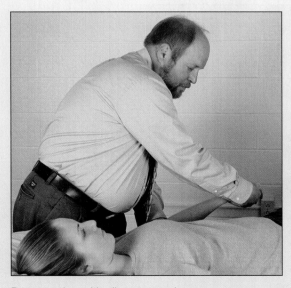

D1 extension with elbow extension.

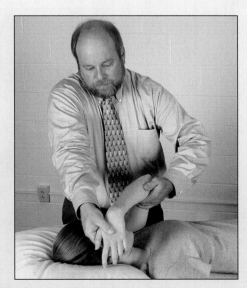

D1 flexion with elbow flexion.

(continued)

Pattern:	PNF diagonal 1 (D1) extension with elbow flexion
	PNF diagonal 1 (D1) flexion with elbow extension
Combining components of motion:	D1 extension with elbow flexion

Combining components
of motion:

D1 extension with elbow flexion
    Shoulder: extension, abduction, internal rotation
    Elbow: flexion
    Forearm: pronation
    Wrist: extension, ulnar deviation
    Digits: extension, abduction

D1 flexion with elbow extension
    Shoulder: flexion, adduction, external rotation
    Elbow: extension
    Forearm: supination
    Wrist: flexion, radial deviation
    Digits: flexion, adduction

Position: Supine

Hand placement: One hand supports the arm. The other hand grasps the hand. When performing ROM of a patient's left upper extremity, the physical therapist's/assistant's right hand controls the patient's left wrist and hand.

Note: In these patterns, motion begins distally and progresses proximally, with the motions occuring more or less simultaneously.

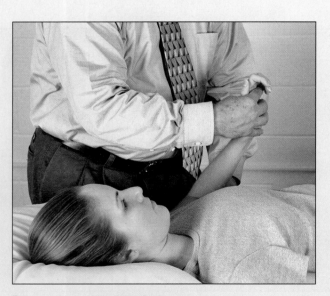

D1 extension with elbow flexion.

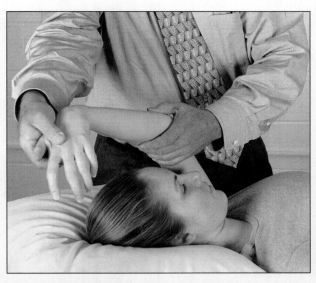

D1 flexion with elbow extension.

Pattern:	PNF diagonal 1 (D1) extension—scapula
	PNF diagonal 1 (D1) flexion—scapula
Combining components of motion:	D1 extension: Scapula: depression, adduction, downward rotation
	D1 flexion: Scapula: elevation, abduction, upward rotation
Position:	Sidelying
Hand placement:	One hand is placed over the scapula. The other hand and forearm support the patient's upper extremity. When performing ROM of the patient's right scapula, the physical therapist's/assistant's left hand is on the right scapula.
Note:	In these patterns, the motion occurs simultaneously.

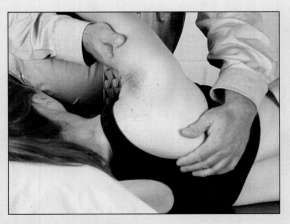

D1 extension—scapula.

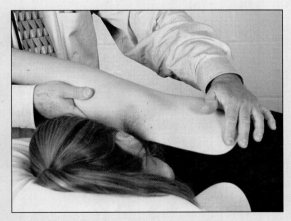

D1 flexion—scapula.

(continued)

Pattern:	PNF diagonal 2 (D2) extension with elbow extended
	PNF diagonal 2 (D2) flexion with elbow extended
Combining components of motion:	D2 extension with elbow extended
	Shoulder: extension, adduction, internal rotation
	Elbow: extended
	Forearm: pronation
	Wrist: flexion, ulnar deviation
	Digits: flexion, adduction
	Thumb: opposition
	D2 flexion with elbow extended
	Shoulder: flexion, abduction, external rotation
	Elbow: extended
	Forearm: supination
	Wrist: extension, radial deviation
	Digits: extension, abduction
Position:	Supine
Hand placement:	One hand supports the arm. The other hand grasps the patient's hand. When performing ROM of the patient's left upper extremity, the physical therapist's/assistant's right hand controls the patient's left wrist and hand.
Note:	*Elbow extended* indicates that the elbow maintains complete extension throughout the movement of both patterns. In these patterns, motion begins distally and progresses proximally, with the motions occurring more or less simultaneously.

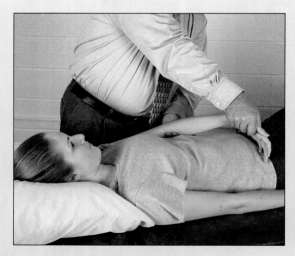

D2 extension with elbow extended.

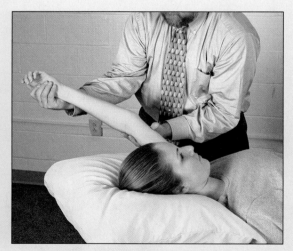

D2 flexion with elbow extended.

Pattern: PNF diagonal 2 (D2) extension with elbow extension
                                PNF diagonal 2 (D2) flexion with elbow flexion

Combining components
of motion: D2 extension with elbow extension
                                    Shoulder: extension, adduction, internal rotation
                                    Elbow: extension
                                    Forearm: pronation
                                    Wrist: flexion, ulnar deviation
                                    Digits: flexion, adduction
                                    Thumb: opposition
                                D2 flexion with elbow flexion
                                    Shoulder: flexion, abduction, external rotation
                                    Elbow: flexion
                                    Forearm: supination
                                    Wrist: extension, radial deviation
                                    Digits: extension, abduction

Position: Supine
Hand placement: One hand supports the arm. The other hand grasps the patient's
                                hand. When performing ROM of the patient's left upper extremity,
                                the physical therapist's/assistant's right hand controls the patient's
                                left wrist and hand.

Note: In these patterns, motion begins distally and progresses proximally,
                                with the motions occurring more or less simultaneously.

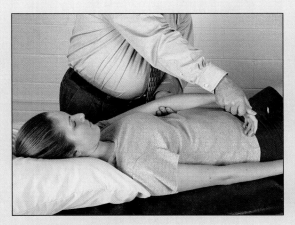

D2 extension with elbow extension.

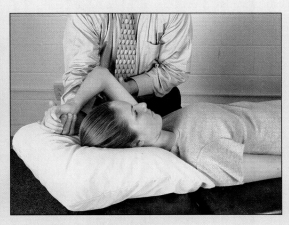

D2 flexion with elbow flexion.

(continued)

Pattern: PNF diagonal 2 (D2) extension with elbow flexion
PNF diagonal 2 (D2) flexion with elbow extension

Combining components
of motion:

D2 extension with elbow flexion
    Shoulder: extension, adduction, internal rotation
    Elbow: flexion
    Forearm: pronation
    Wrist: flexion, ulnar deviation
    Digits: flexion, adduction
    Thumb: opposition
D2 flexion with elbow extension
    Shoulder: flexion, abduction, external rotation
    Elbow: extension
    Forearm: supination
    Wrist: extension, radial deviation
    Digits: extension, abduction

Position: Supine

Hand Placement: One hand supports the arm. The other hand grasps the patient's hand. When performing ROM of the patient's left upper extremity, the physical therapist's/assistant's right hand controls the patient's left wrist and hand.

Note: In these patterns, motion begins distally and progresses proximally, with the motions occurring more or less simultaneously.

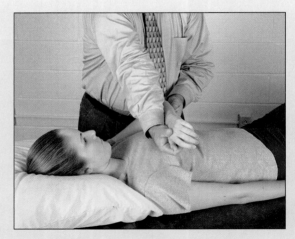

D2 extension with elbow flexion.

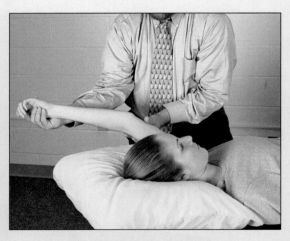

D2 flexion with elbow extension.

Pattern:	PNF diagonal 2 (D2) extension—scapula
	PNF diagonal 2 (D2) flexion—scapula
Combining components of motion:	D2 extension
	Scapula: depression, abduction, downward rotation
	D2 flexion
	Scapula: elevation, adduction, upward rotation
Position:	Sidelying
Hand placement:	One hand is placed on the scapula. The other hand and forearm are used to support the patient's arm. When performing ROM of the patient's right scapula, the physical therapist's/assistant's right hand grasps the right scapula.

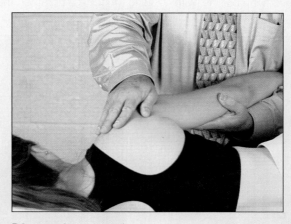

D2 extension—scapula.

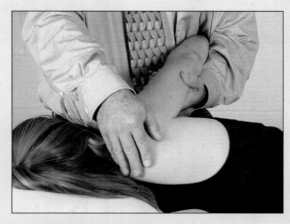

D2 flexion—scapula.

PROCEDURE 9–5   Head, Neck, and Trunk ROM Exercises: Anatomical Planes

Joints: Head and neck (atlantooccipital, atlantoaxial, and successive cervical spine joints)
Motions: Flexion and extension
Position: Supine
Hand placement: One hand grasps each side of the head with the palms above the ears and the fingers spread over the occiput.
Note: When the treatment table does not have a head support that can be lowered, the patient must lie with his or her head over the end of the table.
Precaution: Carefully support the patient's head. Do not force movement. Movement begins with tucking of the chin rather than jutting the chin forward.

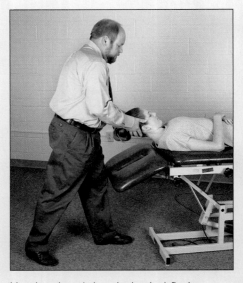

Head and neck (cervical spine) flexion.

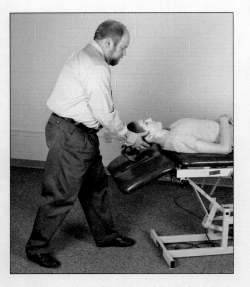

Neutral position of head and neck (cervical spine).

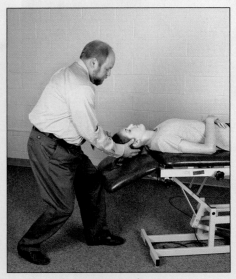

Head and neck (cervical spine) extension.

Joints:	Head and neck (atlantooccipital, atlantoaxial, and successive cervical spine joints)
Motions:	Lateral flexion
Position:	Supine
Hand placement:	One hand grasps each side of the head with the palms above the ears and the fingers spread over the occiput.
Precaution:	Carefully support the patient's head. Do not force movement. Movement begins with tilting the ear to the shoulder rather than pushing the head laterally.

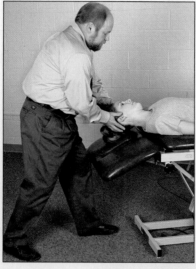

Lateral head and neck (cervical spine) flexion to the left.

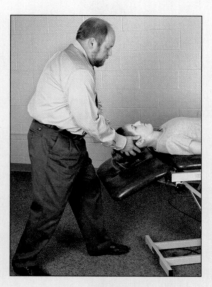

Neutral position of the head and neck (cervical spine).

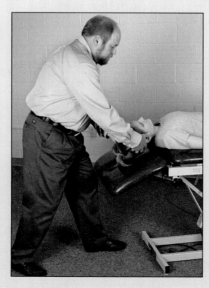

Lateral head and neck (cervical spine) flexion to the right.

(continued)

Joints:	Head and neck (atlantooccipital, atlantoaxial, and successive cervical spine joints)
Motions:	Rotation
Position:	Supine
Hand placement:	One hand grasps each side of the head with the palms above the ears and the fingers spread over the occiput.
Precaution:	Carefully support the patient's head. Do not force movement. Movement should not include flexion/extension or lateral flexion.

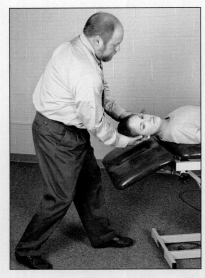

Head and neck (cervical spine) rotation to the right.

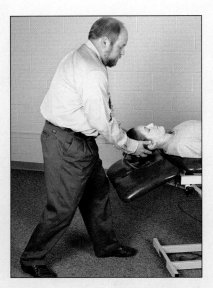

Neutral position of the head and neck (cervical spine).

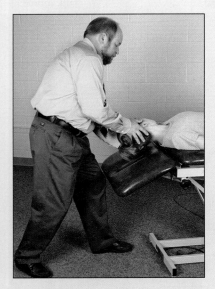

Head and neck (cervical spine) rotation to the left.

Joint:	Lower trunk (lumbar spine) and hip
Motion:	Lower trunk rotation
Position:	Supine, hips and knees flexed such that the patient's feet are resting flat on the supporting surface close to the buttocks
Hand placement:	One hand grasps the knees. The other hand stabilizes the pelvis.
Alternative placement:	Both hands are placed on the knees.
Precaution:	The patient's shoulders remain on the supporting surface as the knees are moved from side to side. When a patient's upper trunk begins to roll, she has reached the end point of lower trunk rotation in that direction.

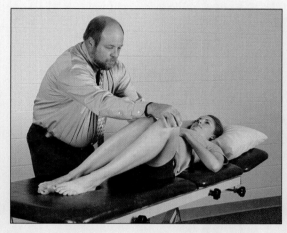

Lower trunk (lumbar spine) rotation to the left.

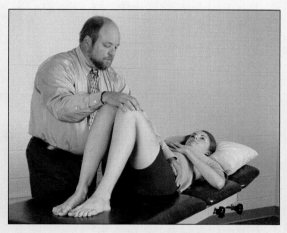

Neutral position of the lower trunk (lumbar spine).

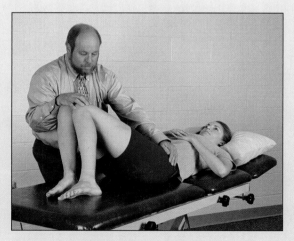

Lower trunk (lumbar spine) rotation to the right.

(continued)

Joint: Lower trunk (lumbar spine) and hip
Motion: Lower trunk flexion
Position: Supine, hips and knees flexed
Hand placement: One arm supports the legs on the posterior aspect of the patient's thighs. The other hand supports the patient's feet as the lower trunk (lumbar spine) is flexed.

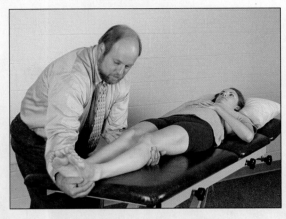

Starting position for lower trunk (lumbar spine) flexion.

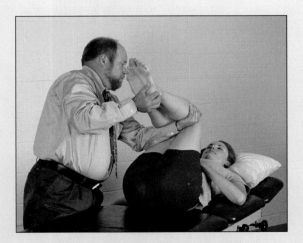

End position for lower trunk (lumbar spine) flexion.

Chapter Review

Review Questions

1. Define passive, active-assisted, and active ROM.

2. How does a physical therapist/assistant support body segments during ROM exercises?

3. What are the differences between joint ROM and muscle ROM?

4. Define the different types of end feel and describe the significance of each.

5. Describe differences in movement when a patient has normal muscle tone, spasticity, rigidity, and pain.

6. Compare and contrast anatomical plane motions and diagonal patterns of motion.

7. List the combining components of motion for each of the diagonal patterns.

Suggested Activities

1. Demonstrate the specific procedures presented in this chapter.

2. Work in pairs to perform the specific procedures. Rotate partners periodically during practice sessions.

3. Identify the type of end feel for selected motions.

4. Practice ROM exercises for all joints and muscles possible in each position—prone, supine, sidelying and sitting, and on different surfaces—mat on floor, treatment table, bed.

5. Practice performing ROM exercises while a partner role-plays various diagnoses (see Case Studies for suggestions). The student role-playing the patient can add "character" to the role by being cooperative, uncooperative, in pain, hard of hearing, or lacking in ROM to enhance the activity. The "patient" must role-play the diagnoses and character consistently.

6. Practice teaching "family and patients" and other health-care providers how to perform ROM exercises.

7. Document range-of-motion interventions.

Case Studies

Use these case studies to complete activity 5 above.

1. Patient is a 22-year-old status posttraumatic brain injury and is in a coma.
2. Patient is an 18-year-old with a complete C6 spinal cord injury, presenting with moderate spasticity in the lower extremities.
3. Patient is a 59-year-old former executive with left hemiplegia with mild spasticity in the lower extremity and moderate spasticity in the upper extremity.
4. Patient is a 44-year-old with multiple sclerosis, presenting with moderate spasticity in the lower extremities.
5. Patient is a 70-year-old with advanced Parkinsonism, presenting with moderate to severe rigidity.
6. Patient is a 12-year-old with cerebral palsy, presenting with severe spastic quadriplegia.

References

1. Knott M and Voss DE. *Proprioceptive Neuromuscular Facilitation,* 2nd ed. New York: Harper & Row, 1968.
2. Root ML, Orien WP, and Weed JH. *Normal and Abnormal Function of the Foot: Clinical Biomechanics—Volume II.* Los Angeles: Clinical Biomechanics Corporation Publishers, 1977.
3. Warwick R and Williams PL. *Gray's Anatomy,* 37th ed. Philadelphia: WB Saunders, 1989.
4. Sullivan PE, Markos PD, and Minor MAD. *An Integrated Approach to Therapeutic Exercise: Theory and Clinical Application.* Reston, Virginia: Reston Publishing Company, 1982.

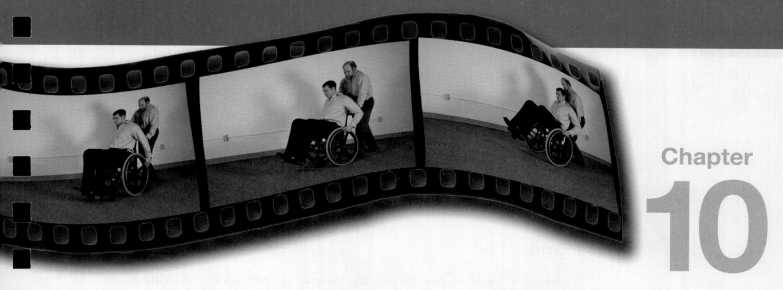

Ambulation with Ambulatory Assistive Devices

Learning Objectives

Upon completion of this chapter, you will be able to:

1. List indications for use of ambulatory assistive devices for ambulation.
2. Describe and discuss the uses of parallel bars during gait training.
3. Describe and discuss the use of the tilt table during gait training.
4. List and discuss the causes of fatigue during gait training and methods to reduce the effects of fatigue.
5. Discuss the effect of patient concentration on gait training.
6. Describe the use of a scale to teach weight-bearing limits.
7. Describe methods of instruction appropriate for gait training.
8. List activities that a patient must master to be independent in ambulation with an assistive device.
9. List assistive-device selection in sequence from those providing most stability to least stability.
10. List assistive-device selection in sequence from those requiring the most coordination to least coordination.
11. List evaluations used to determine appropriate ambulatory assistive devices for different patients and pathologies.
12. List contraindications to the use of ambulatory assistive devices when appropriate.
13. Adjust the height of ambulatory assistive devices properly.
14. Describe various styles of walkers, crutches, and canes.
15. Describe and demonstrate common gait patterns used with ambulatory assistive devices.

Key Terms

Ambulatory assistive
  devices
Full weight bearing (FWB)
Gait pattern
Non–weight bearing
  (NWB)
Partial weight bearing
  (PWB)

Supervision (stand-by)
  guarding
Toe touch weight bearing
  (TTWB)
Weight bearing
Weight bearing as
  tolerated (WBAT)

16. Describe and demonstrate how to guard a patient properly when using ambulatory assistive devices during ambulation on level surfaces, stairs, and curbs; the assumption of sitting from standing and standing from sitting; moving through doorways; falling without injury; and resumption of ambulation after falling.

17. Instruct a patient in the proper method of using various ambulatory assistive devices to perform different gait patterns on level surfaces, stairs, and curbs; moving through doorways; the assumption of sitting from standing and standing from sitting; falling without injury; and resumption of ambulation after falling.

Introduction

Ambulatory assistive devices provide external support for the musculoskeletal system. The ambulatory assistive devices included in this chapter are parallel bars, crutches, canes, and walkers, but not orthotic or prosthetic devices, wheelchairs, or scooters. The ambulatory assistive devices included in this chapter permit some patients with impairments who could not otherwise ambulate to ambulate safely. Three major indications for using ambulatory assistive devices for gait are

1. Structural deformity, amputation, injury, or disease resulting in decreased ability to bear weight through the lower extremities
2. Muscle weakness or paralysis of the trunk or lower extremities
3. Inadequate balance

Ambulatory assistive devices increase a patient's base of support and provide additional support during ambulation. Increasing a patient's base of support creates a larger area within which the patient's center of gravity can shift without loss of balance. Additional support improves balance control and supports or redistributes weight-bearing during ambulation.

Teaching Tips

Training Environment

■ **Take Note**
Motor learning principle—simple to complex environment.

Initial gait training should occur in an environment that is as free of distractions as possible. Physical therapists/assistants should select and monitor the environment to ensure patient safety. Patient rooms or physical therapy departments are usually less distracting than public corridors. When more complex environments are needed to challenge a patient, public corridors can be used for gait training.

Parallel Bars

Gait training with ambulatory assistive devices often begins at the parallel bars. Parallel bars provide maximum stability while requiring the least amount of coordination from patients. Patients can become accustomed to upright posture and learn a gait pattern in the relative safety of parallel bars. Ambulatory assistive devices can be fitted while a patient stands in parallel bars (■ Figure 10–1). When appropriate, a patient can practice standing or a gait pattern while waiting as physical therapists/assistants adjust ambulatory assistive devices, providing efficient use of treatment time.

Initial use of ambulatory assistive devices can be in or alongside parallel bars. Patients are reassured by readily available stability provided by parallel bars. A patient may, however, become too dependent on parallel bars. Physical therapists must progress patients to ambulation with ambulatory assistive devices other than parallel bars as rapidly as is safely possible.

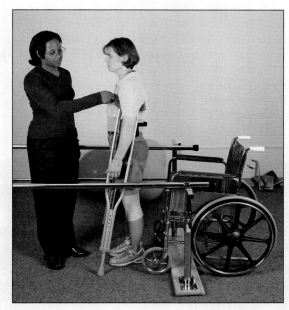

■ **Figure 10–1**   Fitting crutches at the parallel bars.

Fatigue

Fatigue may occur during gait training as a result of

1. Performing an activity that has not been performed for a while
2. Using ambulatory assistive devices during ambulation
3. Greater concentration levels while learning a new gait pattern with an assistive device
4. Physiological responses to the stresses of injury or illness

These factors can cause the patient to feel fatigue rapidly. Frequent rest periods may be necessary during initial gait-training sessions. Several short sessions of gait training, rather than one long session, may decrease the effects of fatigue.

Patient Concentration

When first using ambulatory assistive devices, a patient's need to concentrate can be very high. During initial gait-training sessions, patients require greater concentration to learn a gait pattern properly. Patients often look at their feet and ambulatory assistive devices as they learn gait patterns because visual input of foot and assistive device location with respect to their body is necessary for coordination and safety. Because patients are paying attention to foot and assistive device position, physical therapists/assistants must ensure safety by reducing distraction from other objects and activities in the immediate area.

High levels of concentration exhibited by patients during gait training may interfere with their ability to respond to other inputs, such as conversation. Patients may stop walking to answer questions. Conversation with and around a patient not directly related to gait training should be avoided during initial gait training. Later, however, such additional inputs can be used to test the degree to which patients have mastered use of ambulatory assistive devices and new gait patterns. When gait has again become an automatic activity, patients will be able to respond to questions and attend to other activity in the environment while maintaining appropriate gait patterns. As gait becomes automatic, patients usually start to look around as they ambulate. At this time patients can take over the responsibility of monitoring the environment for themselves, and more complex and distracting environments can be used for gait training.

■ **Take Note**
To monitor fatigue, use vital signs and perceived exertion scales.

■ **Take Note**
Motor learning principle—single task to multi-task.

Weight Bearing

When a patient with a restriction of weight bearing is instructed in gait, bathroom scales can be useful. Placing one lower extremity on a scale can demonstrate different levels of weight bearing and the attendant sensation (■ Figure 10–2).

When using this method, the lower extremity not placed on the scale must be placed on a solid surface. In some cases, two scales may be used, with one lower extremity placed on each scale (■ Figure 10–3).

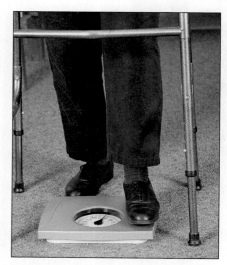

■ **Figure 10–2** Using one scale to measure weight bearing.

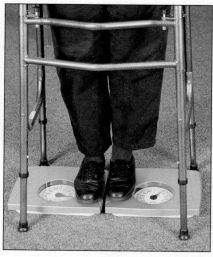

■ **Figure 10–3** Using two scales to measure weight bearing.

Levels of weight-bearing will be discussed later in this chapter with discussion of choosing a gait pattern.

Methods of Instruction

Physical therapists/assistants will not always be available to instruct patients in how to perform tasks outside a rehabilitation setting. Therefore, patients must be assisted in learning how to solve problems on their own when using ambulatory assistive devices. As a teaching method, physical therapists/assistants may challenge patients by presenting novel situations and asking patients how they might proceed in the new situation, prior to a patient attempting the actual maneuver. This method may be indicative of a patient's level of independence prior to discharge.

Before a patient begins ambulating, the physical therapist/assistant must describe and demonstrate proper use of the chosen assistive device and gait pattern. Demonstration is the primary method of instruction. Verbal descriptions reinforce demonstration and must be simple. Observing other patients who are using ambulatory assistive devices *correctly* may also be a useful method of instruction.

Physical therapists/assistants must select specific activities to be mastered in sequence. Ambulation using a chosen gait pattern on level surfaces should be well advanced before gait training in other environments, such as on stairs or in busy corridors, is initiated. A patient's learning capabilities must be balanced with imposed time constraints of treatment sessions or hospital discharge, without compromising patient health and safety.

■ **Take Note**

Motor learning principle—practice in a variety of environments.

■ **Take Note**

Teaching techniques—demonstration and verbal cues.

Content of Instruction

Patients must learn to use the chosen assistive device to move out of and into a chair. Initial instruction will most likely be related to using chairs with armrests. Subsequent instruction for using chairs without armrests, low or soft sofas and chairs, toilets, and car seats, is also necessary. Patients must be taught to sit in a controlled manner, rather than collapsing into a sitting position.

Initial training in the performance of the chosen gait pattern is on level surfaces. When patients can perform safely on a level surface, instruction in the use of stairs, curbs, ramps, elevators, doors, and uneven surfaces is provided, as well as instruction in how to fall safely. Patients should be taught to ascend and descend stairs on the appropriate side. In the United States, this is the patient's right side when facing the stairs.

Uneven surfaces may present specific problems for patients. Gravel, grass, broken sidewalks and paving, and curb cuts may require additional instruction and practice. Patients should be cautioned to avoid small throw rugs that may slip or become entangled with their feet or ambulatory assistive devices. Wet or highly polished floors can be slippery and should also be avoided whenever possible. When ambulating on icy, wet, or highly polished surfaces, smaller movements and shorter step lengths should be used. Taking shorter steps applies forces placed on ambulatory assistive devices more directly downward, which is more stationary and avoids horizontal forces that may cause ambulatory assistive devices to slip.

Patients must be instructed to check that ambulatory assistive devices are in safe working condition. Rubber tips will not grip the floor properly if they become worn excessively or if dirt fills the grooves. Wing nuts on crutches often loosen with use and should be checked regularly to ensure they are tightened appropriately.

> ■ **Take Note**
> Selection of ambulation skills to be taught is based on determination of environment(s) in which patient will be ambulating.

> ■ **Take Note**
> Caution—Crutch and cane tips wear from use on rough and uneven surfaces. Teach patients to check them regularly.

Choosing an Assistive Device

A variety of ambulatory assistive devices is available. Some devices provide more stability and support than others, but some devices require more coordination to use. As abilities increase, patients may change from a device that provides relatively greater stability and support to one that provides relatively less stability and support. Other patients may continue to use the same device throughout the entire time an ambulatory assistive device is required. Patients with progressive disorders change from devices that provide relatively less stability and support to devices that provide relatively greater stability and support as their illness progresses.

Decision-making algorithms (see ■ **Figures 10–4**, ■ **10–5** and ■ **10–6**) are used by physical therapists to determine initial, and subsequent, assistive devices to be used. Deci-

Amount of WB	Unilateral LE WB Restriction	Bilateral LE WB Restriction
PWB almost full WB	1 standard cane	2 standard canes
⇓ PWB	1 crutch	Lofstrand crutches
⇓⇓ PWB	2 canes	2 crutches or walker
⇓⇓⇓ PWB	2 crutches	2 crutches or walker
TT	2 crutches or walker	Unable to walk
NWB	2 crutches or walker	Unable to walk

■ **Figure 10–4** As the amount of weight bearing permitted is reduced and the number of limbs involved increases, the more external support is needed.

Amount of Strength	Unilateral LE Weakness	Bilateral LE Weakness
Minimal weakness	1 standard cane	2 standard canes
⇓ strength	1 quad cane	2 quad canes
⇓⇓ strength	1 crutch	Lofstrand crutches
Significant weakness	2 crutches or walker	2 crutches or walker

■ **Figure 10–5** As strength decreases and the number of limbs involved increases, the more external support is needed.

Balance Impairment	Ambulatory Assistive Device
Minimally impaired	1 cane
⇓	1 Lofstrand crutch
⇓⇓	2 crutches or walker
Significantly impaired	2 crutches or walker and guarding

■ **Figure 10–6** As the balance impairment increases, the more external support is needed.

sions concerning assistive devices to be used are based upon the physical therapy examination results. Physical therapist assistants can implement gait training with assistive devices as directed by a physical therapist.

Different ambulatory assistive devices require the use of different muscle groups. Physical therapists must examine each patient's capabilities to determine which ambulatory assistive device is to be used. Interventions that develop and increase each patient's capabilities must be instituted to ensure that selected ambulatory assistive devices can be used safely and efficiently. Time to improve a patient's capabilities is often limited in hospital environments. This may limit selection of ambulatory assistive devices and may limit a patient's ability to master all necessary skills prior to discharge.

The following list of ambulatory assistive devices is ordered from those providing the most stability and support to those providing the least stability and support:

1. Parallel bars
2. Walker
3. Axillary crutches
4. Forearm (Lofstrand) crutches
5. Two canes
6. One cane

The following list of ambulatory assistive devices is ordered from those requiring the least coordination by a patient to those requiring the most coordination by a patient:

1. Parallel bars
2. Walker
3. One cane
4. Two canes
5. Axillary crutches
6. Forearm (Lofstrand) crutches

Some patients may use one crutch as an intermediate step between two crutches and one cane or instead of one cane.

When selecting an ambulatory assistive device, physical therapists must choose one that will provide the necessary support and that the patient can easily manipulate. The choice of an ambulatory assistive device is based on a patient's impairments and an examination and evaluation of a patient's strength, range of motion, balance, stability, coordination, and general condition. For example, a patient with a fractured lower extremity who must be non–weight bearing may use either crutches or a walker, depending on the results of examination and evaluation. Crutches may be used when necessary strength, stability, and coordination are present. Another patient with the same fracture may require the use of a walker because of poor stability, coordination, or a medically debilitating condition.

A platform for the forearm can be attached to walkers or crutches for patients who are unable to bear weight through their hand, wrist, or forearm, or who have poor grasp (■ Figure 10–7).

■ **Take Note**
Caution—Ensure patient's orientation, alertness, and ability to follow directions.

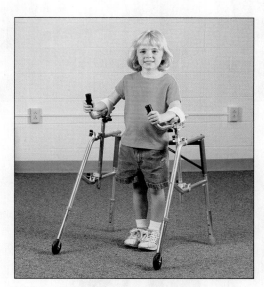

■ **Figure 10–7** Walker with forearm platforms.

Ambulatory assistive devices come in several sizes—tall, standard, junior, and child. Most ambulatory assistive devices are adjustable within a given range, and there is usually some overlap of adjustment between sizes. Some ambulatory assistive devices have ranges of height marked on them by the manufacturer. These markings are estimates only. Accurate measurement must be performed and confirmed by the physical therapist/assistant for each individual patient.

Walkers

Walkers provide a relatively greater degree of stability and are generally easy to use. Walkers are chosen for patients with generalized weakness, debilitating conditions, a need to reduce weight bearing on one or both lower extremities, relatively poor balance and coordination, or an inability to use crutches. This may mean that walkers are used more often with elderly patients.

Walkers may, however, be cumbersome (■ Figure 10–8). A collapsible walker is easier to transport in a car and place out of the way in public places, such as movies and restaurants, than is a noncollapsible walker.

Walkers are usually made of aluminum and are adjustable in height. To adjust the height of a walker, the walker is inverted (■ Figure 10–9). Each leg has a push-button lock with a telescoping leg (■ Figure 10–10). All legs must be adjusted to the same height.

Wheeled walkers are available with either two or four wheels (■ Figure 10–11). Walkers with four wheels should have a brake that is activated during weight bearing on the walker to ensure stability.

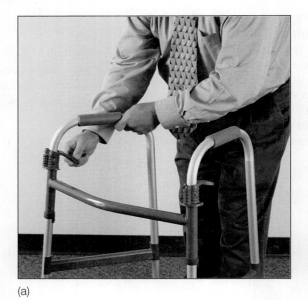

(a)

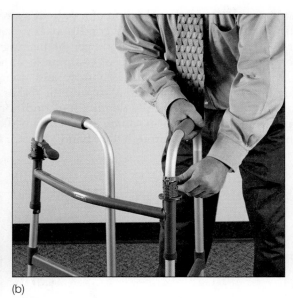

(b)

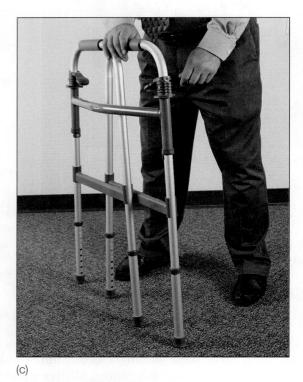

(c)

■ **Figure 10–8**   The sides of a collapsible walker fold flat to allow for easier storage and transporting.

A stair-climbing walker is available for patients who must use stairs frequently. This walker has an additional pair of handgrips on the rear legs to be used when the patient is on the stairs. These handgrips increase the anterior/posterior dimension of the walker, increasing difficulty of maneuvering in small areas. A stair-climbing walker in use is shown on pp. 344–348.

Other special walkers are available. A walker with a trunk support is used for patients who have adequate reciprocal lower extremity movements but lack adequate trunk support. These walkers are called *ring walkers*. Ring walkers are larger than

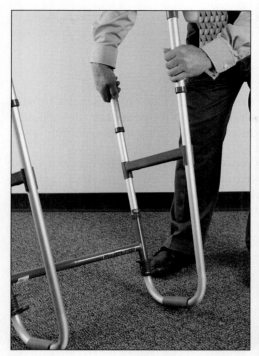

■ **Figure 10–9** Walker inverted for height adjustment.

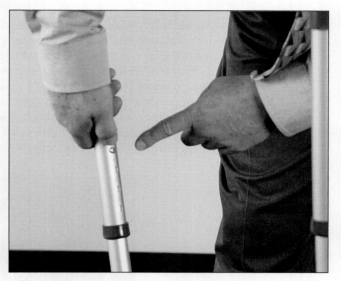

■ **Figure 10–10** Push button for height adjustment on walker.

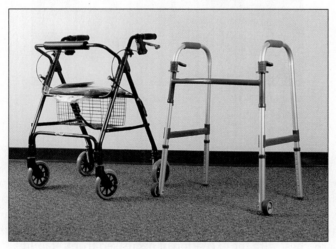

■ **Figure 10–11** Four-wheeled walker with brake (left) and two-wheeled walker (right).

standard walkers in all three dimensions and are not collapsible. An adduction board may be added to a ring walker. *Adduction boards* are suspended from the frame of the walker to prevent a patient's lower extremities from adducting during the swing phase of gait. Although cumbersome, for some patients an adduction board may be the difference between walking and not walking.

A *reciprocal walker* is designed with joints that permit each side of the walker to be advanced independently. A reciprocal walker is used when a patient lacks strength or balance to lift a walker completely to advance the walker during gait.

A *reverse walker,* with or without wheels, is often used by children. Patients stand in the walker with their back to the cross bar. The reverse walker is designed to encourage erect posture. Figure 10–7 shows a reverse walker.

Axillary Crutches

Axillary crutches provide a moderate degree of stability and are slightly more difficult to use than walkers. Axillary crutches are generally chosen for patients with weakness of one or both lower extremities, a need to reduce weight bearing on one or both lower extremities, or a need for some trunk support.

Axillary crutches were traditionally made of wood but now may be made of wood or aluminum. Wing nuts and bolts are used to adjust crutch length and handgrip height of wooden crutches. Push-button locks and telescoping legs may be used on some aluminum crutches. Alternative designs may be found among the many styles and constructions of axillary crutches (■ Figure 10–12).

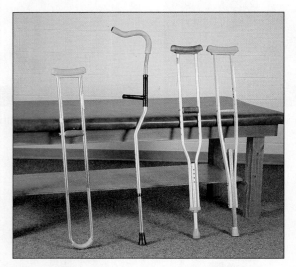

■ **Figure 10–12** A variety of aluminum and wooden axillary crutches.

Forearm (Lofstrand) Crutches

Forearm (Lofstrand) crutches (■ Figure 10–13) are slightly more difficult to use than axillary crutches but provide more ease of movement. The cuff of forearm crutches permits patients to use their hands for manipulating the environment without dropping the crutch. Forearm crutches are recommended for patients with the same problems as would require axillary crutches, with the exception of decreased trunk stability. Patients who will need crutches permanently or for long periods of time may find forearm crutches more desirable because they are lighter and more maneuverable than axillary crutches.

Canes

Canes provide limited stability and weight-bearing capability when used properly. Generally, canes are made of aluminum or wood. Aluminum canes are adjustable using push-button locks and telescoping legs. Wooden canes can be adjusted by cutting them to length, which limits their adjustability. Canes are generally chosen for patients with slight weakness of the lower extremities who need slight weight reduction because of pain or who need assistance with balance while ambulating.

When using one cane to limit weight bearing on one lower extremity, the cane is initially used in the hand on the side opposite the involved lower extremity. Use of a cane on

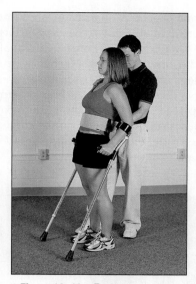

■ **Figure 10–13** Patient using forearm (Lofstrand) crutches.

the uninvolved side reduces the amount of force required by muscles to stabilize the pelvis during stance on the involved lower extremity. This placement also provides a second point of support, which increases the base of support on the uninvolved side. Increasing the base of support on the uninvolved side permits a patient to shift weight to the uninvolved side during stance on the involved lower extremity. When weight bearing on the involved lower extremity is permitted, the cane may be used on the involved side, which increases the base of support on that side. Increasing the base of support on the involved side encourages weight shifting onto the involved lower extremity. Depending upon the severity of a patient's problem, either one or two canes may be required. Two canes are used primarily for bilateral involvement or for assistance with balance.

Several styles of canes are available (■ **Figure 10–14**). The standard cane has a handgrip, shaft, and a single tip. The most common shape of a standard cane has a curved end for the handgrip. This cane style is often referred to as a "J" cane. Another design has an offset shaft and a straight end for the handgrip. This shape allows force applied to the handle to be directly over the tip.

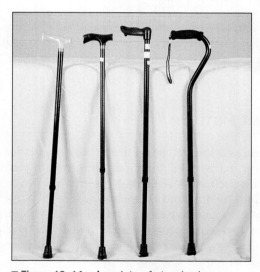

■ **Figure 10–14** A variety of standard canes.

A variation of the standard cane is a quad cane, so named because it has four feet (■ Figure 10–15). Quad canes are available in two base sizes, large and small. The design of a quad cane makes it stable. Quad canes are constructed of aluminum, using a telescoping upper shaft for height adjustment. Offset shaft/handgrip design is available for both quad cane sizes. The outer legs of quad cane bases are angled outward from the base to a greater degree than the inner legs to increase the base of support provided. During use, the wider angled legs are placed away from the patient to avoid interference with a patient's feet during gait. Bases on quad canes can be rotated so the same cane can be used on either the right or left side, maintaining appropriate outward orientation of the larger legs with respect to handgrip orientation.

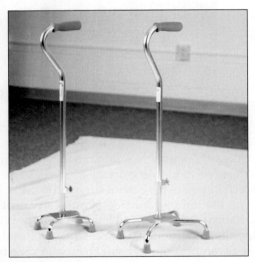

■ **Figure 10–15**   Small-base quad cane (left) and large-base quad cane (right).

Patients can let go of a quad cane without concern that it will fall or slide to the floor as standard canes do. A disadvantage of large base quad canes is that the larger base does not permit it to be placed on a standard stair tread unless turned sideways.

Handgrip designs, particularly for the offset cane, are available in varied shapes and textures to make grasp easier. The variety of handgrip designs are used for both standard and quad canes.

In a variation from standard crutches and canes, a "foot" is attached to the shaft with a moveable joint (■ Figure 10–16). The foot is a flat metal plate with a skid-resistant surface and the "ankle" pivots. As the patient ambulates, the shaft "rolls" over the fixed foot (■ Figure 10–17).

■ **Take Note**

The variety of cane handgrips allows for a selection that can accommodate a patient's hand size and impairments.

Choosing a Gait Pattern

A **gait pattern** is defined as a selected sequence of movements for the ambulatory assistive device(s) and lower extremities. Five gait patterns are commonly used. The gait patterns described in this section are described for forward progression. These patterns, however, are also used for turning and backward progression. A change in the direction of placement of ambulatory assistive devices and lower extremities is necessary when turning or performing backward progression. Choosing a gait pattern is dependent upon several variables, including medical condition, strength, range of motion, balance, and weight-bearing status.

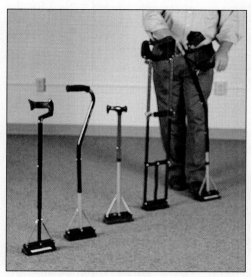

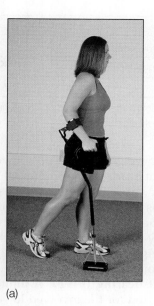

(a)

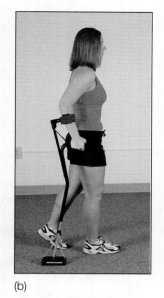

(b)

■ **Figure 10–16** Footpad canes and crutches.

■ **Figure 10–17** Ambulating with a forearm (Lofstrand) crutch with footpad.

Weight-Bearing Status

Weight bearing is the amount of weight that can be borne on a lower extremity during standing or ambulation. The amount of weight bearing permitted is dependent upon the patient's pathology, impairment, and medical management. When ambulating with ambulatory assistive devices, lifting of the body to decrease weight bearing is achieved by shoulder depression and elbow extension.

Decision-making algorithms (see Figures ■ 10–18, ■ 10–19 and ■ 10–20) are used by physical therapists to determine initial, and subsequent, gait patterns to be used. Decisions concerning gait patterns to be used are based upon the physical therapy examination results. Physical therapist assistants can implement gait training with assistive devices and appropriate gait patterns as directed by a physical therapist.

Type of WB	Unilateral LE WB Restriction	Bilateral LE WB Restriction
PWB	3 point	2 or 4 point
TTWB	3 point or swing through	Unable to walk
NWB	3 point or swing through	Unable to walk

■ **Figure 10–18** Choosing a gait pattern by consideration of type of weight bearing and the number of limbs involved.

Amount of Strength	Unilateral LE Weakness	Bilateral LE Weakness
Minimal weakness	3 point	2 or 4 point
Moderate weakness	3 point	Swing through (may need orthoses)
Significant weakness	3 point or swing through (may need orthosis)	Swing through (will probably need orthoses)

■ **Figure 10–19** Choosing a gait pattern by consideration of amount of strength and the number of limbs involved.

Balance Impairment	Gait Pattern
Minimally impaired	3 point
Moderately impaired	2, 3, or 4 point
Significantly impaired	3 or 4 point and guarding

■ **Figure 10–20** Choosing a gait pattern by consideration of the severity of balance.

The amount of weight bearing on a lower extremity can vary from full weight bearing to non–weight bearing. The amount of weight bearing is controlled by the extent to which ambulatory assistive devices are used for weight bearing. There are five commonly used terms to describe weight bearing:

Non–weight bearing (NWB): The involved lower extremity is not to be weight bearing and is usually not permitted to touch the ground.

Toe touch weight bearing (TTWB): The patient can rest the foot of the involved lower extremity on the ground for balance but not for weight bearing.

Partial weight bearing (PWB): A limited amount of weight bearing, such as five pounds, is permitted for the involved lower extremity. When partial weight bearing is required, but a specific amount of weight is not specified, minimal weight bearing should be permitted on the involved lower extremity until a specific amount is confirmed by the referring physician.

Weight bearing as tolerated (WBAT): The patient determines the amount of weight bearing that will occur on the involved lower extremity. The amount of weight bearing permitted may vary from minimal to full, depending upon the tolerance of the patient.

Full weight bearing (FWB): The patient is permitted full weight bearing on the involved lower extremity. Ambulatory assistive devices are not used to decrease weight bearing but may be used for assistance with balance.

Two-Point Gait Pattern

A two-point gait pattern is used when two ambulatory assistive devices, such as two canes or two crutches, are required. This gait pattern is used with patients with impairments such as muscle weakness, pain, or decreased balance.

The patient lifts and moves one ambulatory assistive device and the opposite lower extremity forward simultaneously. When the ambulatory assistive device and lower extremity have been placed on the ground, the patient shifts the weight to these supports. Then the patient moves the other ambulatory assistive device and its opposite lower extremity forward. This two-part sequence is repeated. Each combination of one ambulatory assistive device and the opposite lower extremity is considered "one point." A complete cycle includes "two points," thus the name two-point gait pattern.

Four-Point Gait Pattern

A four-point gait pattern is often described as a deliberate two-point gait pattern. This gait pattern is used when two ambulatory assistive devices, such as two canes or two crutches, are required. A four-point gait pattern is used with patients with the same types of impairments as a two-point gait pattern but for whom the impairments are more severe. A four-point gait pattern may also be used as a starting point to teach a patient the pairing of the opposite upper and lower extremities before graduating to using the two-point gait pattern.

The patient moves one ambulatory assistive device forward and places it on the floor, followed by the opposite lower extremity. The patient moves the other ambulatory assistive device forward and places it on the floor, followed by its opposite lower extremity. Each time an ambulatory assistive device or lower extremity is lifted to be moved forward, weight bearing is shifted to the three supports remaining in contact with the floor. This four-part sequence is repeated. A complete cycle includes "four points."

Three-Point Gait Pattern

A three-point gait pattern is used by patients with impairments of one lower extremity, such as a fracture, muscle weakness, pain, or injury/surgery requiring decreased weight bearing. The levels of weight bearing described earlier may be used by patients ambulating with a three-point gait pattern. This gait pattern requires two crutches, two canes, or a walker. The example that follows assumes the use of two crutches. The use of two canes follows the same pattern. The use of a walker requires that the walker be advanced as a unit, mimicking the simultaneous advancement of two crutches or two canes.

As a patient initially learns this gait pattern, he moves both crutches forward and places them on the floor. The patient moves the involved lower extremity forward between the two crutches such that the ball of the foot is even with the crutch tips. After the involved lower extremity is moved forward, the patient shifts weight bearing to the upper extremities and involved lower extremity if permitted by weight-bearing status. Then the patient moves the uninvolved lower extremity forward past the crutches. The patient shifts weight bearing to the uninvolved lower extremity in preparation for the next forward movement of the crutches and involved lower extremity. This three-part sequence is repeated. Thus, a complete cycle includes "three points."

As patients become more confident, they move the crutches and involved lower extremity forward simultaneously. The shifting of weight bearing and movement of the uninvolved lower extremity follow as before.

Initially, patients may advance the uninvolved lower extremity forward only to the involved lower extremity and crutches. Encourage patients to step beyond the placement of the involved lower extremity and crutches for a faster and more normal gait pattern.

Swing-To Gait Pattern

A swing-to gait pattern requires the use of two crutches or a walker. This gait pattern is used for patients with impairments of the lower extremities such as muscle weakness, paresis, paralysis, or decreased weight bearing on one lower extremity. The levels of weight bearing described earlier may be used by patients ambulating with a swing-to gait pattern. To perform the swing-to gait pattern, the patient must be able to bear full weight on one lower extremity. The example that follows assumes the use of two crutches.

The patient moves both crutches forward simultaneously and places the tips on the floor. The patient shifts weight bearing onto the crutches. The patient moves both lower extremities forward simultaneously to the same point as the crutches were advanced and places them on the floor. The patient shifts weight bearing to one or both lower extremities, as allowed by weight-bearing status, for support so the crutches can be advanced again. This two-part sequence is repeated. Each cycle requires that the lower extremities "swing to" the same point as the ambulatory assistive devices were advanced, thus the name "swing-to" gait pattern.

Swing-Through Gait Pattern

A swing-through gait pattern requires the use of two crutches. This gait pattern is used for patients with the same impairments as would use the swing-to gait pattern, such as muscle weakness, paresis, paralysis, or decreased weight bearing on one lower extremity. The levels of weight bearing described earlier may be used by patients ambulating with a swing-through gait pattern.

As indicated previously, the patient must be able to bear full weight on one lower extremity.

The patient moves both crutches forward simultaneously and places the tips on the floor. The patient shifts weight bearing onto the crutches. The patient swings both lower extremities forward simultaneously beyond the crutch tips. The patient shifts weight bearing to one or both lower extremities, as allowed by weight-bearing status, for support so the crutches can be advanced again. This two-part sequence is repeated. Each cycle requires that the lower extremities "swing through" the crutches, thus the name "swing-through" gait pattern.

PROCEDURE 10–1   Guarding

Guarding is the process of protecting the patient from excessive weight bearing, loss of balance, or falling. Proper guarding requires use of a gait belt. Guarding by holding onto the patient's belt may be uncomfortable for the patient because the narrow belt or belt buckle can bind or pinch the patient. Holding clothing is not appropriate because clothing may tear and does not fit firmly enough to provide control during guarding. A gait belt should fit snugly around the patient's waist. There may or may not be handles for the physical therapist/assistant to grasp the gait belt. Hold the gait belt with the forearm supinated for a stronger grip. Initially the physical therapist/assistant grasps the gait belt with one hand and places the other hand on the patient's trunk over the shoulder girdle on the side to which the physical therapist/assistant is standing.

■ **Take Note**

Proper guarding techniques provide safety for patients and physical therapists/assistants.

In and Out of a Wheelchair

When the patient arises from or sits in a chair, the physical therapist/assistant stands in stride, to one side, and slightly behind the patient. This permits the physical therapist/assistant to move with the patient without blocking the patient's movement. In some instances, the physical therapist/assistant may stand in front of the patient, as for an assisted standing pivot transfer. Standing in front of the patient permits the physical therapist/assistant to provide physical assistance and moves the patient into the physical therapist's/assistant's base of support.

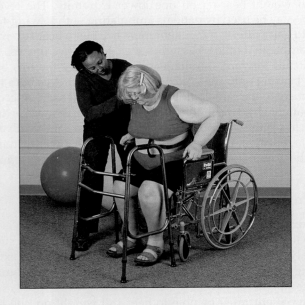

Level Surfaces

1 When the patient ambulates, the physical therapist/assistant stands in stride behind and slightly to one side of the patient. As the physical therapist/assistant grasps the gait belt with a supinated forearm, she places the other hand over the patient's shoulder girdle, not on the upper extremity. If her hand is placed on the patient's upper extremity, it may interfere with free motion needed to control ambulatory assistive devices.

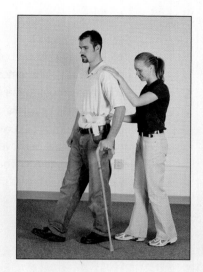

In all situations, the physical therapist/assistant must be positioned in a way that permits the physical therapist/assistant to move as the patient moves. This is extremely important because the physical therapist's/assistant's position must not interfere with the patient's movement. The physical therapist/assistant must be alert to the patient's position and movements and to obstacles in the environment.

During initial gait training, the physical therapist/assistant stands close to the patient to provide increased support and control. As the patient ambulates, the physical therapist/assistant moves with the patient. The physical therapist/assistant moves her "outside" foot (the one most lateral to the patient) when the ambulatory assistive device on that side is moved. The physical therapist/assistant moves her "inside" foot (the one directly behind the patient) when the patient moves the foot on the side the physical therapist/assistant is guarding. Such coordination of physical therapist/assistant and patient movements allows the physical therapist/assistant to move smoothly without kicking or tripping the patient and without interfering with ambulatory assistive devices.

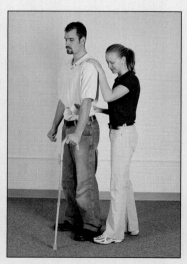

2 When the physical therapist/assistant has both hands on the patient and is behind the patient and ambulatory assistive device, this is described as *close guarding*.

(continued)

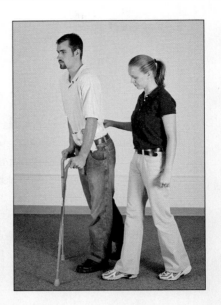

3 As the patient's ambulation skills improve, the physical therapist/assistant removes her hand from the shoulder girdle, stands more to the side of the patient, and continues to grasp the gait belt. This is described as *contact guarding*. As the patient ambulates with this level of guarding, the physical therapist/assistant moves her "inside" foot with the ambulatory assistive device. The physical therapist/assistant moves her "outside" foot with the patient's lower extremity.

Eventually, the physical therapist/assistant walks near the patient without contact or holding the gait belt. This is described as **supervision**, or **stand-by, guarding**.

Falling

If a patient starts to fall, the physical therapist/assistant must decide whether to maintain the patient in an upright position or to permit a controlled lowering to the floor in a manner that will prevent injury to the patient or physical therapist/assistant. Physical therapists/assistants must be alert to a patient's movements at all times and be able to react quickly to prevent or control a fall.

■ **Take Note**

Caution—Be alert to patient balance and movement. Be prepared to prevent or control a fall.

During early stages of gait training, patients usually lean away from weight bearing on an involved lower extremity because they fear pain or further injury if they put too much weight on the involved lower extremity. This is another reason physical therapists/assistants initially guard a patient on the uninvolved or less involved side. By guarding on a patient's uninvolved side, the physical therapist/assistant is on the side to which patients are already leaning as they avoid excessive weight bearing on an involved lower extremity. This positioning, and the tendency of patients to lean in this direction, places physical therapists/assistants in the best position to pull a patient into the physical therapist's/assistant's base of support, reducing the risk of increased weight bearing on an involved lower extremity.

Pulling the patient into the physical therapist's/assistant's base of support is the safer method for both patient and physical therapist/assistant of preventing a fall. The physical therapist/assistant is able to control the patient more completely when the patient's weight is pulled into the physical therapist's/assistant's base of support. If the patient starts to fall, the physical therapist/assistant is better able to provide support and protection of an involved lower extremity by shifting the patient's weight onto the uninvolved lower extremity. This combination of measures is best achieved by guarding a patient on the uninvolved side. For this reason, initial gait training usually begins with the physical therapist/assistant guarding the patient on the uninvolved side.

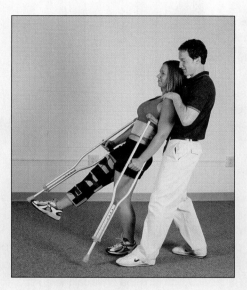

■ **Take Note**
For safety, initial guarding should be from the side of the patient's uninvolved lower extremity.

As the patient's capabilities improve, the physical therapist/assistant guards on the patient's involved side, encouraging upright posture and appropriate use of the involved lower extremity.

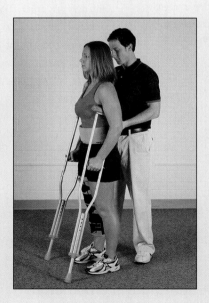

(continued)

Ascending/Descending Stairs

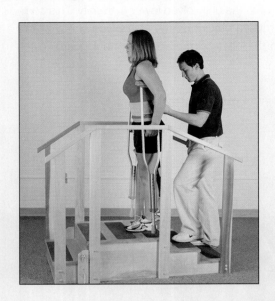 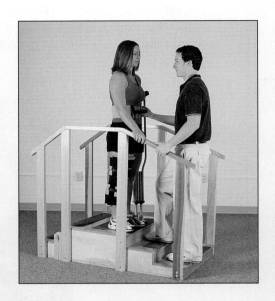

The physical therapist/assistant is positioned below the patient when guarding as the patient ascends and descends stairs. The physical therapist/assistant grasps the patient's gait belt with one hand and a handrail with the other hand. Holding a handrail provides the physical therapist/assistant with a point of stability to halt a fall. The physical therapist/assistant stands in stride on the stairs, placing his feet on different stair treads. A stride position enables the physical therapist/assistant to shift weight and position as the patient moves, permitting the physical therapist/assistant to shift the patient's weight into the physical therapist's/assistant's base of support should the patient begin to fall.

Occasionally a second person is needed to guard a patient learning to ascend and descend stairs. The second person stands in stride on the stairs above the patient and also holds the gait belt and handrail.

■ **Take Note**
When guarding a patient ascending/descending stairs, hold the handrail with one hand for stability to prevent a fall.

PROCEDURE 10–2   Assumption of Standing and Sitting

Preparing the Wheelchair

When the patient is assuming standing from a wheelchair or assuming sitting in a wheelchair, the physical therapist/assistant places the wheelchair against a stable surface, such as a wall or heavy table if possible, and engages the wheel locks. The physical therapist/assistant raises the footplates and removes the footrests and places them out of the way of the physical therapist/assistant or patient.

Positioning the Patient

To ease the assumption of a standing position, the patient moves to sitting at the front edge of the seat, as shown in Chapter 7. The patient places both feet flat on the floor below the front edge of the seat. In this position the patient's knees are flexed to approximately 110 degrees and ankles are in slight dorsiflexion. The patient's center of gravity can be brought over the base of support quickly from this position as the patient assumes standing. The patient may place her feet side by side or in a short stride position. Using a stride position increases the patient's anterior/posterior base of support. When moving to standing with the feet in stride, the patient places the foot of the uninvolved lower extremity slightly behind the involved lower extremity. This allows the patient to use the uninvolved lower extremity efficiently for rising to standing. Having the patient place her hands on the armrests also increases the base of support and provides initial assistance to push to a standing position.

Assumption of Standing

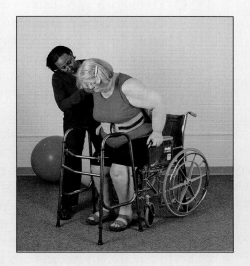

1 To assume a standing position, the patient must lean forward to shift the center of gravity over the feet and extend the knees and hips to rise from the seat.

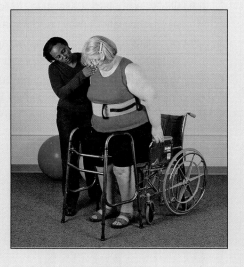

2 Initially, the patient pushes directly downward on the armrests. Pushing at an angle creates a horizontal component of the pushing force vector that does not assist the patient in rising and may also propel the patient horizontally and, thus, off balance.

(continued)

■ **Take Note**

When assuming standing using crutches, place crutches on the side of the patient's uninvolved lower extremity.

Ambulatory assistive devices must be accessible to patients when they are sitting in a chair and after the assumption of standing. Initially, ambulatory assistive devices may not be used during the assumption of standing. During initial learning, the patient places both hands on the armrests of the chair to assist with pushing to standing. In such cases, the ambulatory assistive device must be accessible to the physical therapist/assistant, who hands it to the patient once standing has been achieved. When using ambulatory assistive devices to assume standing, the patient may place one hand on the ambulatory assistive device and the other hand on the armrest. Whichever hand position is used, the movement to assume standing should be a controlled continuous motion.

Assumption of Sitting

❶ To assume a sitting position after walking, the patient must approach the front edge of a chair and then turn away from the chair. When performing this maneuver, the patient may initially feel more confident turning toward the uninvolved side. This occurs because the patient is turning into his or her strength. However, the patient must be able to turn in both directions, toward the involved and uninvolved sides. As the patient approaches a chair, he or she must ensure that the chair is secure and, if the chair is a wheelchair, that the footrests are out of the way.

❷ With the patient standing close to the front edge of the seat and facing away from the chair, the patient's center of gravity can be maintained over the base of support during the assumption of sitting. The patient may place his feet side by side or in a short stride position. Using a stride position increases a patient's base of support. When moving to sitting with the feet in stride, the foot of the uninvolved lower extremity is slightly farther back than the foot of the involved lower extremity. Having patients reach for and use armrests while lowering to the seat also increases a patient's base of support and provides assistance to control the latter stages of lowering.

■ **Take Note**

When assuming a sitting position, the patient's feet are in stride, with the uninvolved lower extremity closest to wheelchair.

Initially, ambulatory assistive devices may not be used for the assumption of sitting. In such cases, the patient may hand the ambulatory assistive device, such as crutches and canes, but not walkers, to the physical therapist/assistant before beginning to lower to sitting. Then the patient uses both hands to grasp the armrests of the chair to assist with the controlled lowering to sitting. When using ambulatory assistive devices during assumption of sitting, the patient places one hand, usually the hand on the side of the involved lower extremity, on the assistive device and the other hand on the armrest. The patient then assumes sitting in a controlled manner.

PROCEDURE 10–3   Ascending and Descending Stairs

Generally, patients ascend and descend stairs on their right side when facing the stairs. When ascending or descending stairs, the patient places the tips of the ambulatory assistive device one-half to two-thirds of the way forward onto the stair tread, in the direction the patient is facing. When two ambulatory assistive devices are used, the patient places them far enough apart to allow room for the patient to move between them. When a stair rail is available, the patient should use it for greater stability. When the patient is using two ambulatory assistive devices, he can place both in one hand to free the other hand for use on the stair rail. When only one upper extremity can be used, the patient can hold the ambulatory assistive device in the hand on the stair rail. If the right upper extremity is unable to be used, patients may use the assistive device only or ascend and descend on the left side when facing the stairs.

■ **Take Note**
The involved lower extremity is never left without support, either from the uninvolved lower extremity or the ambulatory assistive device.

When first learning to ascend and descend stairs, patients usually use a step-to gait pattern. As a patient's condition permits, the patient may progress to a step-over-step gait pattern to ascend and descend stairs.

Ascending Stairs

1. When ascending stairs, the patient moves the uninvolved lower extremity to the next higher stair first because it must lift the body. To do so, the patient shifts weight to the ambulatory assistive device and as permitted to the involved lower extremity, allowing movement of the uninvolved lower extremity.

2. Once the patient has appropriately placed the uninvolved lower extremity on the next stair, he shifts weight to the uninvolved lower extremity. He extends the uninvolved lower extremity to lift the body.

3. The patient advances the involved lower extremity and the ambulatory assistive device to the same stair while he lifts the body.

4. An alternative is to have the patient move the involved lower extremity to the same stair as the uninvolved lower extremity, followed by the ambulatory assistive device.

■ **Take Note**
When ascending stairs, lead with the uninvolved lower extremity.

Descending Stairs

1. When descending stairs, the patient moves the ambulatory assistive devices to the next lower stair first to provide support for the involved lower extremity.

2. The patient shifts weight to the uninvolved lower extremity, permitting the ambulatory assistive devices and involved lower extremity to be lowered to the next lower stair.

3. The patient uses the uninvolved lower extremity to lower the body until the ambulatory assistive device and the involved lower extremity are on the next lower stair.

4. An alternative is to have the patient lower the ambulatory assistive device first, followed by the involved lower extremity once the ambulatory assistive device is in place. The patient shifts weight to the ambulatory assistive device and involved lower extremity when appropriate. Then the patient moves the uninvolved lower extremity down to the same stair.

■ **Take Note**
When descending stairs, lead with the assistive device and then the involved lower extremity.

Curbs

The sequence for ascending and descending curbs is the same as the sequence for ascending and descending stairs. Only ambulatory assistive devices are available for support when ascending and descending curbs because of the absence of handrails.

Moving Through Doorways

There are many combinations of extremity involvement and doorway configurations. A patient may have one or two functional upper extremities, and the impairment of the patient's lower extremities may involve one or both. Doors may open toward or away from the patient, they may be hinged on the left or right, the space around the door available for maneuvering may be ample or limited, and doors may or may not have automatic openers or closers. Each combination of factors will require modifications to the general method of ambulating through doorways. Patient safety must not be compromised regardless of patient level of function and physical configuration of the environment.

■ **Take Note**

Caution—Doorways require movement into spaces where there is no initial visibility because of the door. Proceed carefully when opening and progressing through doorways.

Often balance is a major concern. Patients may be required to lean in all directions, moving their center of gravity with respect to their base of support while pushing or pulling on doors. Another concern is the danger of a door with an automatic closer striking a patient as it closes. Should a door strike a patient, the patient may lose balance control, resulting in more weight bearing on the involved lower extremity than is permitted or the patient falling to the ground. To avoid an automatic closing door from forcefully striking a patient, such doors should be opened wider than the minimal width for a patient to progress through the doorway. This allows the patient time to progress through the doorway before the automatic closing door impedes progress. An alternative technique is to use the tips of ambulatory assistive devices as temporary door stops while progressing through these doorways. Some patients rush to move through such doorways. Rushing can also be hazardous as a patient may not be able to control the ambulatory assistive device or maintain balance when moving at a faster pace.

The physical therapist's/assistant's position for guarding the patient during movement through doorways is the same position as for guarding during ambulation. Recognizing that shorter steps and abrupt turns may be required, the physical therapist/assistant must be prepared to move with the patient, avoiding interference with the patient's freedom of movement or the arc of movement of a door. During initial gait training through doorways, the physical therapist/assistant may need to control opening and closing of the door to protect the patient.

When a door does not have an automatic closer, the door does not have to be opened greater than the width of the patient to prevent the door from closing forcefully on a patient before he has progressed through the doorway. Rapid movement of ambulatory assistive devices to block the door is not necessary. Doors that do not have automatic closers require that the patient turn and close the door after moving through the doorway.

Tilt Table

■ **Take Note**

Use a tilt table to assist patients to achieve and maintain an upright posture. These patients may be non–weight bearing or partial weight bearing.

Some patients must be reacclimated to upright posture in a safe manner before sitting, standing, or ambulation can be initiated. This is usually necessitated by the existence of orthostatic hypotension in patients who have been in bed for extended periods. Accommodation by the cardiovascular system may be necessary to avoid dizziness or fainting as these patients assume an upright posture. Tilt tables are a safe method to provide maximum support for such patients. Support is provided while the patient is raised slowly to an upright position by the tilt table, leaving the physical therapist/assistant free to control the tilt table and monitor the patient. Abdominal binders and elastic wraps or elastic hose on the lower extremities may be used to assist veinous return. Use of lower extremity muscles, such as isometric contractions, often called *muscle setting* exercises, or active range of motion exercises also assists veinous return.

Measure vital signs, as presented in Chapter 5, before, during, and after the process of raising patients to an upright posture (■ Figure 10–21). Lower patients when they report feeling faint. Monitor a patient who is lowered after feeling faint until vital signs return to normal and the patient no longer reports feeling faint. Obtain medical assistance when necessary.

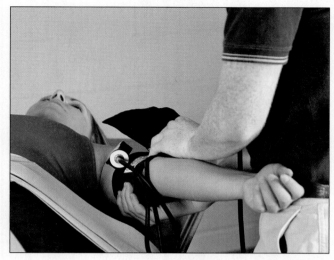

■ **Figure 10–21**   Measuring vital signs before raising tilt table.

Use straps to secure patients on a tilt table (■ Figure 10–22). A variety of styles of straps are available. A bar extends along each side of the tilt table surface. Straps used to secure the patient on the tilt table are attached to the bar on one side of the table.

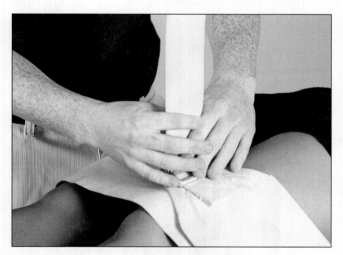

■ **Figure 10–22**   Securing patient on a tilt table.

Straps are passed over the patient and secured around the bar on the other side. The location of the straps across the patient depends on the patient's condition. When upper trunk stability is required, use a chest strap leaving the upper extremities free. A strap over the pelvis stabilizes the lower trunk. Use a strap at knee level when the patient cannot maintain knee extension.

Adjust the angle of tilt to a position the patient can tolerate safely. Perform changes in the position of the table slowly and steadily. Greater degrees of tilt may be assumed as the patient's cardiovascular system adjusts to the demands of an upright posture. For many patients a full upright position provides a sensation of falling forward; therefore, this position is usually avoided.

Patients with non–weight-bearing status on one lower extremity can be placed on a tilt table. Place a lift under the foot of the uninvolved lower extremity, preventing the involved lower extremity from reaching the supporting surface (■ Figure 10–23). Thus, the involved lower extremity is non–weight bearing.

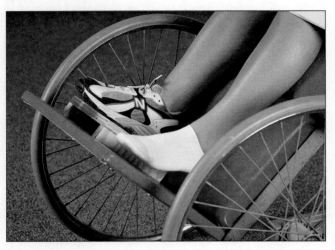

■ **Figure 10–23** A lift under the uninvolved (right) lower extremity avoids weight bearing on the involved (left) lower extremity.

When an exercise program for one lower extremity is to be implemented, loosen the strap across the knees or place it only around the opposite lower extremity. This permits the physical therapist/assistant to implement the patient's lower extremity exercise program. Upper extremity and trunk exercises can also be performed on the tilt table (■ Figure 10–24).

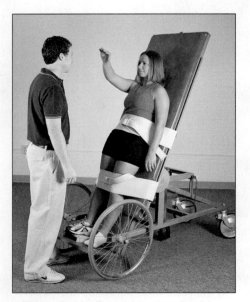

■ **Figure 10–24** Exercising on a tilt table.

A tilt table may also be used when patients have restrictions on sitting or the amount of hip flexion allowed. When individuals move from sitting to standing, the hips ordinarily flex more than 90 degrees. Following total hip replacement, patients are restricted to no more than 90 degrees of hip flexion. For patients unable to assume standing from sitting while maintaining hip precautions, a tilt table can be used to rise to a standing position. Patients can be fitted with ambulatory assistive devices while on a tilt table (■ Figure 10–25) and "walk," with guarding, off the tilt table for ambulation training.

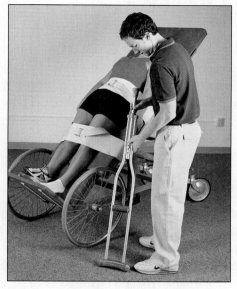

■ **Figure 10–25** Adjusting crutch height while patient is on a tilt table.

Walkers

Fitting

To measure a walker for proper height adjustment, the patient stands upright with the shoulder girdle relaxed within the walker with the crossbar in front. The top of the handgrips should be approximately at the level of the patient's ulnar styloid processes when the upper extremities are relaxed at the side (■ Figure 10–26). This fitting can be done within the parallel bars. When the patient grasps the handgrips with shoulder girdles level and relaxed, the elbows are flexed approximately 20–30 degrees (■ Figure 10–27).

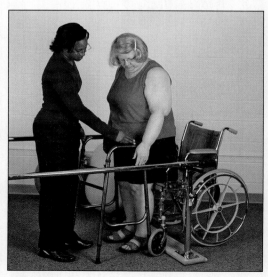

■ **Figure 10–26** Checking handgrip weight when fitting a walker.

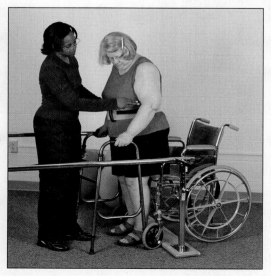

■ **Figure 10–27** Checking elbow flexion angle when fitting a walker.

PROCEDURE 10–4 In and Out of a Wheelchair with a Walker

Two methods of getting in and out of a wheelchair will be described. In both methods, the physical therapist/assistant prepares a wheelchair and positions the patient in the manner presented earlier in this chapter under *Assumption of Standing and Sitting.* Reversing wheelchair desk armrests so the higher portion is at the front of the wheelchair will assist patients in pushing to standing and lowering to sitting. A physical therapist/assistant is positioned in the manner described earlier in this chapter under *Guarding.*

Assuming Standing Using a Walker

The physical therapist/assistant engages wheelchair wheel locks and moves footrests out of the way. The patient is positioned at the front edge of the seat, with her feet in stride or side by side. A physical therapist/assistant is positioned in stride, behind and to one side of the patient. The physical therapist/assistant grasps the patient's gait belt with one hand. The other hand may be on the patient's shoulder girdle if necessary. If a hand is placed on the patient's shoulder girdle, it should not interfere with a patient's ability to move smoothly using the upper extremity.

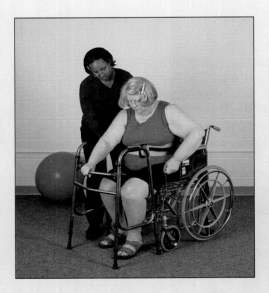

① The patient uses the hand on the uninvolved side to grasp and push down on the crossbar of the walker. The patient places the hand on the involved side on the armrest of the wheelchair. This ensures that the patient is moving into her strength.

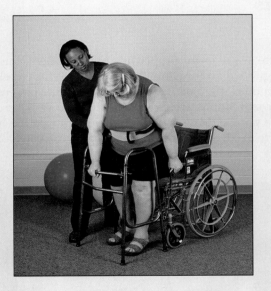

② The patient pushes to standing.

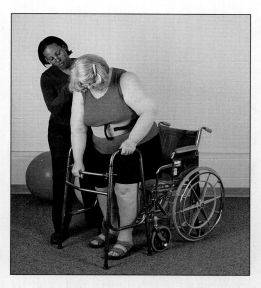

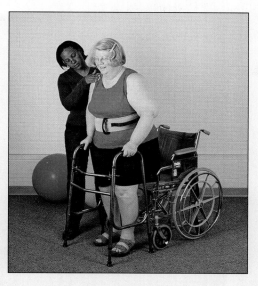

③ The patient moves the hand on the involved side from the armrest of the wheelchair and grasps the handgrip of the walker.

④ The patient moves the hand on the uninvolved side from the crossbar to grasp the other handgrip. The patient is now correctly positioned in the walker to begin ambulation.

Force exerted on the crossbar of a walker must be exerted directly downward to avoid tipping the walker.

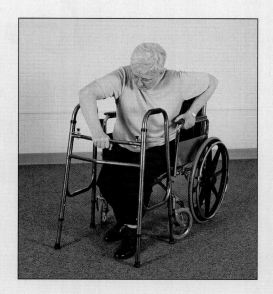

(continued)

If force is not exerted directly downward when a patient's hand is placed on the crossbar of a walker, the walker tips forward.

■ **Take Note**
When a patient uses the crossbar of the walker to assume standing, the force on the crossbar must be directly downward to prevent tipping of the walker.

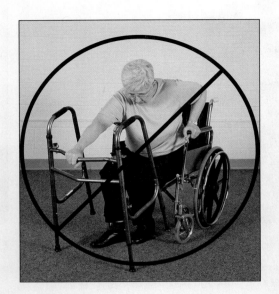

The patient may place the hand on the uninvolved side on the walker's handgrip instead of crossbar. There are two disadvantages to this method. First, a walker's handgrip is higher than the crossbar. The height of the handgrip may make pushing directly downward more difficult for a patient. Second, the handgrip is at the very outside of the walker's base of support. Slight deviation from pushing directly downward will cause the walker to tip sideways.

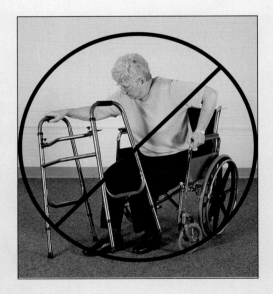

Assuming Sitting Using a Walker

1 The physical therapist/assistant engages the wheelchair wheel locks and moves the footrests out of the way. To sit, the patient is positioned facing away from the wheelchair at the front edge of the wheelchair seat, close enough so she can feel the front edge of wheelchair seat against the back of the lower extremities. The patient can position her feet either in stride or side by side. Positioned in stride behind and to one side of the patient, the physical therapist/assistant grasps the patient's gait belt and shoulder girdle.

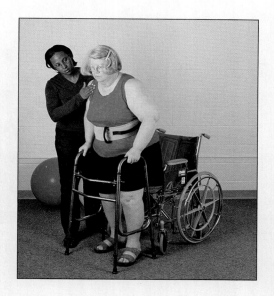

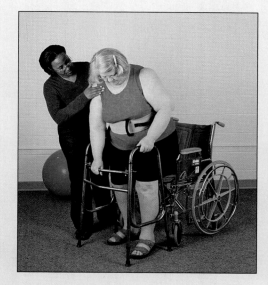

2 The patient grasps the middle of the crossbar with the hand on the involved side.

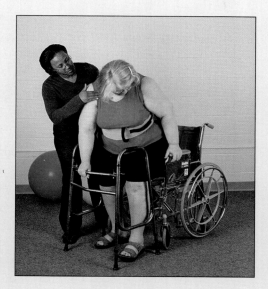

3 The patient reaches backward and grasps the armrest with the hand on the uninvolved side.

(continued)

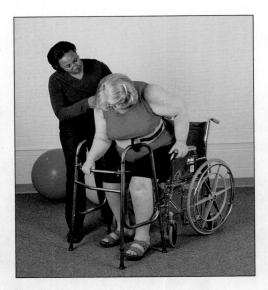

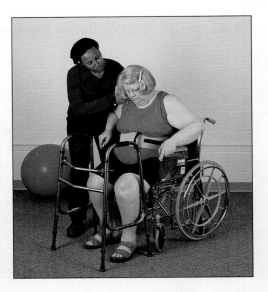

④ The patient lowers in a controlled manner to a sitting position.

⑤ The patient moves the hand from the crossbar to the armrest and adjusts the sitting position in the wheelchair.

Assuming Standing Using Both Armrests

① The physical therapist/assistant engages the wheelchair wheel locks and moves the footrests out of the way. The patient is positioned at the front edge of the seat with the feet in stride or side by side. Positioned in stride behind and to one side of the patient, the physical therapist/assistant grasps the patient's gait belt and shoulder girdle. Sitting on the front edge of the seat, the patient places both hands on the armrests.

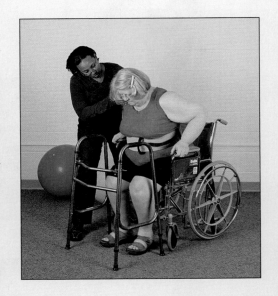

② Using the armrests, the patient pushes to standing.

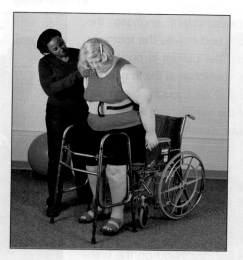

■ **Take Note**
Move the hand on the side
of the uninvolved lower
extremity first.

③ The patient shifts weight completely over the feet. The patient first moves the hand on the uninvolved side from the wheelchair armrest to the handgrip of the walker.

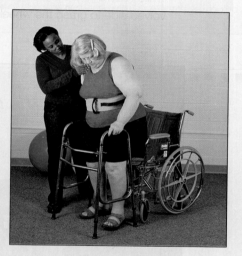

④ Once the patient has the hand on the uninvolved side properly positioned, the patient moves the hand on the involved side from the wheelchair armrest to the handgrip of the walker.

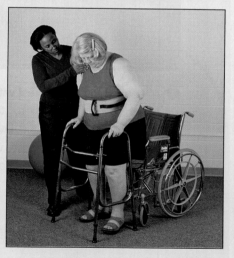

(continued)

3 Extending the uninvolved lower extremity, the patient lifts the body and places the involved lower extremity on the same stair as the uninvolved lower extremity.

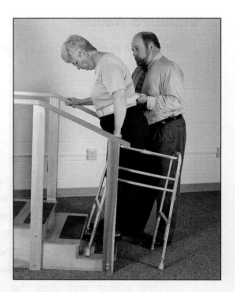

4 The patient advances the walker and the sequence is repeated to ascend the remaining stairs.

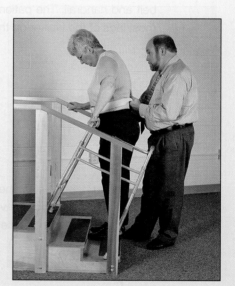

Descending Stairs

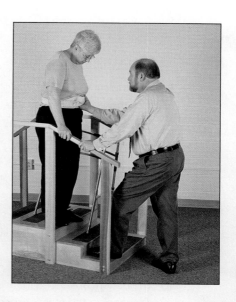

1 To descend stairs using a standard walker, the patient stands facing down the stairs. The patient turns the walker sideways so the crossbar is on the side of the patient away from the handrail. The patient positions the walker with the two forwardmost legs on the next lower step. The patient places her hand closest to the walker on the rearmost handgrip of the walker and uses the other hand to grasp the handrail. Positioned in stride in front of the patient, the physical therapist/assistant grasps the patient's gait belt and the handrail.

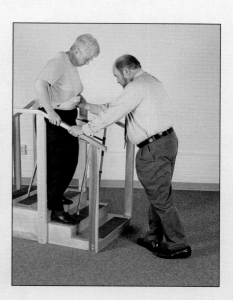

2 Supporting weight on the upper extremities and the uninvolved lower extremity, the patient lowers the involved lower extremity down to the same stair as the forwardmost legs of the walker by flexing the uninvolved lower extremity.

(continued)

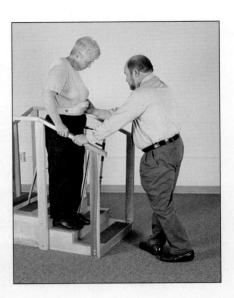

3 Continuing to support weight with the upper extremities, the patient lowers the uninvolved lower extremity down to the same stair as the walker's forwardmost legs and the involved lower extremity.

4 The patient advances the walker and the sequence is repeated until the patient completes descending the stairs. When the patient reaches the landing or floor level, she places the walker in front and grasps both handgrips.

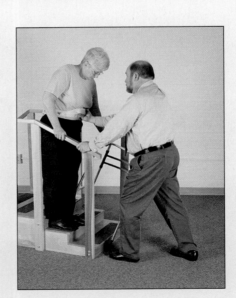

■ **Take Note**
Using a standard walker when ascending/descending stairs is not recommended but is an option when no other alternative is available.

PROCEDURE 10–7 Ambulating Through Doorways with a Walker

Door Opens Toward Patient

Authors' note: In this section, text and photographs depict independent ambulation. This method was used so a physical therapist does not obscure the desired photographic views of the patient.

1 The patient approaches the latch edge of the door, standing outside the arc through which the opening door will move. The patient shifts the weight to the side of the walker away from the hand that will be placed on the door handle. The patient then places the unweighted hand on the door handle.

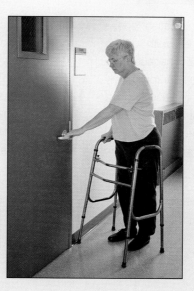

■ Take Note
When a door opens toward the patient, the patient should stand at the latch side of the door.

(continued)

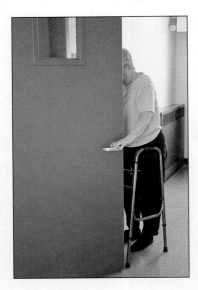

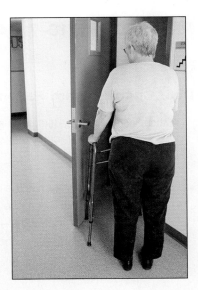

2 Using a pulling motion, the patient opens the door wider than the width of the patient. This is necessary because the door will start to close automatically before the patient can progress through the doorway. The patient must block the door from closing with the walker to allow the patient time to progress through the doorway.

3 The patient quickly returns the hand used to open the door to the walker. The patient lifts the walker and moves it forward into the doorway. The patient places all four legs of the walker on the floor, with the two legs closest to the door serving as door stops. Using this method, the closing door hits the walker's legs, not the patient.

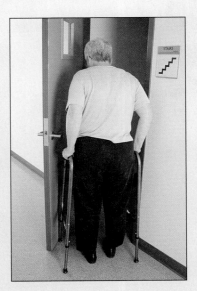

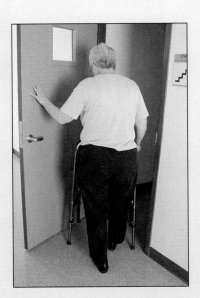

4 Once the walker has absorbed the contact of a closing door, the patient can step into the walker to advance through the doorway.

5 The patient may have to push the door farther open during transit through the doorway to allow a walker to be moved.

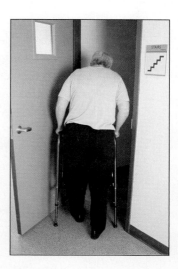

6. The patient should wait until the walker's legs have absorbed the contact of the closing door before moving forward. Once the patient has moved completely through the doorway, the door closes behind the patient.

Door Opens Away from Patient

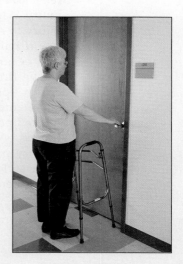

1. When a door with an automatic door closer opens away from a patient, the patient should approach the door and shift the weight to the side of the walker away from the hand that is closest to the door handle. The patient then places the unweighted hand on the door handle.

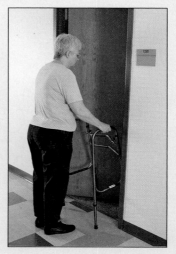

2. Using a pushing motion, the patient opens the door wider than the width of the patient. The patient quickly returns the hand used to open the door to the walker. The patient lifts the walker and moves it forward into the doorway. The patient places all four legs of the walker on the floor, with the two legs closest to the door serving as door stops. Using this method, the closing door hits the walker's legs, not the patient. Once a walker has absorbed the contact of a closing door, the patient can step into the walker to advance through the doorway.

(continued)

3 Using a walker's legs as doorstops, the patient progresses through the doorway. The patient may have to push a door farther open during transit through the doorway to allow a walker to be moved. Whenever this is done, the patient should wait until the walker's legs have absorbed the contact of the closing door before moving forward. Once the patient has moved completely through the doorway, the door closes behind the patient.

Axillary Crutches

Fitting

Axillary crutches are fitted with the patient standing and with shoulder girdles relaxed. Proper adjustment requires appropriate posture because of the potential for injury. When crutches are too long or when a patient rests on the tops of the crutches, injury to nerves and blockage of blood vessels in the axillae can occur. Patients may report pain or tingling in the upper extremities, and muscle weakness or paralysis may occur.

The first adjustment is the overall length of the crutch (■ Figure 10–28). Position crutch tips on the floor, approximately 6 inches away from the toes at a 45-degree angle anterior and lateral to the small toe. With the patient's shoulder girdles in a relaxed position, the physical therapist/assistant should be able to put two or three fingers between the patient's axillae and the top of the crutch on each side. When axillary pads are to be used on crutches, they should be in place during fitting. In some styles of crutches, nuts and bolts should not be tightened completely until all adjustments are completed.

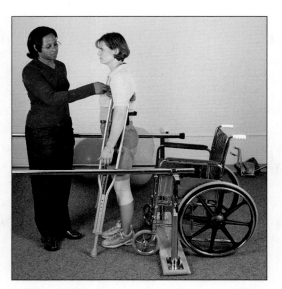

■ **Figure 10–28** Checking overall height of axillary crutches.

Adjust handgrip height after overall length of the crutch is determined (■ **Figure 10–29**). The top of the handgrip should be approximately at the level of the top of the patient's ulnar styloid process when the upper extremities are in a relaxed position at the patient's side. When the patient grasps the handgrips with shoulder girdles level and relaxed, elbows are flexed approximately 20–30 degrees.

■ **Take Note**
When checking for the correct length of axillary crutches, the shoulder girdle must be relaxed.

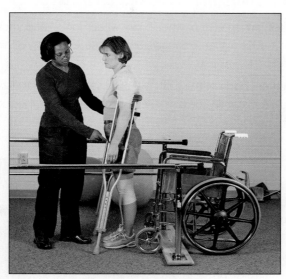

■ **Figure 10–29** Checking handgrip height of axillary crutches.

When all length and handgrip adjustments are made, check all nuts, bolts, and button locks to ensure that they are tightened or fully positioned to maintain crutch integrity during ambulation.

PROCEDURE 10–8   In and Out of a Wheelchair with Axillary Crutches

Assuming Standing—Physical Therapist/Assistant on Involved Side

1 The physical therapist/assistant engages the wheelchair wheel locks and moves the footrests out of the way. The physical therapist/assistant places crutches within reach before the patient starts to stand.

As the patient moves to the front edge of the seat, the physical therapist/assistant may need to support the involved lower extremity the first few times a patient assumes standing.

2 To provide assistance, the physical therapist/assistant squats on the involved side of the patient while supporting the involved lower extremity.

When the patient is unable to flex the knee of the involved lower extremity, an elevating legrest is used for support during sitting. The legrest must be removed or lowered and pivoted to the side before the patient lowers the involved lower extremity to the floor.

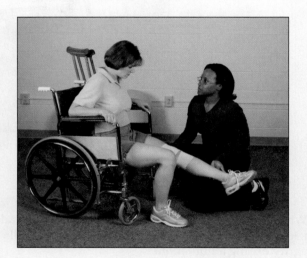

3 The physical therapist/assistant supports the involved lower extremity with one hand and arm while removing the legrest with the other hand. The patient carefully lowers the involved lower extremity to the floor before the patient attempts to stand.

■ **Take Note**
The involved lower extremity is placed on the floor before the patient rises to standing.

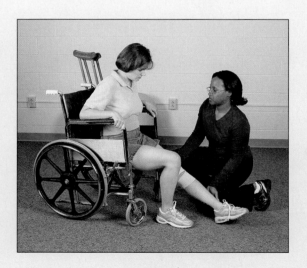

④ Both crutches are placed together in front of and slightly lateral to the patient's foot on the uninvolved side. The patient grasps both crutch handgrips with the hand on the uninvolved side while grasping the wheelchair armrest on the involved side. Positioned in stride to one side of the patient, the physical therapist/assistant grasps the patient's gait belt and maintains contact with the patient's shoulder girdle.

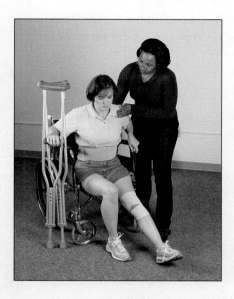

■ Take Note
Caution—The hand on the patient's shoulder girdle should guide, not impede, movement.

⑤ The patient assumes standing using the upper extremities and extending the uninvolved lower extremity. The involved lower extremity must be maintained within the desired weight-bearing status.

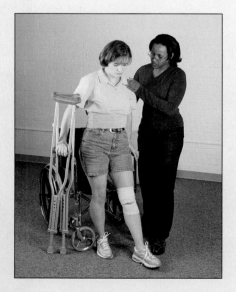

■ Take Note
When a patient requires assistance for the involved lower extremity, the physical therapist/assistant should guard on the side of the involved lower extremity.

(continued)

6 Once the patient has assumed a standing position, the physical therapist/assistant ensures the patient is stable and able to maintain an upright posture. One at a time, crutches are positioned properly under the axillae. The patient reaches across the body with the hand on the involved side for a crutch.

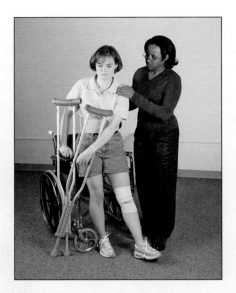

7 The patient first positions the crutch that was retrieved by the hand on the involved side under the axillae.

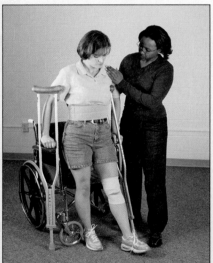

8 The patient positions the crutch that remains in the hand on the uninvolved side. The patient is ready to ambulate.

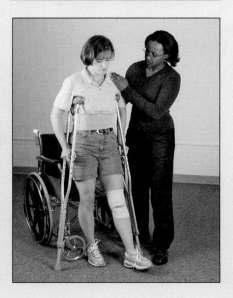

Assuming Sitting—Physical Therapist/Assistant on Involved Side

1 The physical therapist/assistant engages the wheelchair wheel locks and moves the footrests out of the way. To sit, the patient is positioned facing away from the wheelchair at the front edge of a wheelchair seat, close enough so that she can feel the front edge of wheelchair seat against the back of the lower extremities.

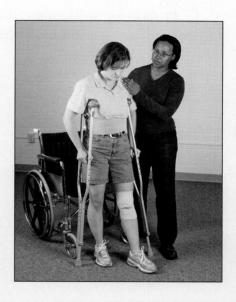

2 The patient can position her feet either in stride or side by side. Positioned in stride behind and to one side of a patient, the physical therapist/assistant grasps the patient's gait belt and shoulder girdle.

3 The patient removes the crutch from the axilla on the involved side and holds it by the handgrip only. The patient removes the crutch from the axilla on the uninvolved side and passes it to the hand on the involved side. The patient holds both crutches by the handgrips and places them in front of and slightly lateral to the patient's foot on the involved side.

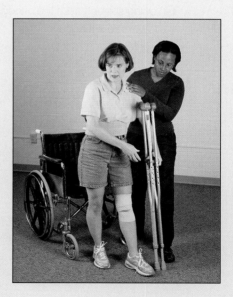

(continued)

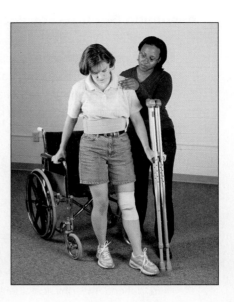

④ Reaching back with the hand on the uninvolved side, the patient grasps the wheelchair armrest.

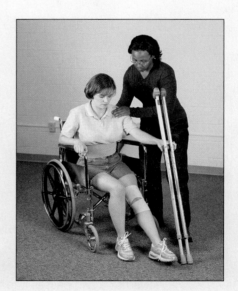

⑤ Using support from the handgrip and armrest, the patient lowers to sitting.

⑥ Setting crutches aside, the patient grasps both armrests and moves completely into the seat. A physical therapist/assistant may or may not need to assist with an involved lower extremity. When necessary, a patient's involved lower extremity is placed on the elevating legrest.

Assuming Standing—Physical Therapist Assistant on Uninvolved Side

When the patient can control the involved lower extremity, the physical therapist/assistant assists the patient to standing from the patient's uninvolved side.

1 The physical therapist/assistant engages the wheelchair wheel locks and moves the footrests out of the way. The patient is positioned at the front edge of the wheelchair seat. Positioned in stride behind and to one side of a patient, the physical therapist/assistant grasps the patient's gait belt and maintains contact with the patient's shoulder girdle.

2 The patient places the crutches together to the front and side of the uninvolved foot. The patient grasps the handgrips of both crutches in one hand and places her other hand on the wheelchair armrest.

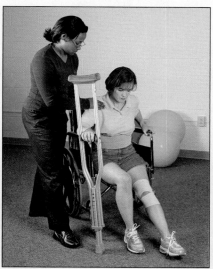

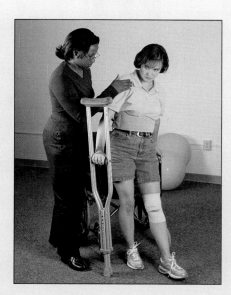

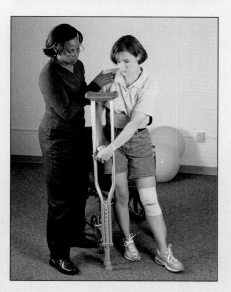

3 The patient pushes to standing using the armrest and the handgrips for support.

4 When the patient has assumed a standing position, the physical therapist/assistant should ensure that the patient can control her balance. Releasing the grasp on the armrest, the patient reaches for one crutch.

(continued)

5 One at a time, crutches are positioned properly under the axillae. The patient first positions the crutch on the involved side.

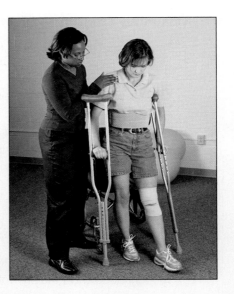

6 Then the patient positions the crutch on the uninvolved side. The patient is then ready to ambulate.

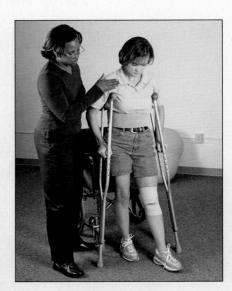

Assuming Sitting—Physical Therapist/Assistant on Uninvolved Side

1 The physical therapist/assistant engages the wheelchair wheel locks and moves the footrests out of the way. To sit, the patient is positioned facing away from the wheelchair at the front edge of a wheelchair seat, close enough so she can feel the front edge of the wheelchair seat against the back of the lower extremities. The patient can position her feet either in stride or side by side. Positioned in stride behind and to one side of the patient, the physical therapist/assistant grasps the patient's gait belt and maintains contact with the patient's shoulder girdle.

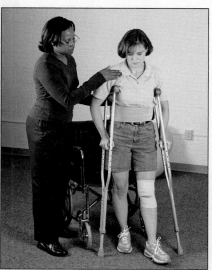

■ **Take Note**

The patient's movements are the same whether the physical therapist/assistant is guarding on the side of the involved lower extremity or uninvolved lower extremity.

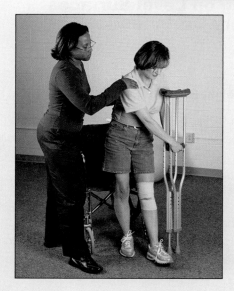

2 The patient removes the crutch from the axilla on the involved side and holds it by the hand-grip only. The patient removes the crutch from the axilla on the uninvolved side and passes it to the hand on the involved side.

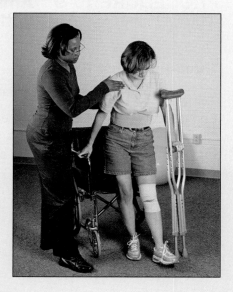

3 The patient holds both crutches by the hand-grips on the patient's involved side. The patient reaches back and grasps the wheelchair armrest with the hand on the uninvolved side.

(continued)

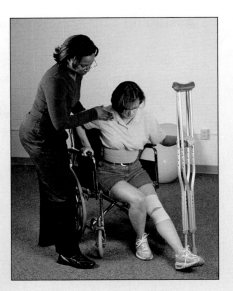

④ Using support from the handgrips and wheelchair armrest, the patient lowers to sitting.

⑤ Setting the crutches aside, the patient grasps both wheelchair armrests and maneuvers completely into the wheelchair seat.

PROCEDURE 10–9   Ambulating on Level Surfaces with Axillary Crutches

Three-Point Gait Pattern

Partial to Full Weight Bearing

When ambulating with crutches, the patent can lift the body to decrease weight bearing by shoulder depression and elbow extension. The patient must also adduct the upper extremities to keep crutches in place under the axillae.

① The physical therapist/assistant is positioned in stride behind and to one side of the patient, grasping the patient's gait belt. When close guarding is required, the physical therapist/assistant maintains contact with the patient's shoulder girdle in addition to the gait belt. In the starting position, the patient stands with crutches approximately 6 inches away from the toes at a 45-degree angle anterior and lateral to the small toe. The patient's feet are side by side.

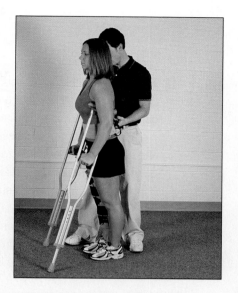

2 To ambulate, the patient advances both crutches simultaneously the same distance. The physical therapist/ assistant advances the outside foot either at the same time or immediately after the crutches are advanced.

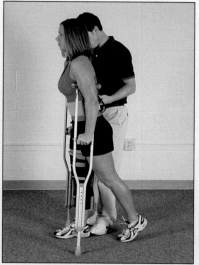

3 The patient advances the involved lower extremity so the ball of the foot is approximately even with the crutch tips. As the patient improves, she may move the crutches and involved lower extremity at the same time, permitting a faster gait.

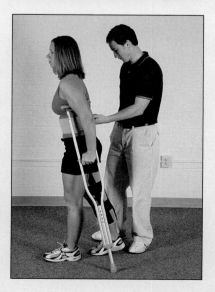

4 Using the upper extremities and involved lower extremity weight-bearing as permitted to support body weight, the patient advances the uninvolved lower extremity beyond the crutches. Initially, the patient may "step to" the involved lower extremity. Stepping through is a normal gait pattern and should be encouraged. The physical therapist/assistant advances the inside foot as the patient moves the uninvolved lower extremity closest to him. The sequence is repeated for continued progression.

(continued)

Non–Weight Bearing

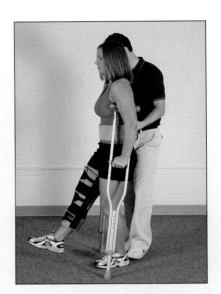

❶ The physical therapist/assistant is positioned in stride behind and to one side of the patient, grasping the patient's gait belt. When close guarding is required, the physical therapist/assistant maintains contact with the patient's shoulder girdle in addition to the gait belt. In the starting position, the patient stands with crutches approximately 6 inches away from the toes at a 45-degree angle anterior and lateral to the small toe. The patient's involved lower extremity is not on the floor. Generally, patients hold the involved lower extremity in front when the knee cannot be flexed, and behind when the knee can be flexed.

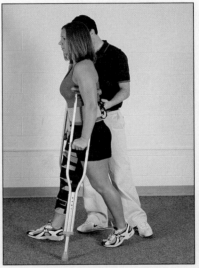

❷ To ambulate, the patient advances both crutches and the involved lower extremity simultaneously the same distance. The physical therapist/assistant advances the outside foot at the same time or immediately after the crutches are advanced.

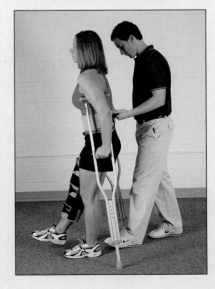

❸ Using the upper extremities to support all body weight, the patient advances the uninvolved lower extremity beyond the crutches. Initially, the patient may "step to" the involved lower extremity. Stepping through is a normal gait pattern and should be encouraged. The physical therapist/assistant advances the inside foot as the patient moves the uninvolved lower extremity. The sequence is repeated for continued progression.

Four-Point Gait Pattern

1 The physical therapist/assistant is positioned in stride behind and to one side of a patient, grasping the patient's gait belt. In the starting position, the patient stands with crutches approximately 6 inches away from the toes at a 45-degree angle anterior and lateral to the small toe. The patient's feet are side by side. To ambulate, the patient advances one crutch. The physical therapist/assistant advances the outside foot when the crutch closest to the physical therapist/assistant is advanced.

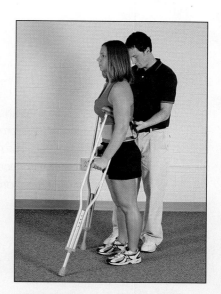

2 The patient then advances the opposite lower extremity so the ball of the foot is approximately even with the tip of the crutch. The physical therapist/assistant advances his inside foot when the patient advances the lower extremity closest to the physical therapist/assistant.

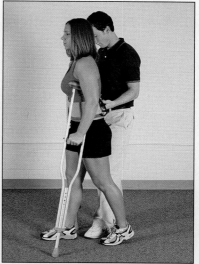

3 The patient shifts weight to the crutch and lower extremity just advanced and then advances the remaining crutch beyond the other crutch.

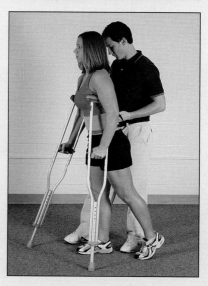

(continued)

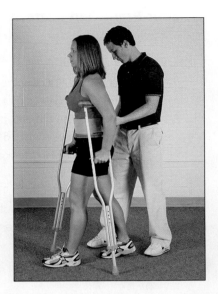

④ The patient advances the remaining lower extremity so the ball of the foot is approximately even with the tip of the crutch just advanced. The patient shifts weight to the crutch and lower extremity just advanced. The sequence is repeated for continued progression.

Two-Point Gait Pattern

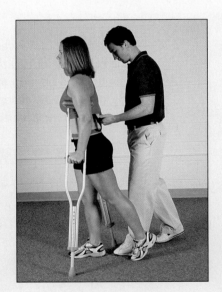

① The physical therapist/assistant is positioned in stride behind and to one side of a patient, grasping the patient's gait belt. In the starting position, the patient stands with crutches approximately 6 inches away from the toes at a 45-degree angle anterior and lateral to the small toe. The patient's feet are side by side. To ambulate, the patient advances one crutch and the opposite lower extremity simultaneously, placing the ball of the foot approximately even with the tip of the crutch. The patient shifts weight onto this crutch and lower extremity as the physical therapist/assistant advances the inside foot.

2 The patient advances the remaining crutch and lower extremity together beyond the first crutch and lower extremity in a normal stride length. The patient shifts weight onto the just-advanced crutch and lower extremity as the physical therapist/assistant advances the outside foot. The sequence is repeated for continued progression.

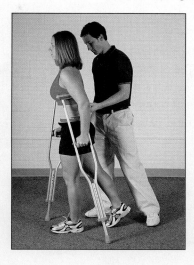

■ **Take Note**
A two-point gait pattern is faster and more automatic than a four-point gait pattern.

Falling

Patients must be taught how to control a fall, as falls may occur during ambulation training or after discharge. When the patient starts to fall, the physical therapist/assistant must decide whether to prevent the fall or to permit a controlled fall in a manner that will prevent injury to the patient or physical therapist/assistant. The physical therapist/assistant must be alert to the patient's movements at all times and be able to react quickly to prevent or control a fall. Proper guarding and attention focused on the patient are required at all times.

■ **Take Note**
Patients should practice falling so they will know what to do if a fall should occur.

1 The physical therapist/assistant prevents a fall by using the biomechanical advantages of standing in stride behind and slightly to the side of a patient. By standing in stride, the physical therapist/assistant is able to shift weight onto the back foot and pull the patient into the base of support.

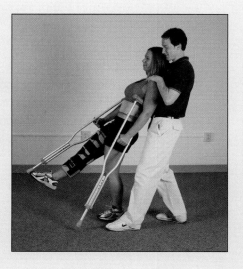

(continued)

2 When the physical therapist/assistant cannot prevent a fall, the fall must be controlled. The physical therapist/assistant instructs the patient to let the crutches fall to the sides, away from the area in which the patient will land, avoiding injury from landing on the crutches. The physical therapist/assistant steps forward in a stride position to widen the base of support while slowing the rate at which the patient falls.

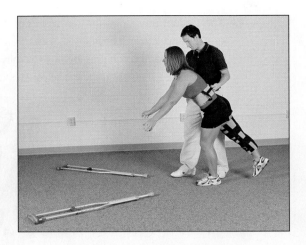

3 Patients can catch themselves on outstretched upper extremities, making sure that the elbows flex slightly to absorb impact. If the elbow is not flexed, the patient's upper extremities may be injured.

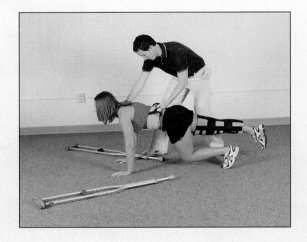

4 The physical therapist/assistant continues lowering the patient to the floor slowly, and the patient turns onto the side of the uninvolved lower extremity to avoid additional injury to the involved lower extremity.

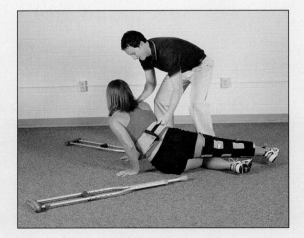

⑤ Turning from the side of the uninvolved lower extremity into a long sitting position, the patient is then in a position to get up from the floor.

The method used to rise from the floor depends on the patient's initial problem and any additional injury the fall may have caused. When the patient is unsure of the ability to arise after having fallen, she should call for assistance. Usually the patient can move on the floor to a sitting position near a chair or couch. Using furniture for stability and assistance, the patient can usually assume standing again. Methods of moving from the floor to a sitting position in a chair are described in Chapter 7, *Independent Transfer from Wheelchair to Floor and Return.*

PROCEDURE 10–10   Ambulating on Stairs with Axillary Crutches

Holding the Crutches

A patient can perform ambulation on stairs using two crutches without the use of a handrail. Use of a handrail, however, provides stability and, thus, is an added safety feature. When using a handrail, it takes the place of the crutch on one side. There are several methods of holding crutches when using a handrail. Whichever method of holding crutches is used, the sequence of movements for the lower extremities and ambulatory assistive devices is the same.

There are three common methods of holding crutches while ambulating on stairs.

The first method of holding two crutches while using a handrail is to place both crutches together under the upper extremity on the side opposite the handrail.

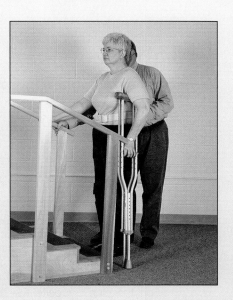

(continued)

The second method of holding two crutches while using a handrail is to hold the crutch on the side of the handrail in the hand that grasps the handrail. The patient holds this crutch by one of its uprights, parallel to the handrail. The patient uses the crutch on the side opposite the handrail in the usual manner.

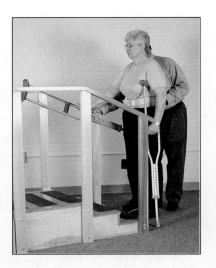

The third method of holding two crutches while using a handrail is to hold the handrail with one hand. The patient holds both crutches in the hand on the side opposite the handrail, one in the usual manner and the other by one of its uprights perpendicular to the first crutch.

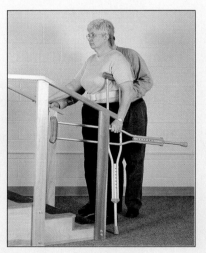

Ascending Using a Handrail

1. To ascend stairs using any of the methods of holding crutches, the patient stands facing up the stairs. Positioned in stride behind the patient, the physical therapist/assistant grasps the patient's gait belt and the handrail. For the method illustrated in this section, the patient places both crutches under the upper extremity on the side opposite the handrail and grasps the handrail with the other hand.

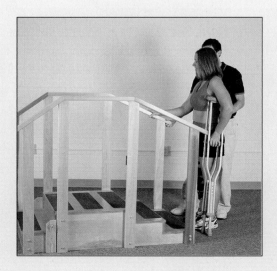

2 The patient places the uninvolved lower extremity on the next higher stair while the body weight is supported by the upper extremities.

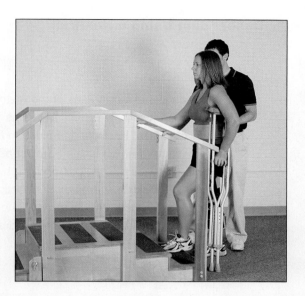

3 The patient shifts weight to the uninvolved lower extremity on the next higher stair. Extending the uninvolved lower extremity, the patient lifts up to the next higher stair. The patient advances the crutches and involved lower extremity to the same stair at the same time.

   The patient must place the crutches midway on the stair tread, and far enough from the handrail or far enough from each other when no handrail is used, to permit movement through the crutches to the next stair. Proper crutch placement on stairs provides stability and space for patients to maneuver.

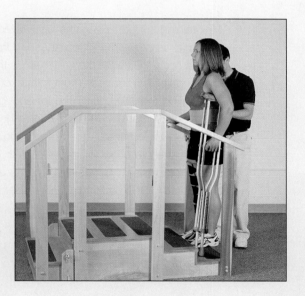

4 The physical therapist/assistant ascends with the patient. This sequence is repeated to ascend an entire flight of stairs.

(continued)

Descending Using a Handrail

1 To descend stairs using any of the methods of holding crutches, the patient stands facing down the stairs. Positioned in stride in front of the patient, the physical therapist/assistant grasps the patient's gait belt and the handrail. For the method illustrated in this section, the patient places both crutches under the upper extremity on the side opposite the handrails and grasps the handrail with the other hand.

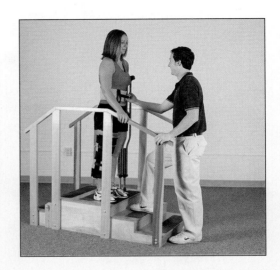

2 Maintaining support using the uninvolved lower extremity and the hand on the handrail, the patient securely places the crutches on the next lower stair. The patient must place crutches midway on the stair tread, and far enough from the handrail or far enough from each other when no handrail is used, to permit movement through the crutches to the next stair. Proper crutch placement on stairs provides stability and space for the patient to maneuver.

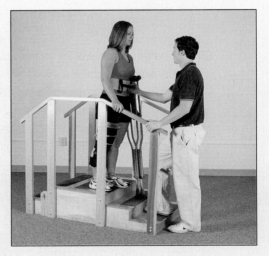

3 With the body supported by the upper extremities and the uninvolved lower extremity, the patient moves the involved lower extremity to the same stair as the crutches.

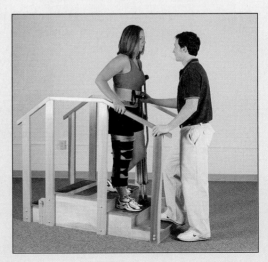

④ Bearing weight on the upper extremities and on the involved lower extremity if weight bearing is permitted, the patient moves the uninvolved lower extremity to the same stair as the crutches and involved lower extremity. The physical therapist/assistant descends with the patient.

⑤ This sequence is repeated to descend an entire flight of stairs.

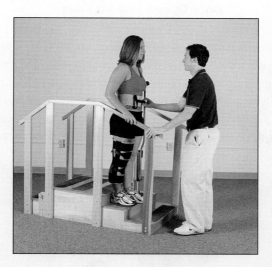

■ **Take Note**
Caution—Physical therapists/assistants must check that the placement of crutches on each stair tread is appropriate for safety purposes.

Ascending and Descending Stairs without Using a Handrail

To ascend or descend stairs without using a handrail, the patient retains the crutches in the same position used for ambulating on level surfaces. Rather than using a handrail for support on one side, patients use one crutch on each side for support. The physical therapist's/assistant's position, and the sequence of moving the crutches and lower extremities, remains the same as for ascending stairs using a handrail and descending stairs using a handrail. The physical therapist/assistant holds the handrail, when available, for stability, whether or not a patient is using a handrail.

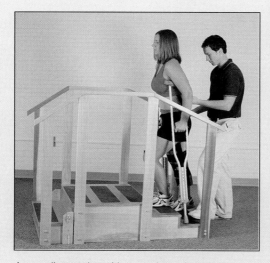

Ascending stairs without using a handrail.

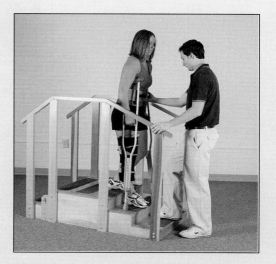

Descending stairs without using a handrail.

PROCEDURE 10–11 Ambulating Through Doorways with Axillary Crutches

Door with Automatic Door Closer

Door Opens Toward Patient

1 The patient approaches the latch edge of the door, standing outside the arc through which the opening door will move. The patient shifts weight onto the crutch on the side away from the hand that will be placed on the door handle. The patient places the unweighted hand on the door handle. Preferably, the patient shifts weight to the side closer to the door handle and uses the hand farther from the door handle to pull open the door. Using the hand farther from the door permits a patient to open a door wider than using the hand closer to the door.

■ **Take Note**
Standing at the latch side of the door, grasp the door handle with the hand farther from the door.

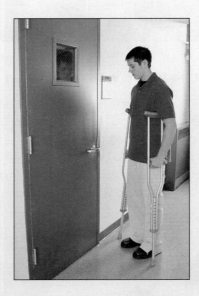

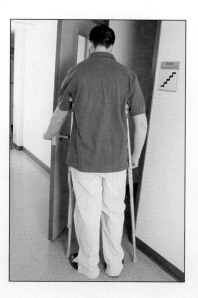

② Using a pulling motion, the patient opens the door wider than the width of the patient. This is necessary because a door will start to close automatically before patients can progress through the doorway.

③ The patient quickly returns the hand used to open the door to the crutch. To block automatic closing of the door, the patient turns into the doorway and places the tip of the crutch closer to the door on the floor in the path of the door. This acts as a door stop, permitting the patient to progress through the doorway without being struck by the closing door.

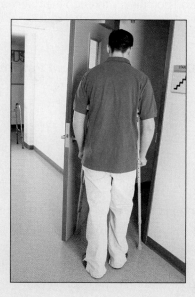

■ **Take Note**
Caution—Have the patient use the crutch tip to block the closing door as the patient passes through the doorway.

(continued)

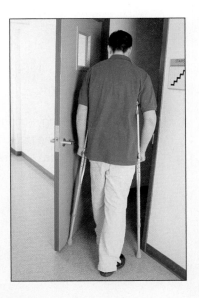

④ Continuing to use the tip of the crutch or shoulder as a door stop, the patient ambulates through the doorway using the appropriate gait pattern.

⑤ As the patient moves through the doorway, the door may have to be pushed open again. The crutch tip used as a door stop is placed progressively closer to the hinge edge of the door. The physical therapist/assistant and patient must be aware that as a crutch tip gets closer to the hinge edge of the door, it becomes more difficult to hold open the door.

⑥ Once the patient has moved completely through the doorway, the door closes behind the patient.

Door Opens Away from Patient

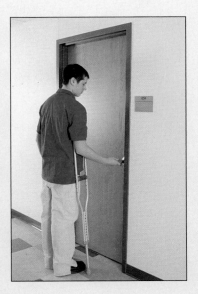

① The patient faces the door and shifts weight onto the crutch away from the hand that is closer to the door handle. Using the hand closer to the door handle permits a patient to open a door wider than using the hand farther from the door. The patient places the unweighted hand on the door handle.

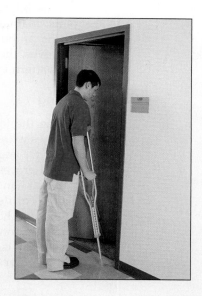

2 Using a pushing motion, the door is opened wider than the width of the patient because the door will start to close automatically before a patient can move through the doorway. Automatic closing of the door must be blocked by the tip of the crutch closer to the door, permitting the patient time to progress through the doorway. The patient quickly returns the hand used to open the door to the crutch. Then the patient advances the crutch closer to the door into the doorway to act as a door stop.

3 As the patient moves through the doorway, the door may have to be pushed open again. Continuing to use the tip of the crutch or shoulder as a door stop, the patient ambulates through the doorway using the appropriate gait pattern.

4 Once a patient has moved completely through the doorway, the door closes behind the patient.

Door without Automatic Door Closer

When a door does not have an automatic closer, the patient's initial rapid movement to place a crutch tip on the ground as a doorstop is not necessary. Extra wide opening of a door is also not necessary. The patient can perform crutch movement more slowly, and the patient is not required to place a crutch tip as a doorstop between a door and a patient. Patients must turn to close the door because the door will not close automatically.

Forearm (Lofstrand) Crutches

Forearm crutches can be used by patients with the same impairments and with the same gait patterns as patients who use axillary crutches. When ambulating with forearm crutches, the patient can lift the body to decrease weight bearing by shoulder depression and elbow extension. The illustrations in this section present the use of forearm crutches for a patient with paraplegia. Patients with paraplegia have paralysis of the musculature of the lower extremities and usually some weakness of trunk muscles. Patients with paraplegia lack sufficient lower extremity and lower trunk muscle strength to support themselves in an upright posture. To overcome this lack of strength, a greater degree of upper trunk and upper extremity strength is required. Ambulation for patients with paraplegia requires upper body movement to control paretic or paralyzed lower extremities.

Patients with paraplegia usually use a swing-to or swing-through gait pattern. They will use bilateral knee-ankle-foot orthoses (KAFOs). KAFOs lock at the knee and ankle joints, maintaining the patient's knees in extension and ankles in slight dorsiflexion during ambulation. Initially, the patient may use a swing-to gait pattern. As ability improves, the patient may progress to the swing-through pattern. The swing-through gait pattern is more efficient, permitting the patient to move more quickly.

Fitting

Setting the length of forearm crutches determines handgrip height. Position forearm crutches with the crutch tip on the floor, approximately 6 inches away from the toes at a 45-degree angle anterior and lateral to the small toe. Handgrips are level with the ulnar styloid processes when the upper extremities are relaxed at the side (■ Figure 10–30).

When handgrips are held with the shoulders relaxed, the elbows should be in 20–30 degrees of flexion. Adjust forearm cuff height after crutch length has been adjusted. Adjust cuff height to a point as high as possible on the forearm without interfering with elbow flexion. Cuff width should be tight enough to stay on the upper extremity when a handgrip is released but loose enough not to bind. Adjust cuff width by squeezing the cuff together or spreading it apart (■ Figure 10–31).

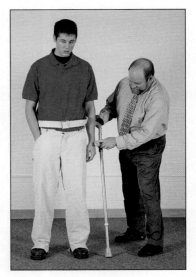

■ **Figure 10–30** Measuring forearm crutch length.

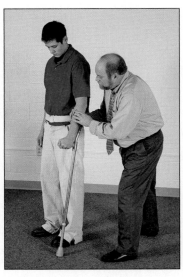

■ **Figure 10–31** Ensuring proper elbow flexion and cuff tightness.

PROCEDURE 10–12   In and Out of a Wheelchair with Forearm Crutches

Two methods, the turn-around method and the power method, may be used to assume standing using forearm crutches and KAFOs. The turn-around method requires less strength than the power method.

❶ The physical therapist/assistant locks the wheelchair wheels and moves the footrests out of the way. The patient is positioned at the front edge of the seat. Positioned in stride behind and to one side of the patient, the physical therapist/assistant grasps the patient's gait belt and shoulder.

❷ The patient positions one forearm crutch on either side of the wheelchair. Crutches must be supported securely enough so they will not fall as the patient moves, yet be accessible to the patient.

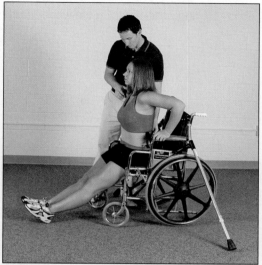

❸ The patient moves forward on the seat of the wheelchair and secures the knee locks of the KAFOs in knee extension.

Assuming Standing Using the Turn-Around Method

For this method, the physical therapist/assistant initially assumes the proper position on the side from which the patient will turn. In the illustrations for this section, this is on the patient's right side. The physical therapist/assistant must be prepared to move with the patient so as not to inhibit the patient's fluid motion. Initially, the physical therapist/assistant may assist by lifting or guiding the patient.

❶ When the patient turns to the left, she begins by hooking the medial upright of the right orthosis over the medial upright of the left orthosis. This aids in placement of the lower extremities as the patient stands. The patient then turns onto the left side. As the patient turns, she reaches behind with the left hand to grasp the right armrest and in front with the right hand to grasp the left armrest.

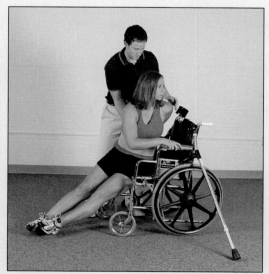

(continued)

2 Using the upper extremities, the patient pushes to standing, completing the turn to assume a standing position facing the wheelchair.

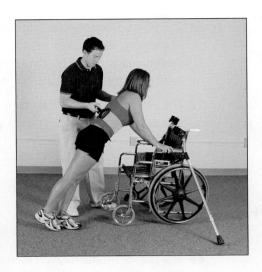

3 Using the armrests for support, the patient performs a push-up, lifting the body to position the lower extremities. Feet must be positioned so the patient is centered in front of the wheelchair at a distance that will permit support with one upper extremity as the crutches are retrieved.

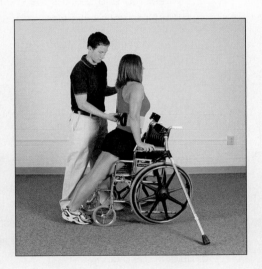

4 The patient shifts weight to one side and grasps and positions the forearm crutch on the side that has been unweighted.

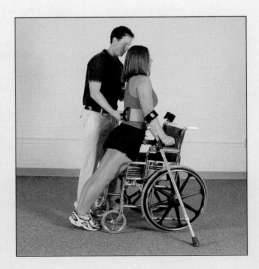

⑤ Shifting weight onto one forearm crutch, the patient grasps the second forearm crutch and places it properly.

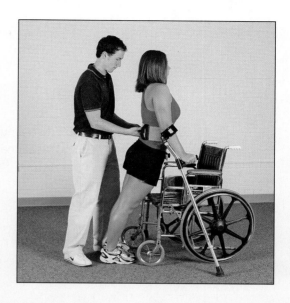

⑥ Using both crutches for support, the patient pushes to a fully upright position, shoulders behind hips to maintain hip extension. This posture is called a "C" curve.

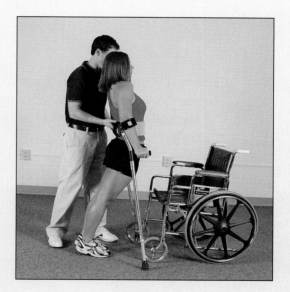

Assuming Sitting Using the Turn-Around Method

① The physical therapist/assistant engages the wheelchair wheel locks and moves the footrests out of the way. Positioned in stride slightly behind and to the side to which the patient will turn, the physical therapist/assistant grasps the patient's gait belt and shoulder. The physical therapist/assistant must be prepared to move as the patient moves to avoid interfering with the patient's fluid motion. Initially, the physical therapist/assistant may guide or control the rate at which the patient turns and lowers into the seat.

(continued)

② To assume sitting using the turn-around method, the patient approaches and faces the wheelchair.

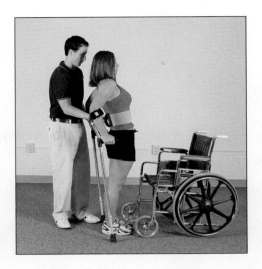

③ Shifting weight onto one forearm crutch, the patient removes the other forearm crutch. The patient places the crutch that has been removed against the wheelchair.

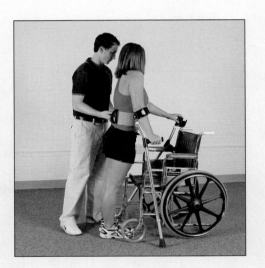

④ The patient then grasps the armrest with the free hand and shifts weight onto the upper extremity that is grasping the armrest. The patient removes the remaining crutch and places it against the wheelchair.

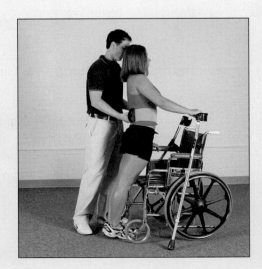

⑤ The patient is then able to grasp the remaining armrest.

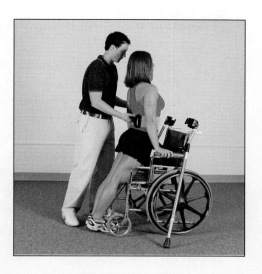

⑥ Turning, the patient then lowers into the wheelchair.

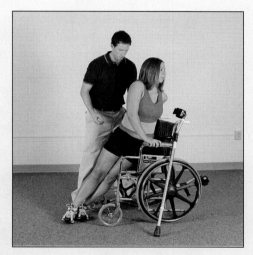

⑦ Repositioning the upper extremities, the patient adjusts her position in the wheelchair. Knee locks on the KAFOs are released. Once KAFO knee locks are released, the patient replaces the wheelchair footrests and assumes a proper sitting position.

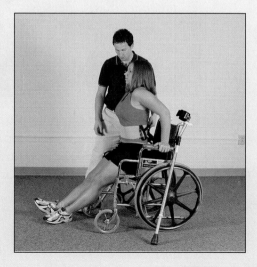

(continued)

Assuming Standing Using the Power Method

1 The physical therapist/assistant engages the wheelchair wheel locks and moves the footrests out of the way. The patient is positioned toward the front edge of the seat. Positioned in stride behind and to one side of the patient, the physical therapist/assistant grasps the patient's gait belt and shoulder. The physical therapist/assistant must be prepared to move as the patient moves to avoid interfering with the patient's fluid motion.

2 With knee locks of the KAFOs secured, the patient grasps one crutch in each hand. The patient places the tips of the crutches on the floor even with the hips in the anterior/posterior direction, one on each side of the wheelchair.

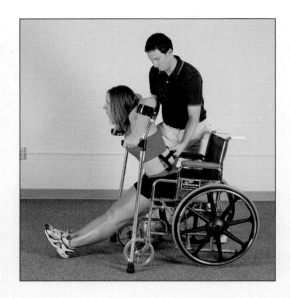

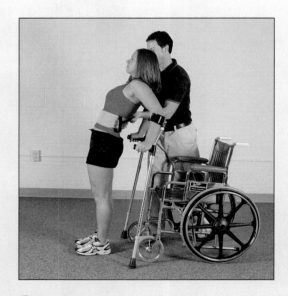

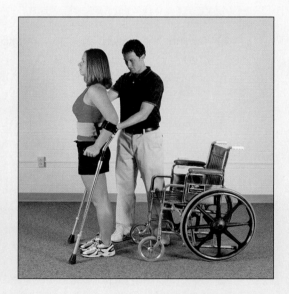

3 Pushing on the crutches, the patient extends the upper extremities and depresses the shoulders, producing a quick thrusting movement to propel the body upward and forward into a standing position.

4 The patient must move the crutches forward quickly to halt the forward momentum. Placing the crutches slightly ahead and to the side of the toes, the patient assumes a "C" curve. The physical therapist/assistant can assist the patient into a "C" curve position by pushing forward on the gait belt and pulling backward on the patient's shoulder.

Assuming Sitting Using the Power Method

1 The physical therapist/assistant engages the wheelchair wheel locks and moves the footrests out of the way. Positioned in stride slightly behind and to the side, the physical therapist/assistant grasps the patient's gait belt and shoulder. The physical therapist/assistant must be prepared to move as the patient moves to avoid interfering with the patient's fluid motion.

2 To sit, the patient stands facing away from the wheelchair with the feet approximately 12–18 inches in front of the front edge of the seat. The position of the feet must permit the patient to end up sitting securely in the seat as she lowers while the knee locks of KAFOs are locked.

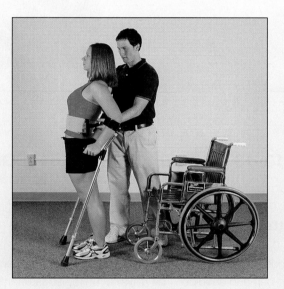

■ **Take Note**
Caution—When using the power method to assume sitting, the wheelchair should be placed against a wall so the wheelchair does not slide backward or tip during the maneuver.

3 Moving the shoulders anterior to the hips, the patient flexes at the hips into a "jackknife" position. The patient starts falling backward, initiating lowering into the wheelchair.

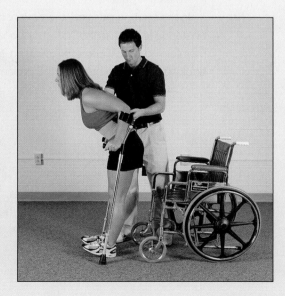

(continued)

4 As the patient sits, she lifts the crutches. After the patient is seated, knee locks on the KAFOs are released. Once the KAFOs have been unlocked, the patient can replace the footrests and assume a proper sitting position.

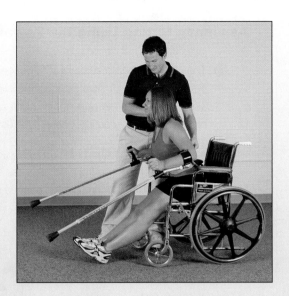

PROCEDURE 10–13   Ambulating on Level Ground with Forearm Crutches

Swing-To Gait Pattern

1 Positioned in stride slightly behind and to the side, the physical therapist/assistant grasps the patient's gait belt and shoulder. The physical therapist/assistant must be prepared to move as the patient moves to avoid interfering with the patient's fluid motion.

In the starting position, the patient maintains her hips in extension by keeping shoulders posterior to hips in the "C" curve posture. The physical therapist/assistant can assist in maintaining a "C" curve by pushing forward with the hand on the gait belt while pulling backward with the hand on the patient's shoulder.

2 To initiate the swing-to gait pattern, the patient advances the crutches one stride length beyond the patient's toes. The physical therapist/assistant advances the outside foot.

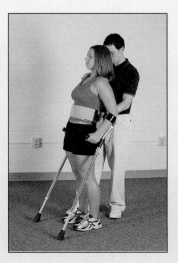

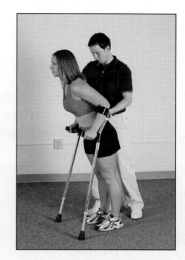

3 Pushing down on the crutches, the patient extends the upper extremities and depresses the shoulders. At the same time, she flexes the trunk to lift the feet off the ground. The physical therapist/assistant may assist by lifting with the hand on the gait belt.

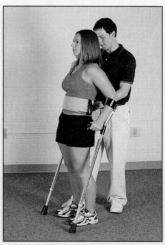

4 With the feet off the ground and trunk flexed, the patient's lower extremities will be swung forward by gravity. As the lower extremities swing forward, the patient begins to extend the neck and trunk to regain a "C" curve. With the feet placed on the floor between the crutches, momentum continues to move the patient's hips anterior to the shoulders. As the patient swings forward, the physical therapist/assistant steps forward with the inside foot. The physical therapist/assistant may assist a patient to regain a "C" curve by pushing forward with the hand on the gait belt and pulling backward with the hand on the patient's shoulder. Once a "C" curve is regained, the patient advances the crutches. The sequence is repeated for continued progression.

Swing-Through Gait Pattern

A swing-through gait pattern is essentially the same as a swing-to gait pattern. The difference is that during the swing phase of the swing-through gait pattern, the patient swings beyond the crutches and lands anterior to the crutch tips.

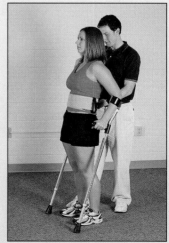

1 In the starting position for a swing-through gait pattern, the patient is in a "C" curve, with crutch tips beyond the toes. The role and position of the physical therapist/assistant is the same as for a swing-to gait pattern.

(continued)

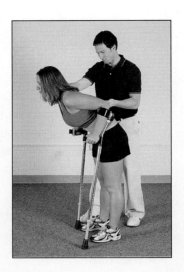

2 Pushing down on the crutches, the patient extends the upper extremities and depresses the shoulders. At the same time, she flexes the trunk to lift the feet off the ground. The physical therapist/assistant may assist by lifting with the hand on the gait belt.

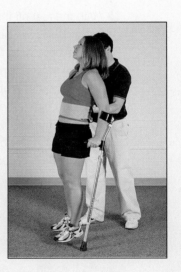

3 With the feet off the ground and trunk flexed, the patient's lower extremities will be swung forward by gravity. As the lower extremities swing forward, the patient extends the neck and trunk to regain a "C" curve.

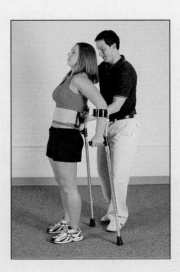

4 The patient lands with the feet anterior to the crutches. As the patient swings forward, the therapist steps forward with the inside foot.

⑤ Because of momentum generated by a larger swing, the patient must advance the crutches quickly to prevent falling. As the patient advances the crutches, the physical therapist/assistant steps forward with the outside foot.

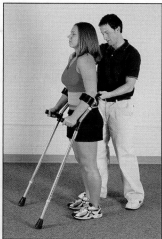

■ **Take Note**

Caution—The physical therapist/assistant must be prepared to move quickly because patients cover a greater distance in less time when using a swing-through gait pattern.

Falling

The patient must be taught how to control a fall, as falls may occur during ambulation training or after discharge. When the patient starts to fall, the physical therapist/assistant must decide whether to prevent the fall or to permit a controlled fall in a manner that will prevent injury to the patient or physical therapist/assistant. The physical therapist/assistant must be alert to the patient's movements at all times and be able to react quickly to prevent or control a fall. Proper guarding and attention focused on the patient are required at all times.

Patients with paraplegia tend to fall when they lose their "C" curve or when momentum into the "C" curve is interrupted, causing them to "jackknife." The most effective method of preventing falls in these situations is for a physical therapist/assistant to assist the patient in regaining the "C" curve. This is achieved by pulling the patient's shoulders backward while pushing forward with the hand on the gait belt.

① When the physical therapist/assistant cannot prevent a fall, he must control the fall. The physical therapist/assistant instructs the patient to let the crutches fall to the sides, away from the area in which the patient will land, to avoid injury from landing on the crutches. The physical therapist/assistant steps forward in a stride position to widen the base of support while slowing the rate at which the patient falls.

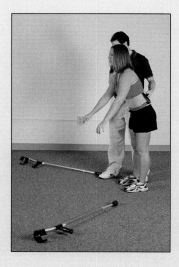

(continued)

2 The patient catches herself on outstretched hands, keeping the elbows flexed to absorb the impact. If elbows are not flexed, the patient's upper extremities may be injured.

■ **Take Note**
Caution—When falling, patients catch themselves with their arms, flexing at the elbows to absorb the force of falling.

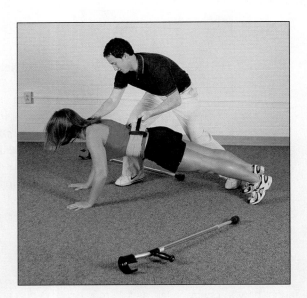

3 The physical therapist/assistant continues to lower the patient to the floor slowly.

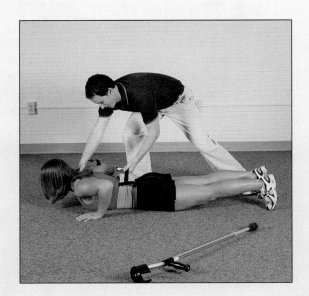

Assuming Standing from the Floor

To assume standing from the floor independently is a difficult maneuver for patients using KAFOs and forearm crutches. The most practical method is to move along the floor to a chair or other sturdy object and then use the object as support to rise from the floor. Methods of moving from the floor to a sitting position in a chair are described in the Chapter 7 section, *Independent Transfer From Wheelchair to Floor and Return.*

1. To assume standing directly from a prone position on the floor, the patient must first retrieve and position the crutches.

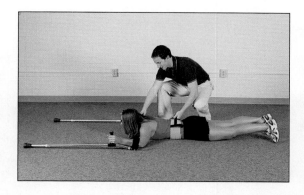

2. Grasping one crutch, the patient places it upright with the tip of the crutch on the floor. The patient places the other hand on the other crutch or on the floor at the level of the shoulder.

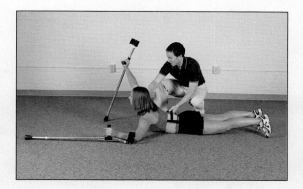

The following sequence of movements must be performed quickly, without pauses.

3. Pushing with the hand on the floor and pulling with the hand on the crutch, the patient raises the trunk. Positioned in stride slightly behind and to the side, the physical therapist/assistant grasps the patient's gait belt and shoulder. The physical therapist/assistant may assist by lifting with the hand on the gait belt.

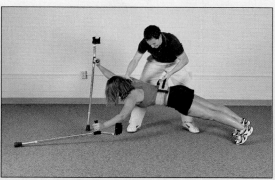

4. With weight shifted onto the upper extremity that is on the floor, the patient pushes down on the handgrip and floor to assume a "jackknife" position. During initial training, the physical therapist/assistant assists by lifting on the gait belt. The physical therapist/assistant may also need to block the patient's feet to prevent them from sliding posteriorly. After shifting weight onto the upright crutch, the patient grasps the handgrip of the remaining crutch.

(continued)

⑤ The patient positions the second crutch upright with the tip on the floor in line with the tip of the first crutch.

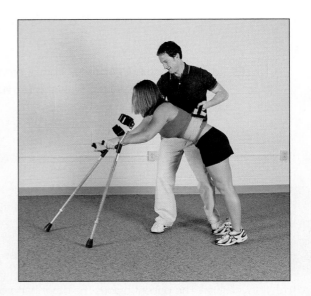

⑥ The patient then uses both crutches to push through an upright position, into a "C" curve. The patient properly positions the crutches, one at a time. The patient is then ready to ambulate.

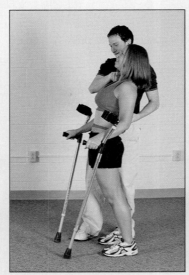
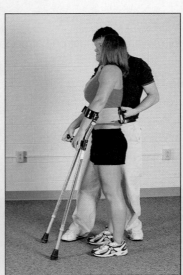
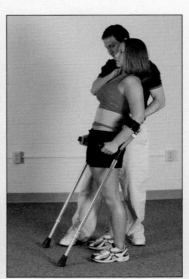

Adjusting first forearm crutch.   Adjusting second forearm crutch.   Ready to ambulate.

Doorways

Patients using forearm crutches maneuver through doorways in the same manner as do patients using axillary crutches.

PROCEDURE 10–14   Ambulating on Stairs with Forearm Crutches

There are two basic methods for patients using KAFOs and forearm crutches to ambulate on stairs: the forward method and the backward method. In both methods, the patient may use a handrail and one crutch or no handrail and two crutches. In both methods, the physical therapist/assistant is positioned in stride on the stairs below the patient and grasps the patient's gait belt and the handrail. Initially, gait training on stairs may require assistance by two people to ensure patient safety.

Ascending—Forward Method

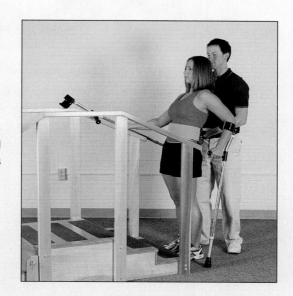

❶ To ascend stairs using the forward method, the patient starts in a "C" curve position facing up the stairs. The patient's feet and crutch tips are parallel with the base of the stair.

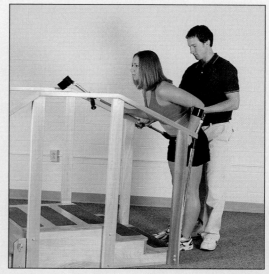

❷ The same motion used to initiate ambulation on level surfaces is used to initiate ambulation on stairs. Flexing the neck and upper trunk, the patient extends the upper extremities and depresses the shoulders to lift the body. As the patient's feet are lifted from the ground, gravity swings the lower extremities forward onto the next higher stair. The physical therapist/assistant may assist by lifting on the gait belt as the patient raises the body.

(continued)

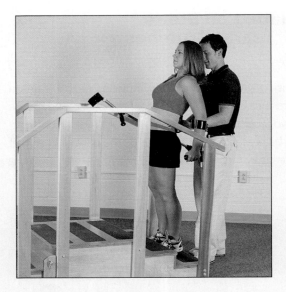

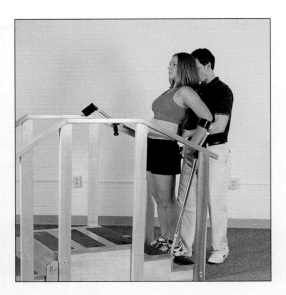

③ The patient then extends the neck and trunk to regain a "C" curve and places the lower extremities onto the next higher stair. The physical therapist/assistant may assist the patient in regaining a "C" curve by pushing forward on the gait belt.

④ The patient advances the crutches to the same stair as the feet. The sequence is repeated to ascend an entire flight of stairs.

Descending—Forward Method

① To descend stairs using the forward method, the patient starts in a "C" curve position facing down the stairs. The feet and crutch tips are parallel with the top of the stairs.

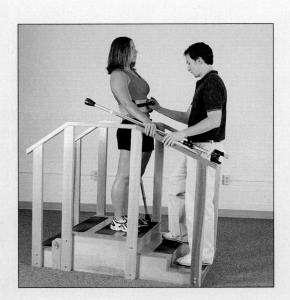

2 The same motion used to initiate ambulation on level surfaces is used to initiate ambulation on stairs. Flexing the neck and upper trunk, the patient extends the upper extremities and depresses the shoulders to lift the body. The physical therapist/assistant may assist by lifting on the gait belt as the patient raises the body. As the patient's feet are lifted from the ground, gravity swings the lower extremities forward over the next lower stair.

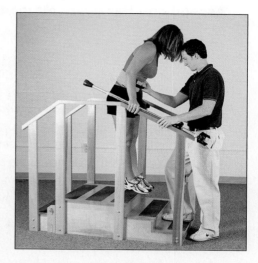

3 As the lower extremities swing over the stair, the patient uses the upper extremities to lower in a controlled manner onto the next lower stair.

   Extending the neck and trunk, the patient regains a "C" curve and places the lower extremities on the next lower stair. The physical therapist/assistant may assist the patient in regaining a "C" curve by pulling forward on the gait belt.

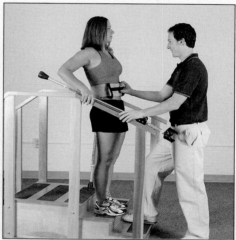

4 The patient advances the crutches onto the same stair as the lower extremities. Patients often descend two steps at a time. The sequence is repeated to descend an entire flight of stairs.

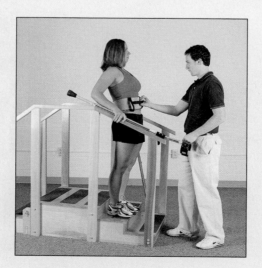

■ Take Note
When descending stairs using the forward method, the patient should not have her movement blocked, so the physical therapist/assistant must move quickly.

(continued)

Ascending—Backward Method

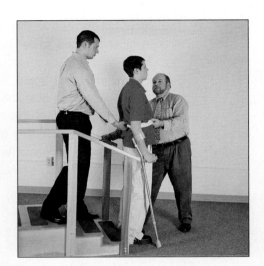

① To ascend stairs using the backward method, the patient starts in a "C" curve position facing away from the stairs. The patient's feet and crutch tips are parallel with the base of the stair. During initial training, two physical therapists/assistants may be positioned on the stairs, one above the patient and one below the patient.

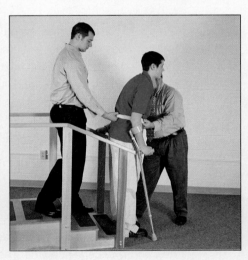

② The same motion used to initiate ambulation on level surfaces is used to initiate ambulation on stairs. Flexing the neck and upper trunk, the patient extends the upper extremities and depresses the shoulders to lift the body. The physical therapist/assistant positioned on the stairs above the patient may assist by lifting and pulling back. The physical therapist/assistant positioned below the patient pushes on the gait belt as the patient raises the body. When the physical therapist/assistant exerts force into the abdominal area to assist patient positioning, he must be careful not to injure the patient.

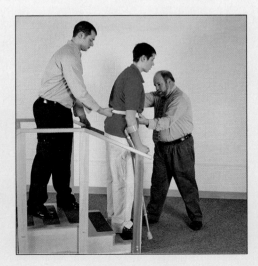

③ As the patient lifts into a "jackknife" position, backward momentum of the lower extremities moves the patient up and over the higher stair. The patient uses the upper extremities to lower onto the next higher stair.

④ Once the patient's lower extremities are on the next higher stair, the patient permits the pelvis to move forward. As this movement occurs, the patient extends the neck and trunk to regain a "C" curve, while moving the crutches onto the same stair as the lower extremities. The physical therapist/assistant positioned below the patient may assist the patient in regaining a "C" curve by pulling forward on the gait belt. The sequence is repeated to ascend an entire flight of stairs.

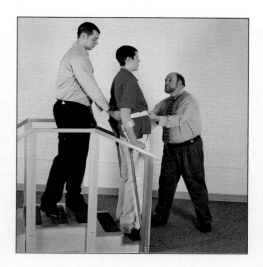

Descending—Backward Method

① To descend stairs using the backward method, the patient starts in a "C" curve position facing away from the stairs. The patient's feet and crutch tips are parallel at the top of the stairs. During initial training, two physical therapists/assistants may be positioned on the stairs, one above the patient and one below the patient.

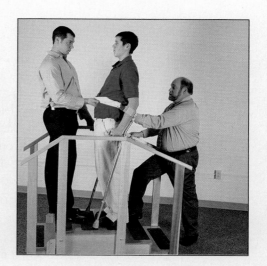

② The same motion used to initiate ambulation on level surfaces is used to initiate ambulation on stairs. Flexing the neck and upper trunk, the patient extends the upper extremities and depresses the shoulders to lift the body. The physical therapist/assistant positioned on the stairs above the patient may assist by pushing on the gait belt and assisting with the lowering. The physical therapist/assistant positioned on the stairs below the patient may assist by lifting on the gait belt as the patient raises the body.

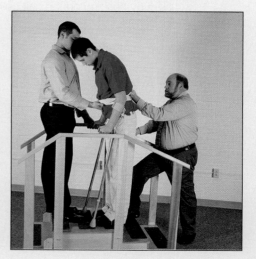

(continued)

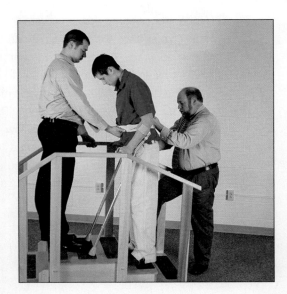

3 As the patient lifts into a "jackknife" position, the backward momentum of the lower extremities moves the patient over the next lower stair. Once the lower extremities are over the stair, the patient uses the upper extremities to lower in a controlled manner onto the next lower stair.

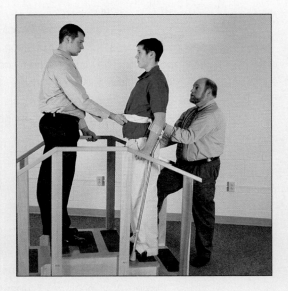

4 After the lower extremities are on the next lower stair, the patient extends the neck and trunk to regain a "C" curve. This movement allows the hips to remain in extension. Then the patient moves the crutches onto the same stair as the lower extremities. The physical therapist/assistant positioned on the stairs above the patient may assist by pulling on the gait belt to assist the patient in assuming a "C" curve. The physical therapist/assistant positioned on the stairs below the patient may assist by pushing on the gait belt.

5 The sequence is repeated to descend an entire flight of stairs.

Canes

Fitting

Canes are fitted with the patient standing with shoulders relaxed. The cane is positioned upright, with the tip on the floor alongside the small toe. With the cane in this position, adjust the top of the cane to be at the level of the patient's ulnar styloid process (■ Figure 10–32). This permits 20–30 degrees of elbow flexion when the cane is held in the patient's hand (■ Figure 10–33). When used properly, forces on a cane should be exerted directly downward.

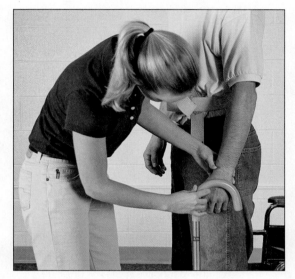

■ **Figure 10–32**   Measuring cane height.

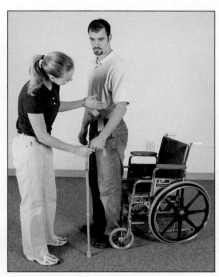

■ **Figure 10–33**   Ensuring proper elbow flexion.

When using a quad cane, the longer legs of the cane are positioned facing away from the patient's lower extremity (■ Figure 10–34). This reduces the risk of the patient's foot becoming entangled in the legs of the quad cane. Quad canes are measured and used in the same manner as standard canes.

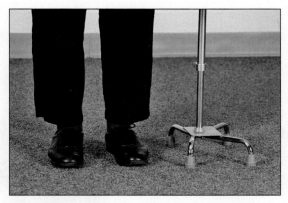

■ **Figure 10–34**   Proper positioning of a quad cane for ambulation.

PROCEDURE 10–15 In and Out of a Wheelchair with One Cane

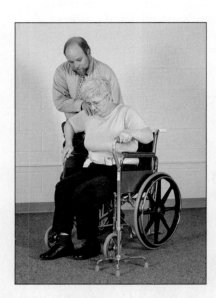

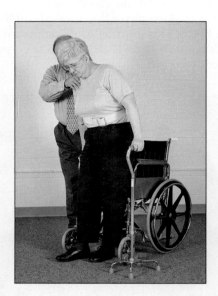

1 The physical therapist/assistant engages the wheelchair wheel locks and moves the footrests out of the way. The patient is positioned at the front edge of the seat, with the feet in stride or side by side. Positioned in stride behind and to one side of a patient, the physical therapist/assistant grasps the patient's gait belt and shoulder.

2 The patient positions the quad cane alongside the foot on the side on which it will be held. The patient may place both hands on the respective armrests or place one hand on the cane and one on the armrest to push to standing. When the patient has only one functional upper extremity, that upper extremity is used on the armrest to push to standing. Once the patient is standing, she grasps the cane.

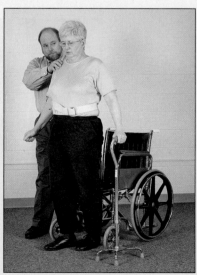

3 The patient pushes to standing and straightens, making sure to be erect and balanced. The patient is then ready to ambulate.

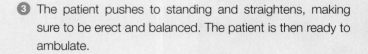

Assuming Sitting—Quad Cane and Armrests

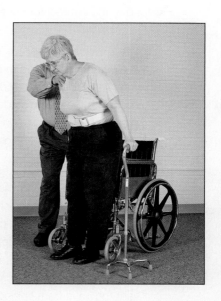

1. The physical therapist/assistant engages the wheelchair wheel locks and moves the footrests out of the way. To sit, the patient is positioned at the front edge of the wheelchair seat, facing away from the wheelchair, so she can feel the front edge of the wheelchair seat against the back of the lower extremities. The patient positions her feet in stride or side by side. Positioned in stride behind and to one side of a patient, the physical therapist/assistant grasps the patient's gait belt and shoulder. The patient reaches for the armrest with one hand while maintaining a grasp on the cane with the other hand.

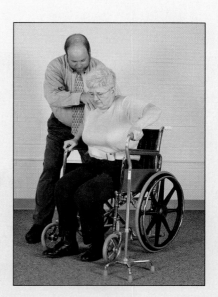

2. While grasping the armrest and the cane, the patient lowers in a controlled manner onto the seat.

   The patient moves completely onto the seat and positions appropriately.

(continued)

Assuming Standing—Quad Cane Only

The patient with sufficient strength and balance may assume standing using a quad cane instead of the armrest for support.

1. The physical therapist/assistant engages the wheelchair wheel locks and moves the footrests out of the way. The patient is positioned at the front edge of the seat, with the feet in stride or side by side. Positioned in stride behind and to one side of a patient, the physical therapist/assistant grasps the patient's gait belt and shoulder.

2. The patient positions the quad cane alongside the foot on the side on which it will be held. She places one hand on the quad cane. When the patient has only one functional upper extremity, that upper extremity is used on the quad cane to push to standing. The patient must push directly downward to prevent the cane from tipping.

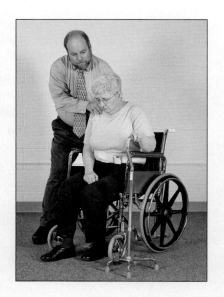

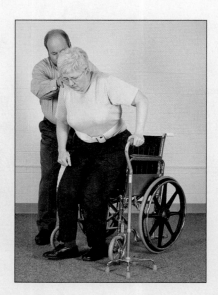

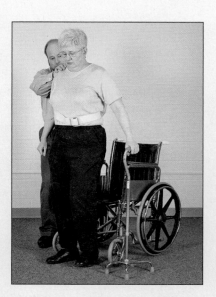

3. The patient leans forward to initiate standing by pushing downward on the quad cane.

4. The patient must be erect and balanced before initiating ambulation.

Assuming Sitting—Quad Cane Only

① The physical therapist/assistant engages the wheelchair wheel locks and moves the footrests out of the way. To sit, the patient is positioned at the front edge of the wheelchair seat, facing away from the wheelchair, so she can feel the front edge of the wheelchair seat against the back of the lower extremities. The patient positions her feet in stride or side by side. Positioned in stride behind and to one side of a patient, the physical therapist/assistant grasps the patient's gait belt.

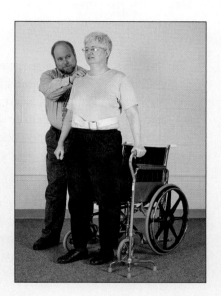

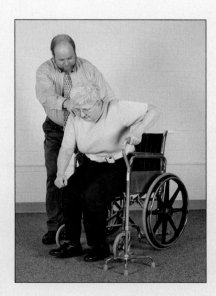

② While grasping the quad cane, the patient lowers in a controlled manner onto the seat.

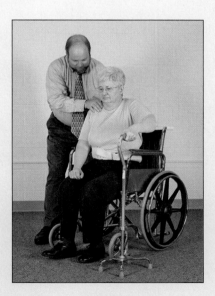

③ The physical therapist/assistant continues to guard the patient until safely seated and appropriately positioned.

(continued)

Assuming Standing—Standard Cane and Two Armrests

Authors' note: In the illustrations for this section, the patient is demonstrating the use of two functional upper extremities.

1 The physical therapist/assistant engages the wheelchair wheel locks and moves the footrests out of the way. The patient is positioned at the front edge of the seat with the feet in stride or side by side. Positioned in stride behind and to one side of a patient, the physical therapist/assistant grasps the patient's gait belt and shoulder.

2 When using a standard cane, the patient places both hands on their respective armrests. The patient grasps the canes in the same hand as will be used for ambulation. Thus, the patient must grasp both the cane and armrest at the same time with this hand.

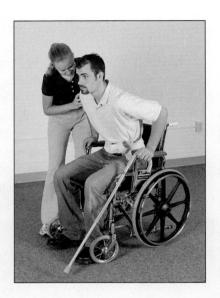

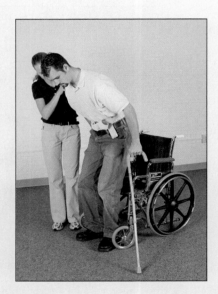

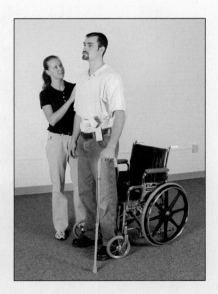

3 Pushing downward on both armrests, the patient pushes to standing.

4 Once standing, the patient releases the grasp on the armrests, stands erect, and positions the cane. The patient is then ready to ambulate.

Assuming Sitting—Standard Cane and Two Armrests

① The physical therapist/assistant engages the wheelchair wheel locks and moves the footrests out of the way. To sit, the patient is positioned at the front edge of the wheelchair seat, facing away from the wheelchair, so he can feel the front edge of the wheelchair seat against the back of the lower extremities. The patient positions his feet in stride or side by side. Positioned in stride behind and to one side of the patient, the physical therapist/assistant grasps the patient's gait belt and shoulder.

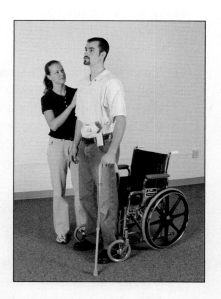

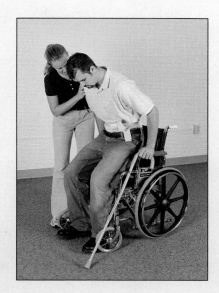

② The patient grasps both armrests. This may be performed with both hands simultaneously or the patient may move the hands one at a time. The patient keeps the cane grasped in the same hand in which it was used for ambulation. The patient holds both the cane and armrest together by the hand that grasps the cane.

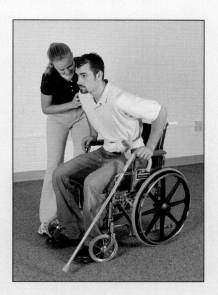

③ The patient lowers in a controlled manner onto the seat. Setting the cane aside, the patient moves completely onto the seat and positions himself appropriately.

(continued)

Assuming Standing—Standard Cane and One Armrest

Authors' note: In the illustrations for this section, the patient is demonstrating the use of two functional upper extremities.

1 The physical therapist/assistant engages the wheelchair wheel locks and moves the footrests out of the way. The patient is positioned at the front edge of the seat, with the feet in stride or side by side. Positioned in stride behind and to one side of the patient, the physical therapist/assistant grasps the patient's gait belt and shoulder.

2 The patient positions the cane alongside the foot on the side on which it will be held. The patient places one hand on the armrest and the other hand on the cane. The patient must push directly downward on the cane to prevent the cane from tipping. When the patient has only one functional upper extremity, that upper extremity is used on the cane to push to standing.

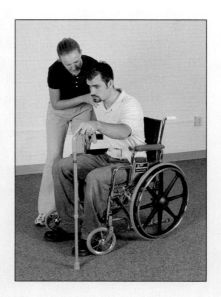

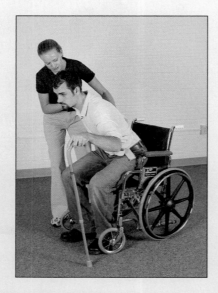

3 The patient then pushes to standing.

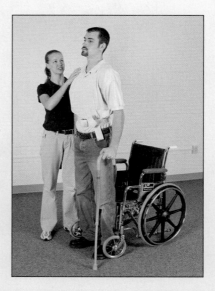

4 Once standing and balanced, the patient releases the grasp on the armrest and stands erect. The patient is then ready to ambulate.

Assuming Sitting—Standard Cane and One Armrest

① The physical therapist/assistant engages the wheelchair wheel locks and moves the footrests out of the way. To sit, the patient is positioned at the front edge of the wheelchair seat, facing away from the wheelchair, so he can feel the front edge of the wheelchair seat against the back of the lower extremities. The patient positions his feet in stride or side by side. Positioned in stride behind and to one side of the patient, the physical therapist/assistant grasps the patient's gait belt and shoulder.

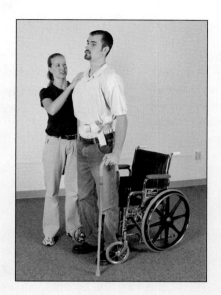

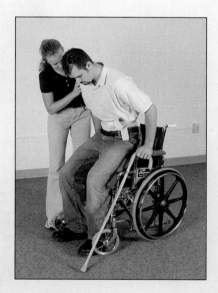

② While continuing to use the cane, the patient reaches back and grasps the armrest with the opposite hand.

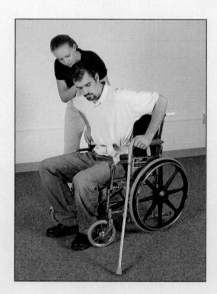

③ The patient then lowers in a controlled manner onto the seat. Setting the cane aside, the patient moves completely into the seat and positions himself appropriately.

PROCEDURE 10–16   Ambulating on Level Surfaces with One Cane

■ **Take Note**
Caution—Initially, have patients use the cane on the side of the uninvolved lower extremity to decrease weight bearing.

The gait pattern and sequence when using one standard cane or one quad cane are the same. To decrease weight bearing on an involved lower extremity, the patient uses the cane on the uninvolved side. This allows a minimal reduction of weight bearing on the involved lower extremity.

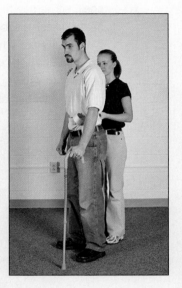

❶ Positioned in stride behind and to one side of a patient, the physical therapist/assistant grasps the patient's gait belt and shoulder. The patient's feet are side by side, with the cane next to the small toe.

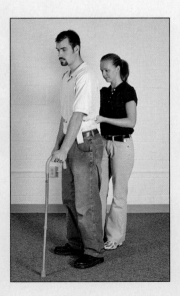

❷ The patient advances the cane first, approximately one stride length ahead. When the physical therapist/assistant is guarding on the side opposite the cane, she steps forward with the outside foot.

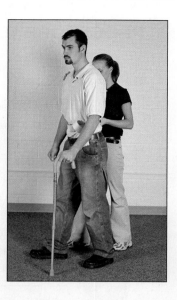

③ The patient advances the lower extremity on the side opposite the cane up to the cane. When the physical therapist/assistant is guarding on the side opposite the cane, she steps forward with the inside foot.

④ The patient advances the lower extremity on the same side as the cane. Initially, the patient may only step to the other lower extremity and cane. However, the patient should be encouraged to step beyond the other lower extremity and cane, to develop a normal gait pattern.

⑤ The sequence is repeated for continued progression. The patient should remain erect during this progression and avoid leaning on the cane.

⑥ As patients improve, they may move the cane and involved lower extremity at the same time, permitting a faster pace of gait. As patients are able, they may use the cane on the involved side, moving the cane and involved lower extremity simultaneously. Using a cane on the involved side encourages weight bearing on the involved lower extremity.

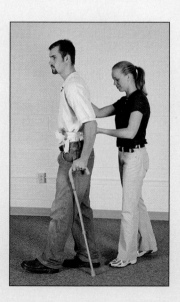

■ **Take Note**
Caution—As patients improve, the cane can be used on the side of the involved lower extremity to increase weight bearing.

(continued)

PROCEDURE 10–17   Ambulating on Stairs with One Cane

Holding the Cane

Initially, the physical therapist/assistant should teach the patient to use a handrail for increased stability. Patients who use a cane on the left side continue to grasp the cane with the left hand and grasp the handrail with the right hand. Patients who use a cane in the right hand must do one of three things: (1) continue to use the cane in the right hand and not use the handrail, (2) switch the cane to the left hand and grasp the handrail with the right hand, or (3) grasp both the handrail and cane with the right hand. Patients with a functional right upper extremity only must either (1) continue to use the cane without using the handrail or (2) grasp both the handrail and cane with the right hand.

There are two methods for grasping both the cane and handrail in one hand. Note that the method is the same whether the patient uses one cane or two.

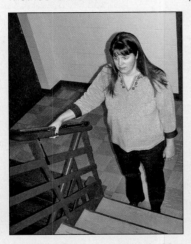

In one method, the patient holds the cane at midshaft, parallel to the handrail.

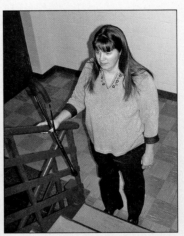

In the second method, the patient holds the cane at midshaft, remaining in a vertical position.

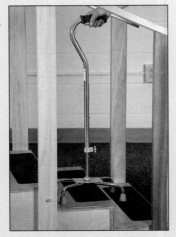

A quad cane's base may be larger than a stair tread.

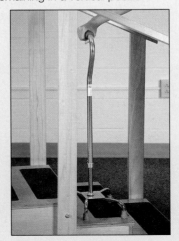

Turning a quad cane sideways permits all four legs to be supported on the stair.

Ascending Using a Cane and Handrail

Authors' note: In the illustrations for this section, the patient demonstrates the use of two functional upper extremities, permitting use of the cane in the left hand while grasping the handrail with the right hand.

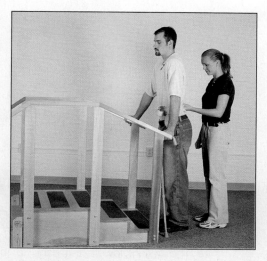

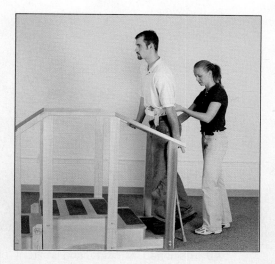

1 Positioned in stride behind the patient, the physical therapist/assistant grasps the patient's gait belt and the handrail. To ascend stairs, the patient stands facing up the stairs with the feet and cane parallel to the base of the first stair.

2 The patient moves the uninvolved lower extremity to the next higher stair and shifts weight onto this extremity.

3 The patient extends the uninvolved lower extremity, lifting the body. The patient places the involved lower extremity on the same stair as the uninvolved lower extremity. The patient advances the cane to the same stair as the lower extremities and places it securely on the stair tread. As the patient's balance and strength improve, he may move the cane and involved lower extremity simultaneously.

4 The sequence is repeated to ascend the remaining stairs.

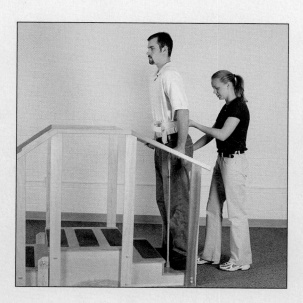

(continued)

Descending Using a Cane and Handrail

Authors' note: In the illustrations for this section, the patient demonstrates the use of two functional upper extremities, permitting the use of the cane in the left hand while grasping the handrail with right hand.

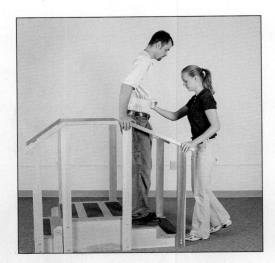

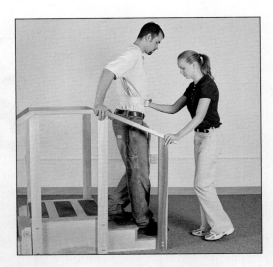

1 Positioned in stride and in front of the patient, the physical therapist/assistant grasps the patient's gait belt and the handrail. To descend stairs, the patient stands facing down the stairs, with the feet and cane parallel to the stair.

2 The patient lowers the cane to the next lower stair and places it securely on the stair tread. The patient lowers the involved lower extremity to the next lower stair by flexing the uninvolved lower extremity. As the patient's balance and strength improve, the patient may move the cane and involved lower extremity simultaneously.

3 The patient shifts weight to the involved lower extremity and cane and lowers the uninvolved lower extremity to the same stair as the cane and involved lower extremity.

4 The sequence is repeated to descend the remaining stairs.

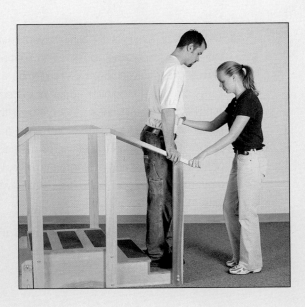

Ascending Using One Cane

Authors' note: In the illustrations for this section, the patient demonstrates the use of only one cane without using a handrail.

When not using a handrail, the gait pattern for ascending stairs with one cane is similar to that used when both a cane and handrail are used. As the patient improves, he should practice using only one cane and no handrail, which prepares the patient for situations in which no handrail is available. Patients who have only one functional upper extremity may have to use this method even if a handrail is available.

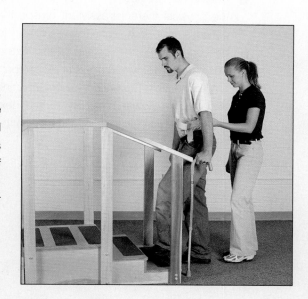

1 Positioned in stride behind the patient, the physical therapist/assistant grasps the patient's gait belt and the handrail. To ascend stairs, the patient stands facing up the stairs with the feet and cane parallel to the base of the first stair. The patient moves the uninvolved lower extremity to the next higher stair and shifts weight onto this extremity.

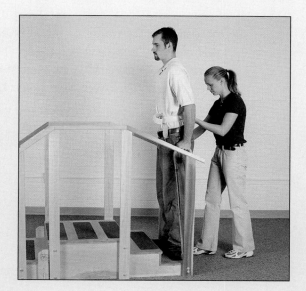

2 The patient extends the uninvolved lower extremity, lifting the body. The patient places the involved lower extremity and cane on the same stair as the uninvolved lower extremity. The patient should move the cane and involved lower extremity simultaneously to avoid leaning backward.

3 The sequence is repeated to ascend the remaining stairs.

(continued)

Descending Using One Cane

Authors' note: In the illustrations for this section, the patient demonstrates the use of only one cane without using a handrail.

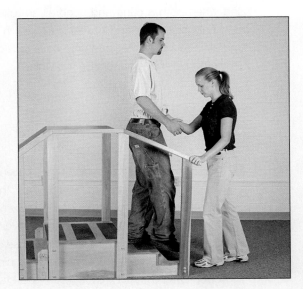

1. Positioned in stride in front of the patient, the physical therapist/assistant grasps the patient's gait belt and the handrail. To descend stairs, the patient starts facing down the stairs, with the feet and cane parallel to the stair. The patient lowers the cane and involved lower extremity to the next lower stair and places them securely on the stair tread.

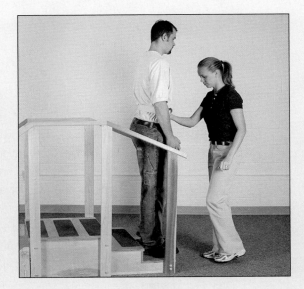

2. The patient shifts weight to the involved lower extremity and cane and lowers the uninvolved lower extremity to the same stair as the cane and involved lower extremity.

3. The sequence is repeated to descend the remaining stairs.

PROCEDURE 10–18   Ambulating Through Doorways with One Cane

Door with Automatic Door Closers

Authors' note: In each of the sections concerning ambulating through doorways with a cane, the patient is demonstrating the use of two functional upper extremities. When patients have only one functional upper extremity, they must hold the cane by the hand of the functional extremity while it manipulates the door handle and door.

Door Opens Toward Patient—Cane at Hinge Edge

Authors' note: In the illustrations for this section, a cane is used in the patient's left hand, the hand closer to the hinge edge of the door when facing the door.

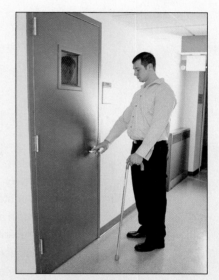

1 The patient approaches the door and stands at the latch edge of the door, out of the arc of the opening door. The patient places his right hand on the door handle.

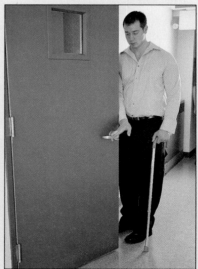

2 The patient opens the door wide enough to permit movement into the doorway before the door closes. Unlike the sequences for a walker or crutches, the patient does not open a door completely in a single motion. Opening a door in a single motion when using one cane is often not possible when patients must move the upper extremity across the body. Attempting to do so can compromise a patient's safety.

(continued)

3 The patient opens the door farther and places the tip of the cane on the floor to serve as a door stop.

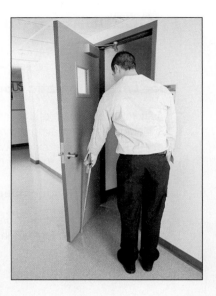

4 As the patient moves through a doorway, he places the tip of the cane progressively closer to the hinge edge of the door to serve as a door stop. The patient may need to use a hand or hip to maintain an open door. The physical therapist/assistant and patient must be aware that as the tip of a cane is placed closer to the hinge edge of the door, the door becomes more difficult to block. Once a patient has moved completely through the doorway, the door closes behind the patient.

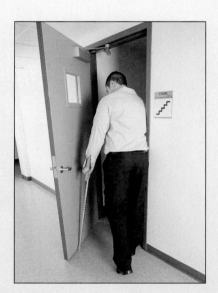

Door Opens Away from Patient—Cane at Hinge Edge

Authors' note: In the illustrations for this section, a cane is used in the patient's left hand, the hand closer to the hinge edge when facing the door.

① The patient approaches the door and places his right hand on the door handle.

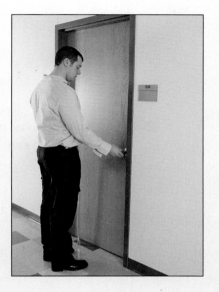

② The patient opens the door wide enough to permit a patient to enter the doorway. The patient places the tip of the cane on the floor to serve as a door stop. A door is not opened completely in a single motion. As the patient moves through a doorway, he places the tip of the cane progressively closer to the latch edge of the door to serve as a door stop. The patient may need to use a hand or hip to maintain an open door. Once the patient has moved completely through a doorway, the door closes behind him.

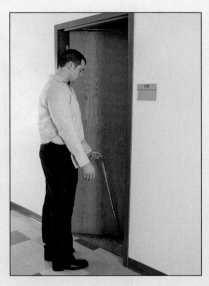

(continued)

Door Opens Away from Patient—Cane at Latch Edge

Authors' note: In the illustrations for this section, a cane is used in the patient's left hand, the hand closer to the latch edge of the door when facing the door.

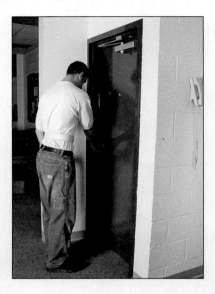

1 The patient approaches the door and places the right hand on the door handle.

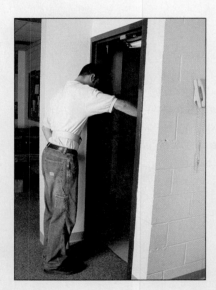

2 The patient pushes the door open wide enough to permit movement into the doorway. The patient moves the right hand from the door handle to the door and uses this hand to hold open the door.

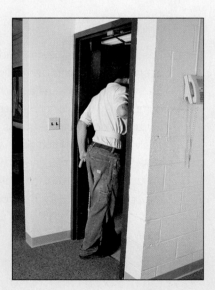

3 The patient continues to move through the doorway, using the hand to hold open the door. Once the patient has moved completely through the doorway, the door closes behind him.

PROCEDURE 10–19   Ambulating on Level Surfaces with Two Canes

Assuming standing and sitting when using two canes is performed in a manner similar to those maneuvers when using one cane.

Three-Point Gait Pattern

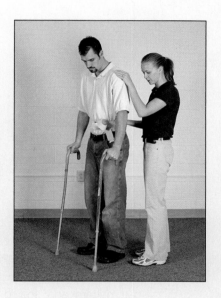

① Positioned in stride behind and to one side of a patient, the physical therapist/assistant grasps the patient's gait belt and shoulder. In the starting position, the patient stands with one cane in each hand in the same position used for measuring cane fit. The patient's feet are side by side.

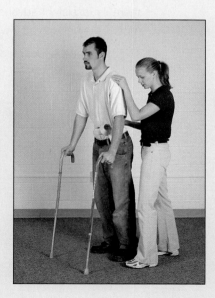

② To ambulate, the patient advances both canes and then advances the involved lower extremity to the canes. As the patient improves, he can advance the canes and the involved lower extremity simultaneously the same amount.

(continued)

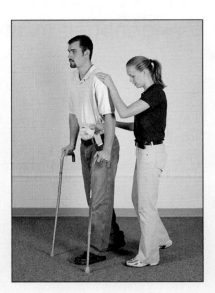

③ The physical therapist/assistant advances the outside foot either at the same time or immediately after the canes are advanced.

④ The patient then advances the uninvolved lower extremity beyond the canes. Initially, the patient may "step to" the involved lower extremity. Stepping through is the normal gait pattern and should be encouraged. The physical therapist/assistant advances the inside foot as the patient moves the uninvolved lower extremity.

⑤ The sequence is repeated for continued progression.

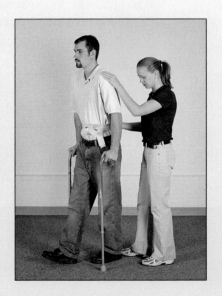

Four-Point Gait Pattern

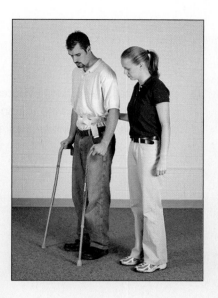

① Positioned in stride behind and to one side of the patient, the physical therapist/assistant grasps the patient's gait belt. In the starting position, the patient stands with one cane in each hand in the same position used for measuring cane fit. The patient's feet are side by side.

② To ambulate, the patient advances one cane. In this example, the right cane is advanced first.

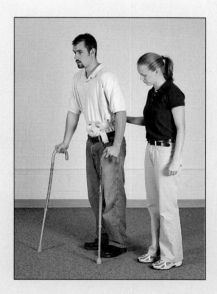

(continued)

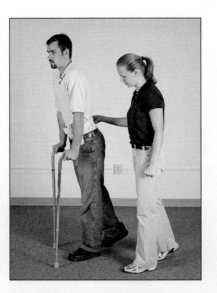

3 The patient then advances the opposite lower extremity to a point even with the tip of the right cane. The physical therapist/assistant advances the inside foot.

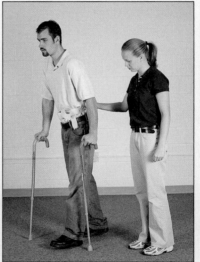

4 The patient shifts weight to the right cane and left lower extremity and advances the left cane beyond the right cane.

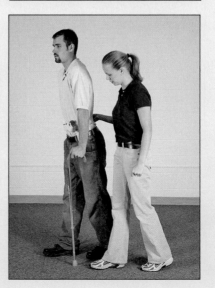

5 The patient then advances the right lower extremity to a point even with the tip of the left cane. The physical therapist/assistant advances the outside foot.

6 The sequence is repeated for continued progression.

Two-Point Gait Pattern

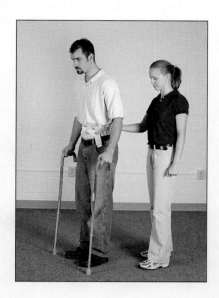

1. Positioned in stride behind and to one side of a patient, the physical therapist/assistant grasps the patient's gait belt. In the starting position, the patient stands with one cane in each hand in the same position used for measuring cane fit. The patient's feet are side by side.

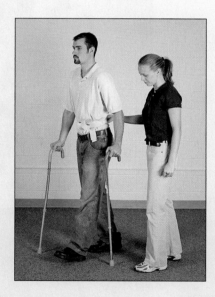

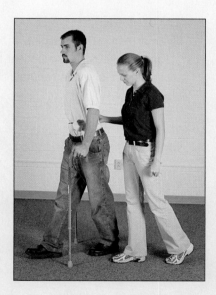

2. The patient advances one cane and the opposite lower extremity simultaneously, placing the toes even with the tip of the cane. The patient then shifts weight onto this cane and lower extremity. In this example, the right cane and left foot have been advanced together. The physical therapist/assistant moves the inside foot at this time.

3. The patient then advances the left cane and right lower extremity together. This cane and lower extremity are advanced beyond the other cane and lower extremity in a normal stride length. The physical therapist/assistant moves the outside foot at this time.

4. The sequence is repeated for continued progression.

PROCEDURE 10–20   Ambulating on Stairs with Two Canes

Holding the Canes

A patient can perform ambulation on stairs using two canes, with or without the use of a handrail. Use of a handrail provides stability and is an added safety feature. When using a handrail, the handrail takes the place of the cane on one side. There are several methods of holding canes when using a handrail. Whatever method of holding canes is used, the sequence of movements for the lower extremities and ambulatory assistive devices is the same.

A practical method of holding two canes while using a handrail is for the patient to place both canes in one hand. There are two methods of holding a cane in the hand that is grasping a handrail and cane simultaneously.

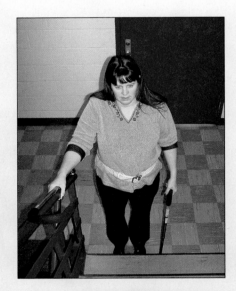

❶ One method of grasping a cane and handrail in the same hand is for the patient to hold the cane at mid-shaft parallel to the handrail.

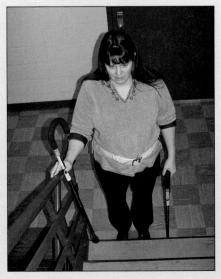

❷ A second method of grasping a cane and handrail in the same hand is for the patient to hold the cane at mid-shaft in a vertical orientation.

The patient uses the cane on the side opposite the handrail in the usual manner.

Three-Point Gait Pattern

Ascending Stairs

Authors' note: For the method presented in this section, the patient grasps one cane in each hand.

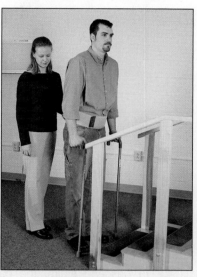

1 To ascend stairs, the patient stands facing up the stairs with feet and canes parallel to the base of the first stair. Positioned in stride behind a patient, the physical therapist/assistant grasps the patient's gait belt and the handrail.

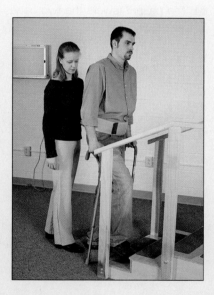

2 The patient places the uninvolved lower extremity on the next higher stair and shifts weight onto this extremity.

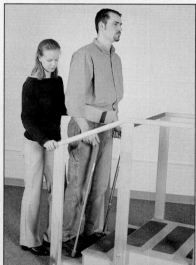

3 The patient extends the uninvolved lower extremity to raise the body. The patient advances the canes and involved lower extremity to the same stair simultaneously. The canes must be properly placed on the stair for stability and to provide room for the patient to maneuver.

4 The sequence is repeated to ascend the remaining stairs.

(continued)

Descending Stairs

Authors' note: For the method presented in this section, the patient grasps one cane in each hand.

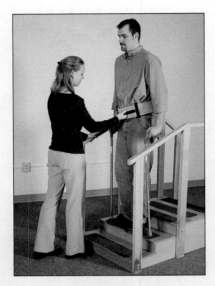

1 To descend stairs, the patient stands facing down the stairs. Positioned in stride in front of the patient, the physical therapist/assistant grasps the patient's gait belt and the handrail.

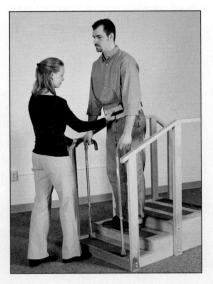

2 The patient lowers the two canes to the next lower stair.

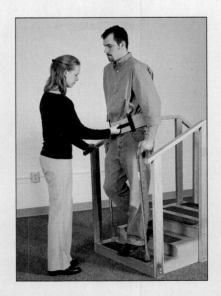

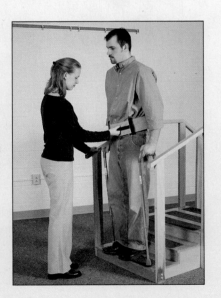

3 The patient lowers the involved lower extremity to the same stair as the two canes. He shifts weight to the involved lower extremity and canes and moves the uninvolved lower extremity to the same stair.

4 The sequence is repeated to descend the remaining stairs.

Four-Point Gait Pattern

Ascending Stairs

Authors' note: For the method presented in this section, the patient grasps one cane in each hand.

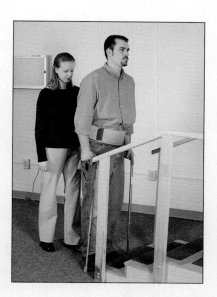

① To ascend stairs, the patient stands facing up the stairs with feet and canes parallel to the base of the stair. Positioned in stride behind the patient, the physical therapist/assistant grasps the patient's gait belt and the handrail.

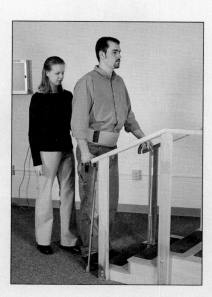

② The patient advances one cane to the next higher stair.

(continued)

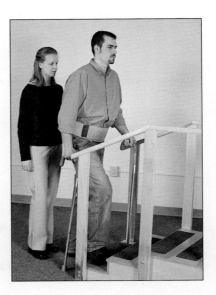

3 The patient then advances the opposite lower extremity to the same stair and shifts weight onto the cane and lower extremity that have been placed on the next higher stair.

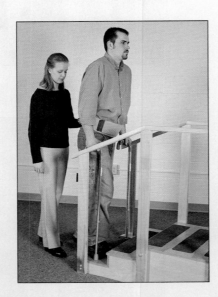

4 The patient advances the second cane to the same stair.

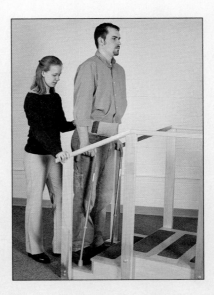

5 The patient then extends the lower extremity on the higher stair to lift the body. The patient places the second lower extremity on the same stair. Thus, both lower extremities and both canes are on the same stair.

6 The sequence is repeated to ascend the remaining stairs.

Descending Stairs

Authors' note: For the method presented in this section, the patient grasps one cane in each hand.

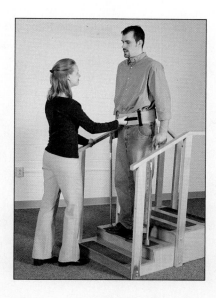

① To descend stairs, the patient stands facing down the stairs. Positioned in stride in front of the patient, the physical therapist/assistant grasps the patient's gait belt and the handrail.

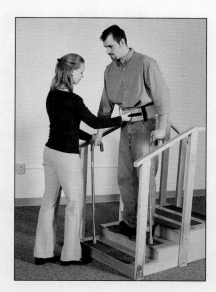

② The patient moves one cane to the next lower stair.

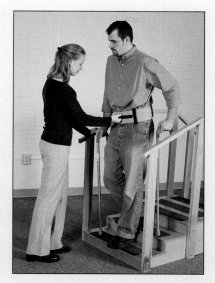

③ The patient flexes the lower extremity on the same side to lower the body, placing the opposite lower extremity on the same stair as the lowered cane.

(continued)

④ Shifting weight onto the cane and lower extremity on the lower stair, the patient moves the second cane to the same lower stair.

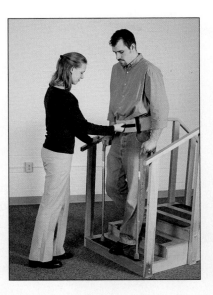

⑤ The patient moves the opposite lower extremity to the same lower stair. Thus, both lower extremities and both canes are on the same stair.

⑥ The sequence is repeated to descend the remaining stairs.

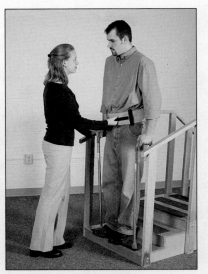

Two-Point Gait Pattern

Ascending Stairs

Authors' note: For the method presented in this section, the patient grasps one cane in each hand.

Ascending stairs using two canes and a two-point gait pattern is very similar to using a four-point gait pattern. The difference is that in a two-point gait pattern, the patient moves one cane and the opposite lower extremity simultaneously.

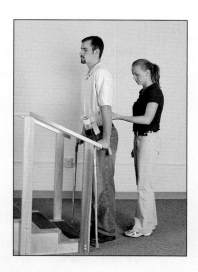

1 To ascend stairs, the patient stands facing up the stairs with feet and canes parallel to the base of the stair. Positioned in stride behind the patient, the physical therapist/assistant grasps the patient's gait belt and the handrail.

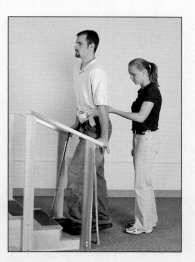

2 The patient moves one cane and the opposite lower extremity to the next higher stair.

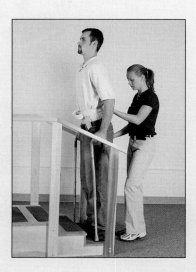

3 Then the patient moves the second cane and opposite lower extremity to the same stair.

4 The sequence is repeated to ascend the remaining stairs.

(continued)

Descending Stairs

Authors' note: For the method presented in this section, the patient grasps one cane in each hand.

Descending stairs using two canes and a two-point gait pattern is very similar to using a four-point gait pattern. The difference is that in a two-point gait pattern, the patient moves one cane and the opposite lower extremity simultaneously.

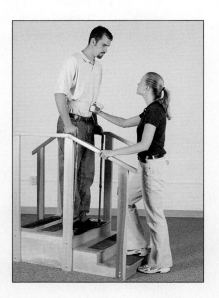

1 To descend stairs, the patient stands facing down the stairs. Positioned in stride in front of the patient, the physical therapist/assistant grasps the patient's gait belt and the handrail.

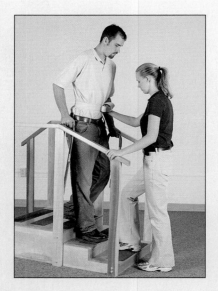

2 The patient moves one cane and the opposite lower extremity to the next lower stair.

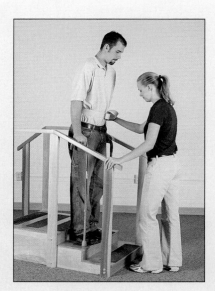

3 The patient lowers the second cane and opposite lower extremity to the same stair.

4 The sequence is repeated to descend the remaining stairs.

PROCEDURE 10–21   Ambulating Through Doorways with Two Canes

Door with Automatic Door Closer

Authors' note: In the illustrations for this section the patient is demonstrating the use of two canes.

When moving through a doorway, patients can use one cane in each hand or may place both canes in one hand. The method of moving through doorways with both canes in one hand is the same as when using one cane.

Door Opens Away from Patient

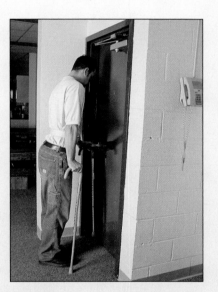

1. The patient faces the door and shifts the weight onto the cane away from the hand that is closer to the door handle. Holding the cane, the patient uses the unweighted hand to grasp the door handle.

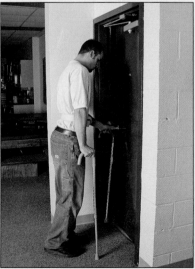

2. Using a pushing motion, the patient opens the door part way and blocks the door the tip of the cane closer to the door.

(continued)

3 As the patient moves through the doorway, he pushes the door open in increments. Continuing to use the tip of the cane as a door stop, the patient progresses through the doorway. The door closes behind the patient.

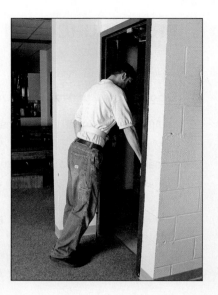

Door Opens Toward Patient

1 The patient approaches the latch edge of the door, standing outside the arc through which the opening door will move. The patient shifts weight onto the cane on the side away from the hand that will be placed on the door handle. Holding the cane, the patient uses the unweighted hand to grasp the door handle. Preferably, the patient shifts weight to the side closer to the door handle and uses the hand toward the hinge edge to pull open the door.

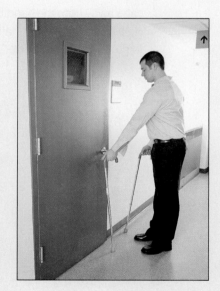

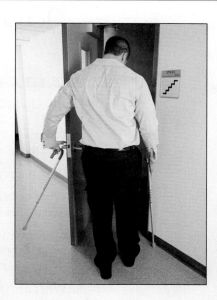

2 Using a pulling motion, the patient opens the door wider than the width of the patient because the door will start to close automatically before the patient can progress through the doorway. To block the automatic closing of the door, the patient moves into the doorway and places the tip of the cane closer to the door on the floor in the path of the door. This serves as a door stop, permitting the patient to move into the doorway without being struck by the closing door.

3 Continuing to use the tip of the cane as a door stop, the patient progresses through the doorway using an appropriate gait pattern. As the patient moves through the doorway, he uses the tip of the cane as a door stop by placing it progressively closer to the hinge edge of the door. The physical therapist/assistant and patient must be aware that as the tip of a cane gets closer to the hinge edge of the door, it becomes more difficult to hold open the door.

4 Once the patient has moved completely through the doorway, the door closes behind the patient.

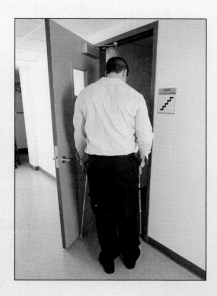

Doors without Automatic Closers

Patients using two canes can negotiate doorways without automatic door closers using the same sequences presented earlier in this chapter in the section *Axillary Crutches*.

Chapter Review

Review Questions

1. What are the general guidelines for instructing a patient in the use of ambulatory assistive devices and gait patterns?

2. Which components of ambulatory assistive devices should be checked for safety?

3. What activities should be taught to a patient learning to use an ambulatory assistive device?

4. List ambulatory assistive devices in the following order: (1) those providing the most stability to the least stability, (2) those requiring the most patient coordination to the least patient coordination.

5. What are the indications for the selection of specific ambulatory assistive devices?

6. Describe the five major gait patterns used with ambulatory assistive devices.

7. Describe which gait patterns can be used with each assistive device.

8. What are the criteria for selection of gait patterns when using ambulatory assistive devices?

9. What is the purpose of using the tilt table in gait training?

10. Describe how to fit each ambulatory assistive device.

11. Describe how a therapist guards a patient ambulating using an assistive device on level surfaces, stairs, and through doorways.

12. How is the wheelchair properly prepared for a patient to move in or out of the wheelchair when using ambulatory assistive devices?

Suggested Activities

1. Working in pairs, practice the procedures presented in this chapter. Rotate partners during the practice session.

2. Practice fitting each assistive device to at least three different people.

3. Practice demonstrating gait patterns with each assistive device.

4. Practice guarding partners using each assistive device with various appropriate gait patterns on level surfaces, stairs, and curbs; the assumption of sitting from standing and standing from sitting; moving through doorways; falling without injury; and resumption of ambulation after falling.

5. Practice teaching partners how to use ambulatory assistive devices on level surfaces, stairs, and curbs, the assumption of sitting from standing and standing from sitting; moving through doorways; falling without injury; and resumption of ambulation after falling, as partners role-play various diagnoses. Students role-playing a patient can add "character" to the role-play by being cooperative, noncooperative, in pain, hard of hearing, or faint, to enhance the activity. The patient must role-play the diagnosis and character consistently (see *Case Studies* for suggested patient roles).

6. Monitor vital signs and check for signs of circulatory problems of the lower extremities as appropriate.

7. Document interventions.

Case Studies

Use these case studies to complete activity 5 above.

1. The patient is a 16-year-old male high school soccer player who sustained a left knee injury in a game the previous night. He is to ambulate using axillary crutches with a non–weight-bearing gait pattern until a diagnosis is determined following an MRI in 2 days.
2. The patient is a 63-year-old female with a left CVA, presenting with right hemiplegia. She has sufficient motor control and balance to ambulate with a small-base quad cane.
3. The patient is a 78-year-old male who had a left total hip replacement one day ago. He is to ambulate using a walker, with weight bearing as tolerated.
4. The patient is a 49-year-old female with severe rheumatoid arthritis who received a right total knee joint replacement 2 days ago. She is to ambulate using a platform walker, with weight bearing as tolerated.
5. The patient is a 21-year-old male with a complete L3–4 spinal cord injury. He is ready to begin gait training using Lofstrand (forearm) crutches and knee-ankle-foot orthoses (KAFOs). His upper extremity strength is adequate for ambulating with these ambulatory assistive devices.

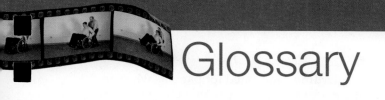

Glossary

A

Abduction movement in the frontal plane that is the result of the limb segment surfaces moving away from the midline of the body; does not include the thumb

Accessible route public path from public transportation, accessible parking spaces, and public streets to building that meets accessibility requirements

Active assisted range of motion (AAROM) exercises performed by a physical therapist/assistant assisting a patient in performing movement

Active pathology part of Nagi model; interruption of normal body function at the cellular level

Active range of motion (AROM) exercises performed independently by a patient, although they may be supervised by a physical therapist/assistant to ensure correct performance

Adduction movement in the frontal plane that is the result of the limb segment surfaces moving toward the midline of the body; does not include the thumb

Afebrile when a patient's oral temperature remains below 100° F (37.8° C)

Airborne precautions prevent transmission of infectious agents that remain infectious over long distances when suspended in the air

Airborne transmission occurs by two modes: (1) airborne droplet nuclei (particle residue 5 μm or smaller in size) that are evaporated droplets containing microorganisms that remain suspended in the air for long periods of time; and (2) in dust particles containing the infectious agent that are dispersed widely by air currents and inhaled by a susceptible host

Alcohol-based hand rub alcohol-containing preparation designed for application to the hands for reducing the number of viable microorganisms on the hands. In the United States, such preparations usually contain 60 percent to 95 percent ethanol or isopropanol

Ambulatory assistive devices provide external support for the musculoskeletal system

Americans with Disabilities Act (1990) (ADA) Public Law 101–336, that contains five titles and provides "a clear and comprehensive national mandate for the elimination of discrimination against individuals with disabilities"

Analysis (SOAP note) list of patient problems and professional opinions concerning a patient's problems and reasoning used as the basis for the plan of care; also includes diagnosis and prognosis related to physical therapy care

Anatomical planes of movement used to move body segments to perform ROM exercises

Anatomical position position in which a person is standing upright, eyes looking straight ahead, arms at the sides with palms facing forward, and the feet approximately 4 inches apart at the heels with the toes pointing forward

Anthropometric measures measurements of physical characteristics such as height and weight

Antimicrobial soap soap (i.e., detergent) containing an antiseptic agent

Antiseptic agent antimicrobial substances that are applied to the skin to reduce the number of microbial flora. Examples include alcohols, chlorhexidine, chlorine, hexachlorophene, iodine, chloroxylenol (PCMX), quaternary ammonium compounds, and triclosan

Antiseptic hand rub applied to all surfaces of the hands to reduce the number of microorganisms present

Antiseptic hand wash washing hands with water and soap or other detergents containing an antiseptic agent

Anti-tipping devices small extensions, with or without wheels, attached to the lower horizontal support bar to prevent accidental backward tipping of a wheelchair

Architectural Barriers Act (1968) (ABA) federal law that requires access to facilities designed, built, altered, or leased with federal funds

Armrests arm supports on a wheelchair

Aseptic technique the methods and procedures used to create and maintain a sterile field

Assisted transfers transfers in which a patient participates actively and requires assistance by additional (one or more) personnel; examples include two-person lift, sliding board transfer, squat pivot, and assisted standing pivot transfer

Audit systematic reviews of documentation that examine the efficacy and efficiency of patient-care outcomes with respect to interventions used

Auscultation monitoring of the heart using a stethoscope; also used to obtain heart rate

B

Bacterial barrier a barrier that keeps microorganisms from coming in contact with sterile items

Basal heart rate pulse rate measured after an extended period of rest; one indication of cardiovascular function in the absence of physical stress

Base of support part of the body in contact with the supporting surface

Biarticular muscles that cross more than one joint

Blanching a noted loss of color of the skin resulting from decreased circulation

Blood pressure a measure of vascular resistance to blood flow

Body mass index (BMI) used to classify a person's weight and height relationship with respect to being underweight, normal, overweight, or obese

Body mechanics requires strength, range of motion (ROM), and motor control to maintain proper skeletal alignment during standing and proper skeletal movement during activity by maintaining the center of gravity within the base of support

Bradycardia a very slow resting heart rate; less than 60 bpm

C

Caster wheels the small front wheels of a wheelchair

Center of gravity the point at which the three cardinal planes intersect

Centers for Disease Control and Prevention (CDC) federal agency responsible for safety and health issues

Cleaning the physical removal of organic material or soil from objects. The process of cleaning is usually performed with water, with or without detergents. Cleaning is the least rigorous of the three levels and is designed to remove microorganisms rather than kill them. Cleaning usually precedes either of the next two levels, disinfection or sterilization

Cleanliness Three levels of cleanliness—cleaning, disinfection, and sterilization—have been established for equipment use in patient care

Clear-space areas include the floor dimensions of an accessible route and clearances for use of certain facilities, such as toilet stalls and drinking fountains

Close guarding indicated for patients who can usually perform an activity without assistance by personnel but have a greater likelihood for needing physical assistance by additional personnel for support or balance

Closed-ended question used to obtain or confirm specific information and often answered with a single word or a brief phrase

Combining components occurs when more than one plane of joint motion is performed simultaneously

Common vehicle transmission applies to microorganisms transmitted by contaminated items such as food, water, medications, devices, and equipment

Compression wrap applied to control edema in a limb segment or to provide some support for a joint

Contact guarding indicated for patients who can usually perform an activity but have a significant likelihood of requiring physical assistance by additional personnel for support or balance

Contact precautions intended to prevent transmission of infectious agents, including epidemiologically important microorganisms, that are spread by direct or indirect contact with the patient or the patient's environment

Contact transmission the most important and frequent mode of nosocomial infection transmission

Contaminated an item, surface, or field whenever it comes in contact with anything that is not sterile

Control mechanisms switches, dial, handles and the like that are used to manipulate or turn a device on/off

Critical items introduced directly into the circulatory system or other normally sterile areas of the body. Surgical instruments, implants, and the blood compartment of a hemodialyzer are examples of critical items

Curb cut a ramp to permit smooth transition from sidewalk to street level

D

Daily note part of POMR method; brief presentation of description of treatment and patient responses for each day

Damp-to-damp dressing application of a moistened gauze pad that is maintained moist until removed or remoistened prior to removal

Damp-to-dry dressing application of a moistened dressing that is allowed to dry before removal

Database part of POMR method; contains subjective and objective information, including medical, family, and social history, and medical examination and test results

Decontaminate hands to reduce bacterial counts on hands by performing antiseptic hand rub or antiseptic hand wash

Department of Justice (DOJ) primary federal criminal investigation and enforcement agency

Dependent transfers transfers in which a patient does not participate actively, or participates only minimally, and additional personnel perform all aspects of the transfer; examples include sliding transfer from cart to treatment table, three-person carry, dependent standing pivot transfer, and hydraulic lift transfer

Detergent compounds that possess a cleaning action. Detergents (i.e., surfactants) are composed of both hydrophilic and lipophilic parts and can be divided into four groups: anionic, cationic, amphoteric, and nonionic detergents. Although products used for hand-washing or antiseptic hand wash in health-care settings represent various types of detergents, the term "soap" is used to refer to such detergents in this guideline

Diagnosis assignment of a label that states the categorization or classification of problems identified and is selected from the practice pattern or diagnostic category that most closely describes a patient's impairments and functional limitations as presented in the *Guide to Physical Therapist Practice*

Diagonal patterns of movement combining components of motion at one joint as well as all the joints of an extremity

Diastolic pressure a measure of the pressure exerted by arterial walls against blood when the heart is not contracting

Direct-contact transmission involves direct body-surface-to-body-surface contact and physical transfer of microorganisms between a susceptible host and an infected or colonized person, such as when turning or transferring a patient or when performing other patient-care activities that require direct personal contact

Disability part of Nagi model; functional limitations that prevent an individual from fulfilling his/her life roles

Discharge note part of POMR method; present the status of patient problems, and the current course of treatment, at the time of patient discharge

Disinfection an intermediate level between cleaning and sterilization. Three levels of disinfection—high, intermediate, and low—have been defined. Disinfection is usually performed using pasteurization or chemical germicides

Documentation medico-legal record of patient care provided by all practitioners for a given patient

Doppler measurements used to examine patency using frequency changes during blood flow

Draping covering a patient appropriately in a manner that maintains patient modesty and comfort

Drive wheels the large rear wheels of a wheelchair; used for propulsion

Droplet precautions intended to prevent transmission of pathogens spread through close respiratory or mucous-membrane contact with respiratory secretions

Droplet transmission theoretically a form of contact transmission but quite distinct from either direct- or indirect-contact transmission, so considered a separate route of transmission; droplets generated from a source person (during coughing, sneezing, talking, performance of certain procedures such as suctioning or wound care) are propelled a short distance through the air and deposited on a host's conjunctivae, nasal mucosa, or mouth

Dry-to-dry dressing application of a dry absorbent or nonabsorbent dressing to cover the wound

E

End feel quality of restriction felt by a physical therapist/assistant when a limit of motion is reached

Equal Employment Opportunity Commission (EEOC) the agency of the United States Government that enforces the federal employment discrimination laws

Evaluation process whereby physical therapists use examination data, professional knowledge, and clinical judgment, to identify impairments and functional limitations and generate diagnoses, prognoses, and a plan of care

Eversion movement of the foot that occurs in the frontal plane about the long axis of the foot such that the plantar surface of the foot faces away from the midline of the body

Examination process of generating a patient/client history, reviewing all physiologic systems, and applying tests and measures

Extension movement in the sagittal plane; does not include the thumb

External (lateral) rotation movement in the transverse plane that results in anterior limb segment surfaces turning outward, away from the midline of the body

F

Febrile when a patient's oral temperature exceeds 100° F

Figure-of-eight wrap started in the same manner as a spiral wrap, but the direction of wrapping changes each time the wrap completes one loop of the figure-of-eight

Fixed frame the wheelchair frame is solid and cannot be folded

Flexion movement in a sagittal plane; does not include the thumb

Folding-frame wheelchair can be folded or collapsed for storage or transport by raising footplates and pulling up on the handles located on either side of the seat

Footrest front rigging with only a footplate

Front rigging consists of a footplate attached to either a footrest or an elevating legrest on a wheelchair; purpose is to provide support for the lower extremities

Full weight bearing (FWB) the patient is permitted full weight bearing on the involved lower extremity

Functional limitations part of Nagi model; loss of a system is sufficient to prevent the performance of routine tasks by an individual, such as performing activities of daily living (ADLs), independently and in a timely manner

G

Gait pattern a selected sequence of movements for the ambulatory assistive device(s) and lower extremities

Gait or transfer belts belts secured around a patient's waist, providing a secure point of contact and control for a physical therapist/assistant

Gauze wrap a type of bandage made of gauze that is used to keep a dressing in place

Generalizability some skills learned for one activity can be used for other similar activities

Grab bar bar to hold onto for support during standing or transitions

Guidelines interpretations for the implementation of laws

H

Hand antisepsis either antiseptic hand wash or antiseptic hand rub

Hand hygiene a general term that applies to handwashing, antiseptic hand wash, antiseptic hand rub, or surgical hand antisepsis

Hand-washing washing hands with plain (i.e., nonantimicrobial) soap and water

Health Insurance Portability and Accountability Act (HIPAA) protects confidentiality of patient medical information and records when stored, when discussed by health-care providers, and as they are conveyed between health-care providers or between health-care providers and insurers

Heel loops constructed of clothstrapping or webbing; attach to footplates and prevent the feet from sliding off the footplates and under the wheelchair

Horizontal abduction movement of the upper extremity posteriorly when the shoulder has already been abducted to 90 degrees in the frontal plane

Horizontal adduction movement of the upper extremity anteriorly when the shoulder has already been abducted to 90 degrees in the frontal plane

Hospital Infection Control Practices Advisory Committee (HICPAC) a federal advisory committee made up of 14 external infection control experts who provide advice and guidance to the Centers for Disease Control and Prevention (CDC) and the Secretary of the Department of Health and Human Services (HHS) regarding the practice of health care infection control, strategies for surveillance and prevention and control of health care associated infections in United States health care facilities

Hyperthermia a rectal temperature greater than 106° F (41.1° C)

Hypothermia a rectal temperature less than 94° F (34.4° C)

I

Identifiers could allow identification of an individual and the individual's medical information and thus are to be protected to prevent inappropriate use of this information

Impairment part of Nagi model; the body cannot compensate or heal itself, so the individual sustains loss of normal function of a system

Independent transfers transfers in which a patient consistently performs all aspects of the transfer, including setup, in a safe manner and without assistance by additional personnel; an example is a sliding board transfer

Indirect-contact transmission involves contact of a susceptible host with a contaminated intermediate object, usually inanimate, such as whirlpool water that is not changed between patient treatments, reuse of self-adhesive electrodes on more than one patient, contaminated hands that are not washed, and gloves that are not changed between patients

Initial note part of POMR method; initial findings and plan of care

Instructions inform patients of what is to be done and provide information as part of the teaching process; may include oral description, visual demonstration, and written description

Internal (medial) rotation movement in the transverse plane that results in anterior limb segment surfaces turning inward, toward the midline of the body

Intervention includes treatment, communication, education, and planning

Interview the process of soliciting information by talking with another person(s)

Inversion movement of the foot that occurs in the frontal plane about the long axis of the foot such that the plantar surface of the foot faces toward the midline of the body

Isolation the separation and placement of patients in environments that reduce the potential for transmission of infectious microorganisms

Isometric muscle contractions contractions of muscles that result in development of muscle tension without joint movement

J

Joint range of motion moving a joint in all planes of motion appropriate for the specific joint

L

Legrest front rigging with a footplate and calf pad support

Levels of assistance stated as stand-by (supervision), close guarding, contact guarding, minimal, moderate, and maximum assistance

Long sitting position in which a person sits with hips flexed to 90° and knees fully extended on a supporting surface

Long-term goals (LTGs) statements describing functional capabilities a patient will have upon discharge

M

Mask A nonactive device that filters environmental air

Maximal heart rate the highest heart rate a person should achieve upon exertion with respect to age and medical condition

Maximum assistance indicated for patients who can perform less than 25 percent of an activity

Minimal assistance indicated for patients who can perform at least 75 percent of an activity

Moderate assistance indicated for patients who can perform at least 50 percent of an activity

Muscle range of motion lengthening a muscle through its available length for all appropriate joint motions

N

Narrative note way for entering patient information that may include headings and subheadings to organize information

Noncritical items do not touch the patient or touch the patient in areas that are normally not sterile, such as intact areas of skin; examples are blood pressure cuffs and crutches

Non–weight bearing (NWB) the involved lower extremity is not to be weight bearing and is usually not permitted to touch the ground

Nosing front edge of a tread

Nosocomial infection infection acquired while hospitalized for treatment of other conditions

O

Objective (SOAP note) verifiable data including examination results, observations by health-care providers, interventions, and patient response to interventions

Occlusive dressing applied to provide a semipermeable barrier to air and moisture penetration

One-arm drive wheelchair has two hand rims on one drive wheel with a linking mechanism between the drive wheels, providing control for both drive wheels using one upper extremity

Open-ended question allows a patient to tell his or her story in his or her own words

Opposition multiplanar movement of the carpometacarpal joint of the thumb that results in approximation of the tip of the thumb and the tip of a finger of the same hand

Orthostatic hypotension the inability of the cardiovascular system to adapt to upright postures after prolonged horizontal positioning

Outcome functional capacity of a patient/client

P

Pain subjective perception described by patients; difficult to measure

Partial weight bearing (PWB) a limited amount of weight bearing, such as five pounds, is permitted for the involved lower extremity

Passive range of motion (PROM) exercise performed with the patient relaxed and a physical therapist/assistant moving the body segment without patient assistance

Patency openness of the peripheral portion of the cardiovascular system; can be determined by measurements of pulse

Patient-care equipment categories three categories of patient care equipment—critical, semi-critical, and noncritical—provide a basis for the level of cleanliness deemed necessary

Patient/client management note developed in response to the implementation of the Physical Therapy Patient/Client Management process; has components of both the narrative and SOAP note formats

Pelvic positioners devices that stabilize a patient's pelvis in the proper position while seated in a wheelchair

Plain soap detergents that do not contain antimicrobial agents or that contain low concentrations of antimicrobial agents that are effective solely as preservatives

Plan (SOAP note) developed by the physical therapist for providing patient treatment

Plan of care statement that specifies outcomes, interventions to be provided to achieve the stated outcomes, and a timeline for reaching the stated outcomes

Platform lifts used for building entrances, in building interiors, and with transportation vehicles

Preferred practice pattern element of evidence-based patient management for specific diagnoses that guides management of patients but doees not prescribe specifics of patient/client management

Problem list part of POMR method; list of the patient's problems identified from information contained in the database; problems may be identified by any professional in a discipline providing patient care and may be listed as an abnormal test result, chief complaint, diagnosis, physical finding, physiological finding, or symptom

Problem-oriented medical record (POMR) method organizes each medical record in a format based on identified patient problems rather than by professional discipline

Prognosis determination of an optimal level of improvement and the time necessary to achieve projected outcomes

Progress (interim) notes part of POMR method; present the progression of treatment, patient responses to treatment, and changes in the plan of care over intervals

Pronation defined differently for the upper and lower extremities; for the upper extremity, pronation of the forearm occurs when the arm is stabilized and the forearm is rotated so that the palm of the hand faces posteriorly; for the lower extremity, pronation of the foot occurs when the leg is stabilized and the foot is rotated about the oblique axis of the subtalar and other midfoot joints

Prone position in which a person lies on his or her stomach on a supporting surface

Proper posture appropriate alignment of the musculoskeletal system such that the stresses and strains placed on bones, muscles, ligaments, and cartilage are as low as possible

Proprioceptive neuromuscular facilitation (PNF) an approach to therapeutic exercise

Protraction multiplanar movement of the scapula around the lateral aspect of the ribs toward the anterior aspect of the thorax; often termed scapular abduction

Pulse a measurement of heart rate in beats per minute

R

Radial deviation when the wrist is moved such that the hand moves away from the midline of the body

Ramp slanted portion of a route

Range of motion (ROM) movement of each joint and muscle through its available arc of motion

Reach range unobstructed space a person can reach controls

Reclining-back wheelchairs type of wheelchair that has a back that can be adjusted from vertical to horizontal and points between

Recommendations ranking scheme CDC's Center for Infectious Diseases has established four categories to indicate the scientific support for their recommendations

Red flag a sign or symptom noted that does not fit with a known medical diagnosis for the specific patient

Regularity evenness of heart rate

Regulations interpretations for the implementation of laws

Respirator a mechanical device that provides a source of air not associated with the immediate environment

Respiratory rate rate of breathing

Resting heart rate pulse rate measured during rest; a measurement of heart rate without imposed stresses

Retraction multiplanar movement of the scapula around the lateral aspect of the ribs as the scapula moves toward the spine; often termed scapular adduction

Rigid dressing provides physical protection to a wound and the adjacent area

Rigidity resistance to passive movement that is not affected by movement velocity

Riser vertical dimension that separates one stair tread from the next stair tread

Rules interpretations for the implementation of laws

S

Sacral sitting occurs when an individual slouches, sliding the buttocks forward and tilting the pelvis posteriorly

Semicritical items devices introduced into body cavities not usually considered sterile, and include, but are not limited to, endotracheal tubes and fiberoptic endoscopes. There is a lower degree of risk of infection associated with semicritical items

Shelf life the length of time an unopened sterilized package is considered to remain sterile

Short-term goals (STGs) more discrete activities a patient will achieve to perform functional activities stated as long-term goals

Sidelying position in which a patient is lying on one side

Signs objective evidence of disease perceptible by a health-care provider and reported in the objective data

SOAP note originated with POMR system and now is used more widely for medical chart notes

Source-oriented method charts are divided into sections for each health profession providing service for a patient, thereby segregating patient information by discipline

Spasticity increased resistance to movement, especially as the velocity of movement is increased

Spiral wrap applied by wrapping gauze in a continuous manner around the limb segment

Standard precautions precautions designed for the care of all patients, particularly hospitalized patients, regardless of their diagnosis or presumed infection status. This is new terminology to replace the term universal precautions

Stand-by assistance indicated for patients who can usually perform an activity without assistance by additional personnel but do not do so consistently; examples include verbal cues, assistance in problem solving during transfer, or assistance if an emergency arises

Sterile an item or environment free from living microorganisms

Sterile field an area considered free from living microorganisms

Sterilization The highest level of cleanliness. Sterilization is the destruction of all forms of microbial life by steam under pressure, liquid or gaseous chemicals, or dry heat

Subjective (SOAP note) relevant data concerning the patient's history that are not verifiable in medical records; includes the patient's description of functional problems, pain, and the date of onset; could also include patient's name, gender, age and date of birth, primary and secondary diagnoses, and physicians

Supervision (stand-by) guarding physical therapist/assistant walks near the patient without contact or holding the gait belt

Supination defined differently for the upper and lower extremities; for the upper extremity, supination of the forearm occurs when the arm is stabilized and the forearm is rotated so that the palm of the hand faces anteriorly; for the lower extremity, supination of the foot occurs when the leg is stabilized and the foot is rotated about the oblique axis of the subtalar and other midfoot joints

Supine position in which a person lies on his or her back on a supporting surface

Surgical hand antisepsis antiseptic hand wash or antiseptic hand rub performed preoperatively by surgical personnel to eliminate transient, and reduce resident, hand flora. Antiseptic detergent preparations often have persistent antimicrobial activity

Symptoms subjective perceptions of patients that may be indicative of disease

Systems review brief or limited examination of (1) the anatomical and physiological status of the cardiovascular/pulmonary, integumentary, musculoskeletal, and neuromuscular systems and (2) the communication ability, affect, cognition, language, and learning style of the patient

Systolic pressure measurement of pressure exerted by blood against arterial walls when the heart is contracting

T

Tachycardia a very fast heart rate; greater than 100 bpm

Target heart rate heart rate that an individual should achieve during exercise for cardiovascular conditioning with respect to age and medical condition

Temperature provides information concerning basal metabolic state, potential presence of infection, and metabolic response to exercise

Tilt-in-space wheelchair has a fixed seat-to-back angle, even when reclined

Toe touch weight bearing (TTWB) the patient can rest the foot of the involved lower extremity on the ground for balance but not for weight bearing

Transitions the act of moving from one position or activity to another

Transmission-based precautions based on the concept of avoiding infection by limiting the potential for transmission of microorganisms, these are designed for the care of only specified patients: patients known, or suspected, to be infected by epidemiologically important pathogens, highly transmissible pathogens for which additional precautions, beyond standard precautions, are needed to interrupt transmission in health-care settings

Tread horizontal dimension of a stair

Trophic physiological sequels to decreased circulation, such as loss of hair, dry or flaky skin, and muscle atrophy

U

Ulnar deviation when the wrist is moved such that the hand moves toward the midline of the body

Uniarticular muscles that cross only that single joint

United States Access Board (USAB) independent federal agency whose primary mission is accessibility for people with disabilities

Unsterile (nonsterile) any item or environment that has not been sterilized, has come into contact with an item that is no longer considered sterile, has entered a field that is not sterile, or has exceeded its shelf life

V

Valsalva maneuver closing of the glottis during heavy exertion resulting in increased intra-thoracic and intra-abdominal pressure, which can cause a rapid increase in blood pressure

Vectorborne transmission occurs when vectors such as mosquitoes, flies, rats, and other vermin transmit microorganisms

Verbal commands auditory cues to patients that are provided during activity performance

Visual analog scale a straight horizontal line with 0 at the left side (representing a complete absence of pain) and 10 at the right side (representing the worst pain a patient can imagine)

W

Waterless antiseptic agent does not require use of exogenous water; after application, the hands are rubbed together until the agent has dried

Weight bearing the amount of weight that can be borne on a lower extremity during standing or ambulation

Weight bearing as tolerated (WBAT) the patient determines the amount of weight bearing that will occur on the involved lower extremity

Wheel locks devices that stabilize the wheels of a wheelchair after the wheelchair has been stopped

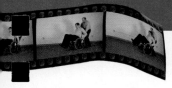

Glossary of Abbreviations

A

A: Assessment
AFO Ankle foot orthosis
ALS Amyotrophic lateral sclerosis
ATNR Asymmetric tonic neck reflex

B

B or bil Bilateral
B/C Because
B/S Bedside
BE Below elbow
BID or bid Twice a day
BK Below knee
BM Bowel movement
BOS Base of support
BP Blood pressure
bpm Beats per minute
BR Bedrest

C

c̄ With
C&S Culture and sensitivity
c/o Complains of
CA Cancer
CABG Coronary artery bypass graft
CAD Coronary artery disease
CAT Computerized axial tomography
CBC Complete blood cell count
CC or C/C Chief complaint
CG Contact guard
CHF Congestive heart failure
CNS Central nervous system
Cont. or cont'd continue; continued
COLD Chronic obstructive lung disease
COPD Chronic obstructive pulmonary disease
COTA Certified occupational therapy assistant
CPM or cpm Continuous passive motion
CPR Cardiopulmonary resuscitation

CPT Chest physical therapy
CS Close supervision

D

D/C Discontinue or discharge
DJD Degenerative joint disease
DM Diabetes mellitus
DME Durable medical equipment
DNR Do not resuscitate
DO Doctor of osteopathy
DOB Date of birth
DOE Dyspnea on exertion
DTR Deep tendon reflex
DVT Deep vein thrombosis
Dx or dx Diagnosis

E

ECF Extended care facility
ECG or EKG Electrocardiogram
EEG Electroencephalogram
EENT Ear, eyes, nose, throat
EMG Electromyogram
eval Evaluation
ex Exercise
ext. Extension; external
e-stim Electrical stimulation
ER External rotation

F

F Fair (as a muscle grade)
FBS Fasting blood sugar
FES Functional electrical stimulation
FEV Forced expiratory volume
FH Family history
fl or flex Flexion
FRC Functional residual capacity
FUO Fever, unknown origin
FVC Forced vital capacity

F/U Follow-up
FWB Full weight bearing
Fx Fracture; function

G

G Good (as a muscle grade)
GCS Glasgow Coma Scale
GI Gastrointestinal
G-tube Gastrointestinal tube
GSW Gun shot wound
GYN Gynecology

H

H or hr. Hour
H&P History and physical
H/A or h/o History of
HA or H/A Headache
HEENT Head, ear, eye, nose, throat
HEP Home exercise program
HHA Home health aide
HNP Herniated nucleus pulposus
HOB Head of bed
HR Heart rate
HTN Hypertension
hs At bedtime
ht. Height
Hx or hx History

I

I or indep Independent
I&O or IO Intake and output
ICU Intensive care unit
Imp. Impression
inf Inferior
int rot or IR Internal rotation
IP Interphalangeal joint
IV Intravenous

J

J-tube Jejunsotomy tube

K

KAFO Knee-ankle-foot orthosis

L

L or Ⓛ Left
Lat Lateral
LBBB Left bundle branch block
LBP Low back pain
LBQC Large base quad cane
LE Lower extremity
LLL Left lower lobe
LLQ Left lower quadrant
Lig Ligament
LMN Lower motor neuron
LOB Loss of balance
LOC Loss of consciousness; level of consciousness
LOS Length of stay
LTG Long-term goal
LTC Long-term care
LUL Left upper lobe
LUQ Left upper quadrant
LVH Left ventricular hypertrophy

M

Max Maximum; maximal
MCA Middle cerebral artery
MCP Metacarpal phalangeal joint
MD Medical doctor
MED Minimal erythemal dose
Meds. Medications
min Minimum; minimal
MMT Manual muscle test
mod Moderate
MRI Magnetic resonance imaging
MS Multiple sclerosis
MVA Motor vehicle accident
mvt Movement

N

N Normal (as a muscle grade)
N/A Not applicable
NBCQ Narrow base quad cane
NDT Neurodevelopmental treatment
neg. Negative
NG Nasogastric
NICU Neonatal intensive care unit
nn Nerve

noc   Night; at night

NPO **or** npo   Nothing by mouth

NSR   Normal sinus rhythm

N/T   Not tested

NWB   Non-weight bearing

O

O: Objective

OA   Osteoarthritis

OB   Obstetrics

OBS   Organic brain syndrome

od   Once daily

OOB   Out of bed

O.P.   Out patient

O.R. **or** OR   Operating room

ORIF   Open reduction internal fixation

OT **or** OTR   Occupational therapy; occupational therapist

P

p̄   After

P   Poor (as a muscle grade)

P: Plan

P.A.   Physician's assistant

PA   Posterior/anterior

para   Paraplegia

pc   after meals

PCA   Posterior cerebral artery

PE   Pulmonary embolus

per   by/through

PERRLA   Pupils equal, round, reactive to light, and accommodation

PET   Positron emission tomography

PF   Plantar flexion

PH   Past history

PIP   Proximal interphalangeal joint

PMH   Past medical history

PNF   Proprioceptive neuromuscular facilitation

PNI   Peripheral nerve injury

PO   Per oral (by mouth)

POMR   Problem-oriented medical record

pos.   Positive

post   Posterior

post op   Postoperative

PRE   Progressive resistive exercise

pre op   before surgery

prn   As often as necessary

PROM   Passive range of motion

prox   Proximal

Pt   Patient

PT   Physical therapy; physical therapist

PTA   Physical therapist assistant; prior to admission

PVD   Peripheral vascular disease

PWB   Partial weight bearing

Q

q   Every

qd   Every day

qh   Every hour

qid   Four times a day

qn   Every night

quads   Quadriceps

R

R **or** Ⓡ   Right

RA   Rheumatoid arthritis

RBBB   Right bundle branch block

re   concerning; about

RBC   Red blood cell

R.D.   Registered dietician

Rehab   Rehabilitation

reps   Repetitions

resp   Respiratory; respiration

RLL   Right lower lobe

RLQ   Right lower quadrant

RML   Right middle lobe

RN   Registered nurse

R/O **or** r/o   Rule out

ROM   Range of motion

ROS   Review of systems

RR   Respiratory rate

RROM   Resistive range of motion

R.T.   Respiratory therapy; respiratory therapist

R/T   Related to

RUQ   Right upper quadrant

Rx   Prescription; treatment; orders; intervention; therapy

S

S   Supervision

s̄   Without

S: Subjective
SAQ Short arc quads
SBA Stand by assist
SBQC Small base quad cane
SCI Spinal cord injury
SED Suberythemal dose
SLE Systemic lupus erythematosus
SLP Speech language pathologist
sig Significant
SLR Straight leg raise
SNF Skilled nursing facility
SOAP Subjective, objective, assessment, plan
S/O Standing order
SOB Short of breath
SOS Step over step
s/p Status post
stat Immediately; at once
STG Short-term goal
STNR Symmetrical tonic neck reflex
sup Superior
surg Surgical; surgery
sx Symptoms

T

T Trace (as a muscle grade)
TBA To be assessed
TBI Traumatic brain injury
TDWB Touch down weight bearing
temp Temperature
TENS Transcutaneous electrical nerve stimulator
ther. ex Therapeutic exercise
THR Total hip replacement
TIA Transient ischemic attack
tid Three times a day
TKA Total knee arthroplasty
TKR Total knee replacement
TMJ Temporomandibular joint
TNR Tonic neck reflex
t.o. Telephone order
T/O Throughout
TPR Temperature, pulse, and respiration

TTWB Toe touch weight bearing
Tx Treatment; traction

U

UA Urine analysis
UE Upper extremity
U/L Unilateral
UMN Upper motor neuron
URI Upper respiratory infection
US Ultrasound
UTI Urinary tract infection
UV Ultraviolet

V

VAS Visual analog scale
VC Vital capacity; verbal cues
v.o., VO or V/O Verbal orders
vol. Volume
v.s. or VS Vital signs
Vtach Ventricular tachycardia

W

WB Weight bearing
WBAT Weight bearing as tolerated
WBQC Wide base quad cane
w/c Wheelchair
WBC White blood cell
wk. Week
WFL Within functional limits
WNL Within normal limits
wt. Weight

X

x Times

Y

y/o or y.o. Years old
yr. Year

Z

Z Zero (as a muscle grade)

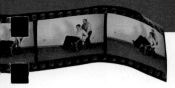

Index